PANDEMICS, POVERTY, AND POLITICS

Pandemics, Poverty, and Politics

DECODING THE SOCIAL
AND POLITICAL DRIVERS
OF PANDEMICS FROM PLAGUE
TO COVID-19

TYLER B. EVANS, MD, MS, MPH

Forewords by Peter J. Hotez, MD, PhD, and David Mabey, MD, CBE

JOHNS HOPKINS UNIVERSITY PRESS | *Baltimore*

© 2025 Johns Hopkins University Press
All rights reserved. Published 2025
Printed in the United States of America on acid-free paper
9 8 7 6 5 4 3 2 1

Johns Hopkins University Press
2715 North Charles Street
Baltimore, Maryland 21218
www.press.jhu.edu

Library of Congress Cataloging-in-Publication Data is available.

A catalog record for this book is available from the British Library.

ISBN 978-1-4214-5178-7 (paperback)
ISBN 978-1-4214-5179-4 (ebook)

Special discounts are available for bulk purchases of this book. For more information, please contact Special Sales at specialsales@jh.edu.

EU GPSR Authorized Representative
LOGOS EUROPE, 9 rue Nicolas Poussin, 17000, La Rochelle, France
E-mail: Contact@logoseurope.eu

CONTENTS

PART III. HOW CAN WE DO BETTER?   315

COVID-19 taught many Americans (and many more people globally) about the multiple facets of a deadly pandemic. As it turned out, the public health impact was just one key aspect. Equally important were the significant financial effects that brought many economies to a screeching halt and the ability of the virus to promote global insecurity and political unrest. In turn, politics thwarted public health interventions.

Misled by Russian health disinformation on social media and political targeting by elected officials in the United States in concert with Fox News, thousands of Americans perished because they falsely believed that either the pandemic was a hoax or that COVID-19 vaccines were intended as a form of political control. We faced an unprecedented situation in which the US government, in cooperation with multinational pharmaceutical companies, accelerated the production of COVID-19 vaccines, antiviral drugs, and home diagnostic tests—and yet these deliverables often were not accepted by the American people or were used insufficiently or inappropriately. Our technical ability to design and develop new and exciting interventions for biomedicine could not counter the political and social institutions that blocked their uptake.

This failure means we need to pay greater attention to the sociopolitical aspects of pandemic threats and epidemic infectious diseases, and this is why this new book by Dr. Tyler B. Evans is so vitally important.

We have another urgent reason to study the social science and politics that accompany infectious disease threats—namely, poverty. During the COVID-19 pandemic, the essential workers and their families living in my state of Texas were the first to succumb to SARS-CoV-2 when it arrived here in the summer of 2020. I subsequently testified to the US Congressional Hispanic Caucus to express the horrors of young adults from low-income communities becoming exposed to the virus while working in family-oriented businesses and then taking COVID-19 back to multigenerational homes, where many grandparents in their 70s and 80s, as well as parents in their 40s, 50s, and 60s, became infected and lost their lives. Poverty became a major predictor of COVID-19 deaths, especially in 2020 before the vaccines became widely available. Even afterward, when vaccines first rolled out from Operation Warp Speed, launched by President Donald J. Trump, it quickly became apparent that low-income neighborhoods lacked the infrastructure, especially pharmacy chains or hospital systems, to deliver adult immunizations at scale. This became a major task of President Joseph R. Biden's administration in the first quarter of 2021.

Likewise, it is almost always the poor who disproportionately suffer from HIV/AIDS, tuberculosis, and malaria, as well as the so-called neglected tropical diseases such as human hookworm infection, schistosomiasis, Chagas disease, or leishmaniasis—all diseases for which my research group at Texas Children's Hospital is working to develop new vaccines. Though we may refer to them as neglected tropical diseases, these conditions are overwhelmingly associated with crushing poverty. Show me extreme poverty, and I will show you endemic infectious diseases. This is true both in the United States and the rest of the world.

A good example of the influence of poverty occurred in 2016 when I became concerned that a new Zika virus epidemic affecting Brazil and neighboring countries in Latin America and the Caribbean could emerge in my city of Houston. One could not help but notice the depressed conditions in Houston's low-income neighborhoods, which included poor housing and discarded car and truck tires strewn about. Old tires collecting rainwater are notorious for breeding the mosquitoes that transmit the Zika virus, and I worked with city officials to focus their attention on these impoverished areas of Houston. I even wrote a book (with Johns Hopkins University Press) titled *Blue Marble Health* to address the neglected tropical diseases that become embedded among the poor who live in high-income nations.

During the early 2000s, Sir Michael Marmot championed the idea that social inequalities represented an understudied yet essential element of poor health, especially in the United Kingdom. Marmot's books on the social determinants of health helped to galvanize and expand a new field of study in this area.

Now Dr. Evans taps into his extensive experience as an infectious diseases-trained public health physician on the front lines of both the HIV/AIDS and COVID-19 pandemics to apply those principles to current and future pandemic threats. His effort to look at infectious disease epidemics through a sociopolitical lens is welcomed. Exactly what will happen when the next major pandemic strikes either North America and Europe or the world's low- and middle-income countries is anyone's best guess, but a few elements must be considered.

First, we might see populations walking, not running, to vaccination centers, assuming we can develop a new vaccine for the next emerging virus. After 80% of adult Americans took the full primary two-dose immunization in the first two years of the COVID-19 pandemic, by the third year only 20% were willing to take the new bivalent booster that became available in fall 2022. That low number reflected inadequacies in the public messaging about vaccines from health agencies, but overwhelmingly it was an inundation of health disinformation that convinced the US population that the booster was either unnecessary or unsafe. If a major pandemic occurs within a few years of the COVID-19 pandemic, we might expect vaccine acceptance to more closely resemble that of 2022–2023 than of 2020–2021.

We should also expect greater pushback the next time around from mask mandates, stay-at-home measures to prevent patient surges at hospitals, and a general distrust of government public health recommendations. We should anticipate, too, that once again the heaviest disease burden—at least until vaccines become available—will affect the working poor or the essential workers who haven't the luxury of conducting their business while secure in their homes, working online and videoconferencing.

From COVID-19 we have learned a lot about how to advance health care technologies, including new point-of-care diagnostics, antiviral drugs, and vaccines. We remain perplexed, however, about how to address the social and political determinants of pandemic threats. This aspect has become perhaps the toughest part of all. For this reason, I expect Dr. Evans's book to become an important and useful tool for those of us who aspire to prevent the next pandemic, which will surely arrive.

Peter Hotez

Professor of Pediatrics and Molecular Virology
and Microbiology Texas Children's Hospital
Endowed Chair in Tropical Pediatrics Dean,
National School of Tropical Medicine,
Baylor College of Medicine, Houston, Texas

In 1943 Charles-Edward Amory Winslow, professor of public health at Yale University Medical School, published a book called *The Conquest of Epidemic Disease*, a fascinating historical account of what he called "the great sanitary awakening" in which bacteria and viruses, rather than miasmas and the wrath of God, were shown to be the causes of plague, cholera, and other epidemic diseases. With the causes of epidemics and their modes of transmission finally identified, he assumed it would be possible to develop vaccines and other public health interventions to ensure that no epidemics occurred in the future. Around the same time, Howard Florey and others proved penicillin to be the first effective treatment for serious bacterial infections, reinforcing the view that epidemic diseases were to become a thing of the past.

Sadly, this has not been the case. In 1994 Laurie Garrett published her best-selling book *The Coming Plague* with the subtitle *Newly Emerging Diseases in a World Out of Balance*, a comprehensive account of recent epidemics of Lassa fever, Ebola, and Marburg viruses in Africa; the 2009–2010 Swine Flu pandemic; and the emergence of the worldwide HIV/AIDS pandemic in the 1980s. She pointed out that urbanization, insecurity leading to displaced populations, and air travel made it inevitable that new infectious disease pandemics would occur in the future. The COVID-19 pandemic proved her right.

The whole world is now aware of the devastating impact of pandemic infectious diseases but not necessarily of the reasons underlying the continuing circulation of preventable infectious agents in human populations. This book on the sociopolitical determinants of pandemics, by Dr. Tyler B. Evans, explores these reasons.

Dr. Evans is an American doctor specializing in infectious diseases and public health with many years' experience in the treatment and prevention of infectious diseases in a wide variety of settings. He has worked in Mexico, Uganda, South Africa, South Sudan, Sierra Leone, the Dominican Republic, Haiti, Peru, Brazil, Myanmar, Korea, Japan, Thailand, India, Pakistan, Ethiopia, Kosovo, Macedonia, Nepal, Cuba, the Democratic Republic of the Congo, Israel, and the Palestinian territories and was the chief medical officer in New York City during the COVID-19 pandemic.

He has seen firsthand that poor people and disadvantaged groups such as refugees, asylum seekers, ethnic minorities, homeless people, and people with mental health problems are far more likely to die during an epidemic than educated middle-class people in both high- and low-income countries. These groups not only lack access to health care but also experience discrimination that makes them less likely to trust health care providers appointed by the government and accept vaccinations or other preventive measures.

Yet this need not be so. In the 1980s Kenneth Warren, director of health sciences at the Rockefeller Foundation, launched a program for the control of what he called the "Great Neglected Diseases of Mankind." Soon afterward the World Health Organization set up a program for controlling, eliminating, and eradicating neglected tropical diseases (NTDs), defined as those that disproportionately affect populations living in poverty, causing significant morbidity and mortality, as well as stigma and discrimination, and thus justifying a global response; NTDs are amenable to broad control, elimination, or eradication and are relatively neglected by research. Former president Jimmy Carter persuaded the chief executive of Merck pharmaceutical company to donate its recently patented drug ivermectin for the control of one of these diseases: river blindness. A number of other drug donation programs followed. In the 1990s I and my colleagues in The Gambia showed that a single dose of azithromycin, a new antibiotic manufactured by Pfizer, effectively treated trachoma, an NTD that remains the leading infectious cause of blindness. Since then Pfizer has donated more than 1 billion doses of azithromycin, eliminating trachoma as a public health problem from the Gambia and 17 other countries and reducing the number of people at risk from 1.5 billion to 116 million.

Evans's book *Pandemics, Poverty, and Politics* brings together his worldwide personal experience with a fascinating historical review covering the 3rd Plague and 6th Cholera epidemics in Europe in the 19th century, the Spanish Flu and other flu pandemics of the 20th century, the HIV/AIDS and Ebola epidemics in West Africa and the Democratic Republic of Congo, and the COVID-19 pandemic.

The development and rollout of an effective vaccine against COVID-19 within two years of its identification was an unprecedented achievement, and, as Tyler Evans points out, never before have so many resources been available worldwide for research and development to increase life expectancy. Yet every day about 25,000 children die of diseases that could have been cured or prevented, most of them among the 1 billion people living on less than one dollar a day.

Evans feels passionately that this should not be allowed to continue, and this beautifully written book aims to raise awareness of the relationship among social deprivation, stigma, and health and to suggest ways to improve health and life expectancy worldwide. His passion comes across clearly in the book, which will appeal to all of us who share his view of the world and are committed to reducing inequality worldwide.

David Mabey
Emeritus Professor of Communicable Diseases
Clinical Research Department
London School of Hygiene & Tropical Medicine
United Kingdom

We're living in a world where millions of people are dying every year of their impoverishment—both in the United States and beyond. Yet the paradox is that we're also living amid the greatest wealth and technological capacity in the history of the world, the combination of which has rendered these deaths absolutely unnecessary and entirely avoidable. It is this stark reality that led me to write this book.

This book is a manifestation of the vision I have developed over four decades of working on multiple continents, traveling to over 110 nations, and living in many of them. When people see me, their judgment is generally overshadowed by the phenotype in front of them. Let me be clear: I have so much privilege—as a white, heterosexual, cisgender American male physician leader—that I clearly check nearly every box of privilege. The difference is that I don't see the world the same way as others who look like me. Here is why . . .

My life experiences growing up were varied—and oftentimes calamitous. My mother's long battle with alcoholism and depression, my father's ill health, and our financial struggles throughout my youth made life tougher than any child should have to endure. Consumed with the immortality of youth, I never offered much thought to the concept of death. This mindset came to a dramatic halt with the unrelated yet concentrated deaths of all my older family members by the time I was 22—deaths that occurred beginning at age 17 with the loss of my father and maternal grandparents. My experience as an orphan began.

The combination of my mother's struggles with behavioral health and the financial challenges we faced in my youth caused me to act out. Growing up in Los Angeles and New York led to further identity confusion, and I began to reach out to other kids who seemed to accept me. Many of these were not healthy relationships and contributed to a series of poor sophomoric decisions. This led to a number of high school expulsions and a series of juvenile incarcerations. In fact, my first was at the tender age of 15 when the police thought it would be appropriate to place me with some of the most violent youth offenders in the South Bronx. The other kids naturally assumed I was Puerto Rican because no other white kids were being held there. I quickly made a few key friends.

I learned from some of these poor decisions after facing some very serious responsibilities. While still reeling from the shock of my losses, I discovered that my life lessons were just beginning. Due to economic pressures in conjunction with these family tragedies, I was forced to drop out of high school at the young age of 16. Less than nine months after my father's death, I was a father myself while still just a child of 17. Though the hardship of acknowledging such a responsibility can never be denied, not long after I recognized that life clearly had an upside. This concept was to be further developed six years later with the birth of my second daughter. My children have proven to be one of the most rewarding aspects of my life (and have grown to follow very ambitious paths themselves—one as a nurse practitioner and the other as a social worker—both embracing a similar cause).

Understanding the importance of education, and wanting to offer my daughter a fruitful life, I decided to sit for the GED exam. Given my work schedule, I wasn't afforded much time to study, so suffice it to say I was relatively surprised when I scored in the 99th percentile after studying for two days. After others continued to push me, I decided to enroll in community college the following semester.

At this point I was completely alone, both emotionally and financially, as my entire family had ceased to exist—save one. My daughter (who was soon to have a sister) gave me the incentive to overcome these hardships. I was given a choice: to surrender or to fight for my dreams of education in medicine and public health. I chose the latter, which has made all the difference. These tragic realities unfortunately influence thousands of other youths. You have a ticket for success and an associated fork in the road. For some, it's not really a choice. I was fortunate.

Based on numerous child-labor laws and the need to financially support a mother and child, I was awarded legal emancipation and afforded the opportunity to work 50 hours per week while attending junior college. Seven years later I was attending graduate school at an Ivy League university. Twenty years after that, I would become the first chief medical officer for New York City during the deadliest pandemic this country had seen in 100 years. Clearly, this was no easy path.

The adverse experiences I collected in my youth were soon matched by the number I witnessed in my travels around the world. I immersed myself in communities with which I felt spiritual connections. I didn't just want to help them . . . I deeply empathized with them.

This was my life—like it or not. Pain and adversity are relative, and we all have bled. The question is, How do you apply this positively toward your future? Life is about choices, and I chose to use these experiences to better empathize with people's pain. But as Johann Wolfgang von Goethe pointed out: "Knowing is not enough—we must apply." And that is the new meaning my life has taken on—to help alleviate that pain worldwide.

So my life has not been easy, but for this I am fortunate. I understand pain, resilience, and relentlessness, the virtues best known by those who struggle most. While working in impoverished settings around the world, I have found that this "street credibility" somehow radiates through my interactions with the people there. My experiences have allowed me to relate, empathize, and resonate with those from all walks of life—my greatest talent.

These experiences are what formed my overwhelming dedication to helping others in pain. It is through service in medical humanitarianism that I feel I am best able to do so. Because of my own youth, I believe I can truly empathize with the discomfort felt by the populations I have elected to be my patients. I have been given a "voice" (which I did not earn) and have decided to dedicate my career to lending this agency to the "voiceless," historically marginalized communities throughout the world. This book is a sounding board for the conditions that lead to unnecessary pain and suffering, and I am grateful that you are now reading these words.

Since completing my education and training in gerontology, internal and preventive medicine, infectious diseases and tropical medicine, public health, and epidemiology from universities across the world, including the University of Southern California (USC), Columbia University, the University of Arizona, the University at Buffalo (State University of New York), Tel Aviv University, and the London School of Hygiene and Tropical Medicine, I have dedicated my career to the service of others through the work of public health and community medicine. My career has mostly been geared toward engineering the ideal interface between clinical medicine and public health, focusing on infectious disease (specifically HIV/AIDS, tuberculosis, sexually transmitted infections [STIs], viral hepatitis, and tropical medicine), primary care / community health, substance use, refugee health, LGBTQIA+ health, Indigenous health, and homeless health).

My background has been heavily invested in international health and development. I have worked in a health care capacity in several countries, including Mexico, Uganda, South Africa, South Sudan, Sierra Leone, the Dominican Republic, Haiti, Peru, Brazil, Myanmar, Korea, Japan, Thailand, India (including Kashmir), Pakistan, Ethiopia, Kosovo, Macedonia, Nepal, Cuba, the Democratic Republic of the Congo (DRC), Israel, and the Palestinian territories. Much of that work has been with Doctors Without Borders, UNICEF, Physicians for Human Rights, and Partners in Health, as well as smaller grassroots nongovernmental organizations. In 2014 I led a medical team for Doctors Without Borders in South Sudan, where we built a pediatric malnutrition hospital, and I was the only physician responsible for the care of over 29,000 refugees. I also worked on the Ebola response twice—in Sierra Leone in 2015 and in the DRC in 2019.

Domestically, I have worked serving Native Americans with the Indian Health Service at the Wind River Reservation in Wyoming and at a large federally qualified health center in New York City, where I established one of the first refugee/asylee integrated primary care and mental health programs. Also in New York, I helped develop a clinical program focusing on transgender women of color, created a hepatitis C training program, and helped found the New York City Refugee and Asylee Health Coalition. As the national director of infectious disease for the AIDS Healthcare Foundation (the largest community-based HIV organization in the United States), I oversaw the implementation of all hepatitis C programs, more than 25 STI centers across the United States, and behavioral health programs having an impact on thousands of people living with HIV across the nation. In addition, I led a number of integrated behavioral health programs in primary care centers, focusing especially on the implementation of street medicine and substance use programs across New York and California. I previously served as the medical director for Alameda County's (including Oakland, California) Health Care for the Homeless, where I oversaw over a dozen street medicine programs.

During the COVID-19 response, I held a number of positions, including as the first chief medical officer for New York City, overseeing all COVID-19 operations in 2020, as well as the deputy public health officer and chief of the COVID-19 vaccination branch at Marin County Health and Human Services Agency. I was also one of the operational leads for the COVID-19 vaccination rollout with the Association of Bay Area Health Officers and the chief executive and medical officer for Curative Medical Associates, which administered over 2 million doses in 10 states, with a focus on health equity. I currently serve as the chief executive officer and cofounder for Wellness Equity Alliance, a national group of population and public health experts committed to transforming the intersectional systems of community and public health care delivery to historically marginalized communities.

My research interests are in HIV/AIDS, hepatitis C, tropical and travel medicine, STIs, refugee health, and transgender health. I am a research associate professor at the USC Institute on Inequalities in Global Health within the Keck School of Medicine's Department of Population and Public Health Sciences as well as at the Leonard Davis

School of Gerontology. I am also a clinical associate professor in the Department of Medicine at the University of California, San Francisco, where I conduct my research on sexual and gender-based violence in the DRC, collaborating with the 2018 Nobel Peace Prize laureate, Dennis Mukwege. I am a fellow of the Infectious Disease Society of America and have served on a number of boards and executive committees, including that of the HIV Medicine Association, representing >12,000 HIV providers in the United States.

My service to historically marginalized communities is founded on one core driving principle: social justice. My life experiences (starting in my youth) provided a path that would ultimately furnish the vision needed to connect with people suffering injustices in this nation and beyond. They are what drove me to write this book.

I cut my teeth in HIV/AIDS care. Every day it kills thousands, mostly indirectly, and has collectively infected over 70 million, with over 35 million dead. But HIV is only one infectious killer. Every year, approximately 300–500 million people are infected with malaria, and over 3 million die as a result. In fact, it is the world's leading cause of both morbidity and mortality—most victims being African children less than five years old and their pregnant mothers. Tuberculosis is the largest killer overall. With each heartbreaking year, about 11 million children die in total, many from infectious diseases and mostly before their fifth birthday. More than half of those succumb to malnutrition, and more than 25,000 die every day of avoidable diseases and deficits, including malaria, tuberculosis, diarrhea, and pneumonia, yet these are mostly abstract terms to many of us living in the privileged Global North.

Never before in the history of mankind have we seen such significant advancements in technological developments as have occurred in the past 200 years. Never before have so many resources been spent worldwide on research and development to increase life expectancy. Progress is undeniable, but people can only benefit from technological progress if they have access to its results. Unfortunately, this is not the case for so many. Increasingly, we are gaining resources but fail to apply them to the countries most desperately in need. Why? Because research institutions organized by private industry conversely pour their resources into solving the problems of those with the purchasing power to pay for the solutions. Low- and middle-income countries make up over 80% of the world's population but less than 10% of the world's pharmaceutical market. Since 1975, less than 1% of patented medications were directed for the tropical diseases that kill millions of people each year. (This includes antibiotics for bugs that have acquired such broad resistance that they are nearly immortal in certain contexts.)

Even after nearly seven decades of national and international development efforts, more than a billion people still have to eke out their daily struggle to survive with the purchasing power equivalent of less than a dollar a day. They live in absolute poverty, or rather, misery. Moreover, millions of people are needlessly dying largely due to policies that systematically exclude them. So why is nothing done?

The failure to put into practice what I see as right has to do with a detachment from these problems, both in space and time (the temporospatial paradox). People may read about distant regions of the globe afflicted with astounding morbidity, mortality, poverty, and human rights violations and may simply pass it off as abstraction. Sickness and death are perceived with horror and pain when they affect our nearest and dearest, but people remain relatively unmoved by statistics telling them that every day about 25,000 children die of avoidable diseases and deficits. These tragic realities make one wonder for whom scientific advances are made. Attempts to limit access to medicine and technology based on "purchasing power" may be reasonably construed as the quintessential crime against humanity.

Over a decade of work in the Global South in my 20s and 30s, the structural realities of both "worlds" became indefensible to me. Initially, I eschewed the disparities that existed within the United States because I found that they paled "statistically" (and emotionally to a degree) in comparison with those that operated globally. The more that I worked within US systems and became more familiar with the stark realities in the fields I was working (including a mean survival into the 40s or

50s among certain American Indian communities in the Pacific North-west or people experiencing homelessness in Los Angeles's Skid Row or in Oakland, California), however, the more I recognized the universal needle that stitches a thread through these tattered cloths.

I eventually realized that managing Ebola around the diamond mines in eastern Sierra Leone, countering sexual and gender-based violence on the eastern border of the DRC, and curbing methamphetamine use and a rise in syphilis among transgender women in the South Bronx all had a common social denominator. The majority of the people experiencing these adverse health outcomes were marginalized as the result of a number of seemingly arbitrary factors, including the color of their skin, their tribal lineage, the languages they spoke, their zip codes, their immigration status, the gender they identified with, or the type of people they found sexually attractive. The composition of their tribal "makeup" didn't necessarily matter; what did was whether it differed from that of the ruling "class." In Sudan, those would be Arabs, but in South Sudan, they would be Dinkas; in Wyoming, this would be the Eastern Shoshone; and in the general United States, it would be cis white educated urban males. The social and political determinants were universal. Understanding how these universal conditions are deterministic in facilitating the conversion from infectious disease outbreaks to syndemics (don't worry, I'll explain this in due time) to public health emergencies of international significance and pandemics has been a core driver of my thinking for years. It took the most recent pandemic (COVID-19) for me to commit these thoughts to writing. Here is my story . . .

ACKNOWLEDGMENTS

This book has indeed been a labor of love and has spanned over two decades. To be clear, the list here is not exhaustive. There are seemingly not enough pages to name all the people to whom I owe a debt of gratitude for this book ever to have made it to the finish line.

First and foremost, I thank my incredibly talented wife, Nancy, who tolerates and supports my dedication to my work and provided me with our two effervescent balls of joy—Zion and Zen. You are my heart. Thank you to my recently deceased brother, Scott, who is survived by his wife, Deborah, for their relentless support of me and my ambitions over the years. Without parents or sufficient credit in my 20s, you stepped in and cosigned for my student loans for medical school. Without you, this book could not have been written. I would be remiss if I did not acknowledge my deceased family—namely, my mom for her (Italian) passion; my biological father, Niels Laursen, a dedicated obstetrician / gynecologist, for his work ethic; and my stepfather for his kindness and tolerance. Thank you to my two beautiful and talented daughters—Giselle and Alyssa—who have had to share their dad with the rest of the world. Thank you for your understanding. I am so proud of your accomplishments—mostly your respective commitments to the underserved.

Thank you to Jessica Perlin, who stood by my side and supported me when I was living through some of my darkest years of losing my mother and everything associated with her. Somehow, I matriculated at one of the top universities in the nation (University of Southern California) with a GED and made it into an Ivy League graduate school as you were by my side. I would surely have lost my way without your dedication. Thank you to Elaine Trebek-Kares, who stepped in to support me as a "second mother" and help me find my way at a vulnerable age. I was at rock bottom, and you helped redirect me onto the right path. Without your encouragement of my talents and determination, this book would not have been written.

Thank you to all the professors and mentors who helped guide and inspire me and nurture my academic talents throughout the years. A particular acknowledgment goes to Paul Farmer, who inspired me to pursue a path of medical humanitarianism (at a time when such a path was not well-known) after meeting him in Haiti in my 20s. A special mention for John Walsh, my undergraduate neuroscience professor, who also encouraged me to cultivate my talents and has continued to cheerlead from the sidelines over the years.

I would be remiss if I did not recognize those whom I especially value in the current state. My present personal "board of advisors" (Woody Myers, Ben Young, and Jeremy Veatch) have been supremely helpful in refining my leadership skills. I want to acknowledge my business partner and cofounder at Wellness Equity Alliance, Abinash Achrekar, who has helped me affirm the notion that our organization is necessary to serve the most historically marginalized and that a bunch of doctors could actually run a business. Thank you to Jeff Klausner, who introduced me to Curative and always had my back. Thank you to members of the prestigious boards of Wellness Equity Alliance and Wellness Equity Institute, including Howard Hu, George Rutherford, Maureen Lichtveld, Marsha Zimmerman, Judith Feinberg, Dominique McDowell, Ricky Bluthenthal, and Jim Withers. Thank you to my former boss in New York City, Deanne Criswell, who supported my ideas to invest in addressing the social determinants during some of the city's darkest hours of the pandemic.

The production of this book took several years, and I want to acknowledge all of those who helped contribute. A big shout-out to Robin Coleman and the team over at Johns Hopkins University Press for affirming and developing the ideas manifested in this book. Thank you to the incredible team of interns who helped with all the nuts and bolts in order to get this book out of the proverbial garage—especially

Laura Shepherd, Kimia Ghasemian, and Nancy Yang. Thank you to my "little sister," Antonella Sturniolo, for coordinating much of the interns' efforts and editorial revisions.

In addition, thanks to our marketing/communications teams at Wellness Equity Alliance—especially Mari Anixter and Aaron Mabry. A special tribute to Marsha Zimmerman, our chief development officer, who has cultivated an expertise in speaking "Tyler" and shepherding so many of our projects to successful outcomes. Thank you to all my friends and colleagues whom I did not mention but who have been there either directly (or peripherally) in the struggle to help support the health care needs of the most historically marginalized.

Finally, at its core this book is dedicated to the millions who struggle every day to make ends meet and find access to quality health care for themselves and their families. I hope it will inspire your communities and the change-makers within who can address the needless inequities. Light up the darkness . . .

Introduction

In such a world of conflict, a world of victims and executioners, it is the job of thinking people, not to be on the side of the executioners.

　—ALBERT CAMUS

COVID-19 is very bad (I write from the present tense). This book is not about that. This book is about how COVID-19 has been transformative. This pandemic has engaged living rooms across the world with the chambers of public health. Never before have we had so many "armchair epidemiologists" with strong opinions about public health policy and practice. Most public health professionals have historically dealt with diseases that were arcane, seemingly impacting communities with little or no connection to ones they lived and operated in. Case in point: The average American does not feel deeply concerned about how malaria may place them or their loved ones at risk. While HIV/AIDS may seem more familiar, most communities in the West chalk it up as a disease of "the other." This is what is known as temporospatial dissonance, and it is unfortunate that after decades of advocacy—of the "Ryan Whites" of the world showcasing the universal threat that it poses for all—it remains the case.[1]

The issue of vaccine hesitancy long preceded COVID-19 and remains universal, although it is far more dominant in areas with poor health literacy. While this phenomenon has spread given recent information platforms, which we'll discuss below, let's be honest: There is something particularly visceral experienced in the psychological reaction to injections that may be associated with an adverse event (or side effect).

I have an example from my time working with Doctors Without Borders (Médecins sans Frontières) on a pediatric malnutrition program in South Sudan from 2013–2014, where I was the only physician for >29,000 internally displaced people, or refugees, who cannot cross a border because of fear of retaliation. We stood up (launched) a number of mass immunization program initiatives for children, principally for measles. Many of these people had never seen a medical doctor before, but there seemed to be a situational awareness of this "evil medicine," and associated hesitancy (or outright resistance) remained high. Through the "magical powers" of local community health workers (CHWs) who had the faith and trust of these communities, we were able to work through many of these concerns. As I reflected on the COVID-19 vaccine hesitancy demonstrated among Latinx communities in the Bay Area, California, over a decade later, the world started to feel a lot smaller to me, conceptually.

In addition to the sociopolitical trappings that have created a radically unequal understanding of our access to essential services, there is a very real constellation of factors that impede people's ability to access health care services. These are what we in public health call the *social determinants of health*. The Centers for Disease Control and Prevention defines them as nonmedical factors that influence health outcomes, factors that could be as simple as transportation networks or child care availability. The common denominator is poverty—and it disproportionately impacts Black, Indigenous, and people of color (BIPOC). If the associated health systems do not address these social conditions, administrators will continue to see grave disparities in their data sets.

Less than 10 years after my time in South Sudan, I was leading COVID-19 vaccine operations in Northern California, including one in

Marin County that *The New York Times* described as one of the most effective programs in the United States.[2] Even so, we found that access was largely "restricted" to what we ultimately coined the "triple C's": Caucasians with cars and computers. In the early months of COVID-19 vaccine availability in December 2020 and January 2021, my team and I analyzed the data and determined that >90% of those vaccinated were white, with personal transport and digital access, while the people that we were missing were those most at risk of the greatest adverse health consequences. In other words, access to a lifesaving medication was largely sociopolitically determined. In frustration, as we strategically adapted our thinking to address the most vulnerable communities, we realized that it was not simply about access. It was about changing sociopolitical thought that had manifested in health behavior for centuries. This was a prominent feature of COVID-19 vaccine hesitancy.

Public health is arguably one of the most politicized professionalized fields, as it touches on core issues such as choice and access. In US public health, it is difficult to avoid the correlation of the word "choice" with the hotly contentious discussion of abortion. Otherwise, the word "choice" is deeply branded in the American spirit and is commonly correlated with "freedom." Access, on the other hand, seems to connote entitlement, which is certainly a provocative concept for the politically conservative. Toggling between these concepts and trying to find the right balance that optimizes health equity is the career goal of many public health professionals, including myself.

In my field, which is infectious disease and primary care medicine for vulnerable communities, we simply want the best for our patients. We see when the system does not work. It affects our "spiritual" wellness, despite our best efforts to create a professional distance. It bothers us. The Venn diagram of economics and ethics should simply overlap as it just makes sense to invest in a strong public health infrastructure that is accessible for all—from white and Asian suburban communities to BIPOC urban communities. (I draw a distinction between equity and equality, which I'll discuss later). The absence of such egalitarian (mindful to avoid the dreaded *socialist*) health policies that promote the principles of primary care and prevention leads to polarizing patterns of health care consumption, from underutilization to "superutilization" (first described by the Camden Coalition). While overseeing homeless health programs, I've had some patients visit the emergency department more than 500 times per year—that is, more than once per day. To be clear, excluding certain communities from quality-based health care does not mean that they will not access it. What it does mean is that they will not access it well, which ultimately leads to higher costs, sicker populations, and a greater likelihood of magnified communicable disease transmission (i.e., epidemics→ syndemics→pandemics). Got it? This book explains why this chain of causality occurs.

The tragedy is that BIPOC communities (I'm generalizing) are the least likely to have the foundational knowledge that they need to access primary care regularly, optimize their health behavior (e.g., avoiding obesity, smoking), and have the confidence and security to seek out services, some of which may be government-sponsored ("public charge"), for fear of government retaliation.[3] They will also be least likely to have access to essential services, including medical insurance, paid time off from employment, transportation, childcare, and quality-based local health care, including behavioral health. Finally, and perhaps most crucially, they will be least likely to have the necessary attitudes and beliefs that support the principles of primary care and prevention, including vaccinations.

The combination of these cascading elements—or what has been increasingly referred to as *syndemics* (the focus of part II)—leads to unhealthy and possibly even toxic population health patterns, which in turn fuel spikes of infectious disease outbreaks and compromise the capacity of the health system to care for all community residents (including the most privileged).

This book, *Pandemics, Poverty, and Politics*, performs a deep dive into this topic and how those social determinants relate to the further production of pandemics. Many global public health professionals have felt that tackling infectious disease in the Global South was aspirational at best, as policymakers and influencers of the Global North could not connect to the lives of people living so far away or to health crises that did not seem to pose a viable threat to them in real time. The aim of this book is to bring all changemakers together: from public health professionals to aspiring students to political activists to community leaders to policymakers to cultural influencers to donors. We all need to be reading the same proverbial sheet of music and all must play our part. Deep public health objectives cannot just be accomplished by the experts. It truly takes a village. HIV/AIDS and COVID-19 will be particularly compelling arguments for these folks, as they pierce the temporospatial paradox and any potential argument that boils down to "not my problem." It is our problem, and here is why . . .

While HIV/AIDS has been the global health unifier (for the converted) for several decades, and will be the subject of substantive discourse in the book, I want to spend some time on the front end discussing how COVID-19 has—for the first time in contemporary history—united the world to address unparalleled mortality and disruption as the result of an infectious disease. For the first time in recent history, an infectious disease has disproportionately impacted the Global North, with >15% of global cases and attributable mortality taking place in the United States alone. Never before did public health become the conversation in so many living rooms in the United States. People are engaged and apparently informed, but what is their source of information? We have rapidly transitioned from an era of minimal health information to over- and misinformation: an infodemic. Health literacy in the United States is poor, with an average fifth-grade reading level. Many people's worldview is determined by their social media feeds. Anti-science has seemed to guide large-scale communities on how to respond to the existential elements of fear. Together, these factors form a toxic recipe that has led to far more morbidity and mortality than the United States should have ever endured.

During the first COVID-19 surge, the rise in excess mortality exceeded that of the 1918 Spanish Influenza pandemic. While serving as the first ever chief medical officer for New York City in that surge, overseeing the Office of Emergency Management, the amount of misinformation that we encountered was unprecedented. That misinformation was disproportionately identified in BIPOC communities such as the South Bronx, where I practiced for years and where decades of systematic discrimination and ensuing distrust made it very challenging for the city to penetrate this misinformation. As a result, incidence rates were far higher in zip codes housing poorer communities of color. The ironically named Corona, Queens, had the highest reported incidence rate until May 2020.

At the time, we lacked sophisticated capacity for testing, treatment, or contact tracing, armed mostly with an arsenal of high-rise hotels to isolate and quarantine infected and exposed residents. What the city really needed was not more sophisticated facilities but simply a more democratic distribution of basic facilities in the most at-risk communities. We did not need more emergency medicine (EM) physicians. Despite my deep respect for my EM colleagues in standing up the COVID-19 field hospital at the Billie Jean King Tennis Center, where the US Open is played, the stadium was replete with passionate EM docs looking for someone to intubate. Instead, we needed CHWs, social workers, and mental health professionals who had the trust and faith of the communities at risk. *We needed to navigate access.*

The city spent >$500 million on this project, but because of the historical patterns of access (including the knowledge and trust around those access points), we found these hotels largely vacant. That COVID-19 field hospital alone cost >$50 million. While we never performed the forensics on this poor utilization, we speculated that the most at-risk populations (e.g., communities of color living in poorer, multigenerational homes) were immobilized by fear—either of the actual disease or of the government attempting to create refuge against it. As misinformation continued to thrive, it became increasingly challenging for us to discharge patients, as both individual homes and community shelters were afraid to receive them, despite our reassurances. Of course, this spiked rate of transmission clustered in areas with historically poor access, overwhelming the public hospital capacity in Queens,

Brooklyn, and the Bronx. More privileged Manhattanites made a mass exodus for the safety of their "sterile" homes in the Hamptons or Catskills. Privilege followed the Darwinian maxim—survival.

This is the world in which we're living: one where cracks in the proverbial population and public health pavement are further widened by the corresponding socioeconomic fault lines that lie beneath. While the majority of these fault lines were created in the Global South throughout the 19th, 20th, and early 21st centuries, certain pandemics, including HIV/AIDS to some extent and particularly COVID-19, have created a reckoning for wealthy nations that have not invested in the necessary foundational social and economic conditions that would alleviate disparities in chronic health access and associated outcomes. The political activation of these proverbial tectonic plates during times of population stress continues to widen these cracks, and the most vulnerable are swallowed up first.

Public health should not be politicized. It is a system established to create foundational services accessible to all (equality) and to support a healthy, functional, and productive society. Population and public health should be equitable (note: not necessarily equal) in terms of their operational efforts, meaning those most at risk need the most attention. This book makes a case for a rational system that depoliticizes our communal need to address the root causes of disease; outlines a road map for the future of infectious disease detection, prevention and control; and creates a call to action for all global citizens to do their part in addressing the social determinants of future pandemics. We can do better. We must do better.

While this book is intended to depoliticize public health, we cannot ignore the current political carnage taking place in Washington, which is hurting folks on both sides of the political divide in real time as well as in a predicted heap of downstream consequences. During the time of writing, Donald J. Trump was recently sworn in (again) as the 47th president (previously the 45th) of the United States. Within the first few weeks of office, he raced to blow up as much infrastructure as he possibly could—from appointing the richest man in the world (an

Afrikaner, or white South African descending from predominantly Dutch settlers, who had grown up in Apartheid South Africa) to decimate as many foundations of already tenuous social service and health systems, including that of foreign aid (US Agency of International Development) to appointing a staunch vaccine denialist without any health care experience to the head of the largest health agency in the country: the US Department of Health and Human Services. These profoundly devastating actions will likely precipitate a rabid spike in inequities between the haves and the have-nots, and the principles as well as the overall thesis of this book will have become even further concretized. The readers of this book will therefore have even a more compelling duty to act.

This book is a call to action. It is written by someone who has been on the proverbial "front lines" and in the public health "foxholes" and wishes to share some of these experiences firsthand. Health care is a human right for all. When you have the "right" conversation with most folks, they will often come to that same conclusion. I will do my best to avoid political "land mines" (e.g., human rights) for my reader, but my intention is to create a common understanding for all readers to acknowledge a common call to action.

This book is not political and is not intended for any particular partisan camp. It's a conversation about how inequities in systems during times of stress spill over into communities across the world and disrupt their access to systems, even when they previously had privilege. I often hear how "blue skies" (nonemergency, I'll explain later) arguments, rooted in nimbyism, spill over from high-risk communities into low-risk ones. I have been in many rooms where people argue about providing clean syringes/needles, since people who inject drugs are at higher risk for HIV and viral hepatitis, among other infectious diseases. These harm reduction services mitigate risk of infectious disease not just for those at highest risk but for all surrounding communities. Even if the moral argument is not convincing enough, the economic argument is compelling. The same principle applies to COVID-19. Investing in systems that allow us to effectively disrupt disease transmission from a systems standpoint requires us to think deeply about the root causes and force multipliers that amplify risk. Most of these are sociopolitically determined.

This book is divided into three parts. The first (chapters 1–4) lays down the conceptual framework of the nuances of health systems across the world, with a focus on the United States, and how access is largely determined by social and political forces. The second part covers how sociopolitical determinants have moved scalable diseases across borders for over 100 years, by providing examples of historical and contemporary pandemics or public health emergencies. The third part explains how we can take this information and translate it into positive impact at the community level. This book is intended to inform a crossover audience—from students to health care professionals to academics to policymakers to influencers to concerned community members. The point is not to preach to the proverbial choir but to awaken the lay community and students enough to make a difference. The silver lining of COVID-19 is that we have a more activated global audience to better understand and address the conditions that manufactured it. With this knowledge, we can have a formidable impact on the next emerging infectious disease outbreak. While COVID-19 was very bad, it is far from the worst. If we do not address the core elements that precipitate and amplify these outbreaks, COVID-19 will be a mere appetizer for a far more lethal entrée in the years to come.

PART I

THE FOUNDATIONAL PRINCIPLES OF SOCIAL MEDICINE

CHAPTER 1

A Primer in Health Systems

When morality comes up against profit, it is seldom that profit loses.
—SHIRLEY CHISHOLM

Many people discuss systems as some abstract or purely philosophical concept. In health care, they are very real. Unfortunately, we live in a society where many of these health systems are fragmented. While I have worked in many nations, most of the examples in this part will be drawn from US systems.

Broken systems naturally lead to dysfunction in service delivery. US health care systems are built on market-driven models (notably with the highest spending in the world). As a result, these systems revolve around competitive elements that naturally lead to their failure to align with one another. Consequently, deep silos emerge, and collaborative models are mostly selected against, unless there is a market advantage. The result is the highest health care spending in the world. While certain recent models like accountable care organizations (ACOs) set up by the Centers for Medicare and Medicaid Services (CMS) are intended for cooperative outcomes through contracts and market incentives, they are still fraught with a number of institutional challenges that prevent them from acting as a true systematic unit.

Even defining the concept of "health systems" in the United States is challenging. The Agency for Healthcare Resource and Quality (AHRQ) attempts to but still struggles, often including a hospital as an essential component.[1] Others disagree. The RAND Corporation, for example, defines a health system as more than one organization with a shared payment or service delivery model.[2] The latter seems to make more sense as a common denominator for a "system" yet should certainly not be a setting primarily focused on inpatient care. This is likely pathognomonic of the US health care model, where we see health care delivery through the lens of the most infirm. That should not be our system.

Alternatively, I define a health system as one similar to RAND's but going a step further to include effective information sharing and a common mission. Information and data sharing is far from ideal in the United States, as it is a snake pit of competitive vendors incentivized to avoid working together. Epic Systems Corporation is one of the most successful, and we will be discussing this further in this chapter. These challenges notwithstanding, some health information–sharing platforms and exchanges (Health Information Exchange) successfully bridge these divides.

When it comes to funding health care systems, they tend to be broken up into four models globally:

- Beveridge
- Bismarck
- National health insurance
- Out-of-pocket

The Beveridge model is a centralized government-controlled system in which all aspects of health care delivery (including public health) are streamlined, and most health care staff are government employees. It was first established in the United Kingdom, where it evolved into the National Health Service.[3] Similar adaptations can be found in countries like Spain and New Zealand, with Cuba demonstrating the purest form of this model. In the United States, similar examples would be the Veterans Administration or the Indian Health Service. I've worked for both.

The Bismarck model was first established in Germany and is more decentralized.[4] It is largely funded by the employment sector and deducted from payroll in "sickness funds." Several permutations of this model exist with respect to how insurers are set up and their respective level of competition, but the common denominator is that all are controlled by rates and policies set by the national government. Belgium, Japan, and Switzerland have similar models. In the United States, the Affordable Care Act (ACA; colloquially referred to as Obamacare, a reference that generated considerable political challenges) and general employer-based insurance are largely based on this principle.

The National Health Insurance model is a hybrid of both the Beveridge and Bismarck models, with a single payer (i.e., government insurer) but with health care staff who are not directly employed by the national government.[4] The most well-known example of this system is in Canada, but Taiwan and South Korea have similar permutations. In the United States, CMS is set up with similar foundational principles.

Finally, the out-of-pocket model is market driven and lacks any central coordinating policies, thereby creating universal fee-for-service systems.[3] We see this model in most low- and middle-income countries in the Global South. In the United States, it is how the uninsured generally access health care, with a few important exceptions. The health care safety net, including policies such as the Emergency Medical Treatment and Labor Act, is set up to provide clinical services regardless of one's ability to pay, but in theory it is still structured as an out-of-pocket financial paradigm.

Consequently, the US health care system is a mosaic of all four funding models. For the purposes of this book, we are going to categorize health systems based on the mechanisms and associated intentions of clinical service delivery. I would outline some of the key systems as the following:

- Hospital networks
- Community health networks
- Population health
- Safety networks
- Public health

Hospital Networks

This is the most straightforward (albeit incomplete) way of thinking about a system from a public-facing standpoint. According to the AHRQ's definition described above, many would argue that systems must necessarily include hospitals in what we can illustrate as a "hub-and-spoke" model. Think of this model animated as a bicycle wheel, with the hub at the center and the spokes radiating out into the periphery—all connected by one single hub (figure 1.1). In this setting the hospitals or set of hospitals would be the hubs, with ambulatory centers and mobile services serving as the spokes. These systems, by definition, will have more than one hospital and are often quantified by the number of hospitals or beds they operate (note quantify a system based on how much "sickness" and not "wellness" they can manage). Globally, the largest hospital networks are in the United States, with Germany, Malaysia, the Philippines, Taiwan, India, and China also ranking high according to the rubric.[5]

Expanding beyond the community health concept, "health care safety nets" are officially defined by the National Academy of Medicine, formerly the Institute of Medicine, as "those providers that organize and deliver a significant level of healthcare and other needed services to uninsured, Medicaid and other vulnerable patients."[6] In the United States, this is a patchwork of providers, funding, and programs tenuously held together by the power of demonstrated need, community support, and political acumen.[7] These include everything from free clinics to citywide direct access programs, a critical part of the system that has undergone a transformation since the implementation of the ACA.[8] Unofficially, these safety networks typically consist of publicly funded

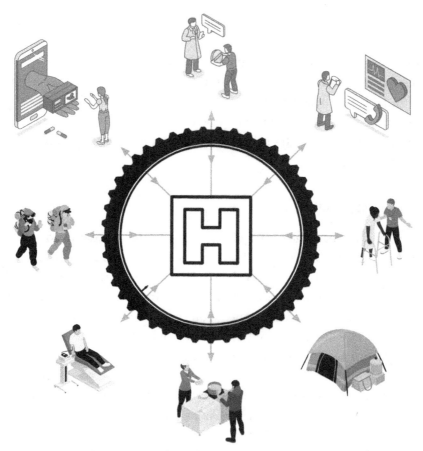

FIGURE 1.1. Models of operational distribution often seen among hospital networks. The hub-and-spoke model applied to health care. *Source:* Sofia Gallo, post to LinkedIn, December 2, 2018, https://www.linkedin.com/pulse/hub-spoke-model-applied-healthcare-sofia -gallo/.

infrastructure with a tertiary care facility (or county / city hospital) often serving as the hub. While some researchers may describe these terms interchangeably, I would argue that the hospital hub is a discerning element between community health and safety networks. These "safety-net hospitals" are set up to serve all populations but disproportionately serve low-income communities and are well-known for maintaining an open-door policy for their services.[9]

The idea of a "safety net" originated in social welfare studies, classically referring to providing benefits as a last resort.[10] The safety-net system plays a fundamental role in filling coverage gaps that the traditional insurance system creates and ensures that health care is accessible and affordable for those who are historically marginalized.[11] While safety-net programs are a critical component of health care access, they are not a substitute for the protection often afforded by comprehensive health insurance.

Community Health

Community health also struggles to follow a uniform definition, but I would describe it as a service delivery model intended to meet the needs of key communities in a given area. In the United States, confusion often arises regarding the definitions of community and population health. I will aim to create some distance between the two.

How do we define "community" in this context? MacQueen describes community as "linked by either social ties, common perspectives, and engage[d] in joint action in geographical locations or settings; venues or areas that are identified with key activities, such as residence, work, education, and recreation; and venues or areas that are physically, geographically, culturally, and administratively, or geopolitically-defined."[12]

An effective community health model really strives to understand the target community's needs, both real and perceived—often starting with a community health needs assessment. Funding is often an issue. In the United States, much of that funding is delivered through federally qualified health centers (FQHCs), created in 1991 to accept groups that are usually excluded in most conventional private clinics—namely those with low income, the underinsured/uninsured, seasonal and migrant farmworkers, migrants, and people experiencing homelessness.[13,14] Importantly, patient funding depends on the patient's ability to pay and can often be on a sliding scale if the patient is under/uninsured.

FQHCs currently serve >30 million patients a year in more than 13,000 communities (both urban and rural) in the United States.[15] This number is increasing rapidly, with 5.3 million patients seen in 2019, up from 3.4 million in 2013, an increase of nearly 40% in just four years.[16] The vast majority of these patients are low-income individuals, >70% of whom have family incomes below the established federal poverty level.[17] Approximately 10% of patients are insured by Medicare and 38% by Medicaid; 36% have no insurance.[18] They are overseen and largely funded by the Health Resources Services Administration. The genesis of the construction of FQHCs was spearheaded by Dr. Jack Geiger, an internist, civil rights activist, and revolutionary who concretized the delivery system of community health. In 1991 FQHCs were added as an important Medicare benefit—soon to be added to Medicaid—yet many didn't know what to do with them at the time.[19,20] In 1996 the Health Center Consolidation Act was passed and focused on very clear historically marginalized communities to begin with—that is, migrants and people experiencing homelessness.[21] In 2010 the standing of FQHCs was further advanced when the ACA started including them. Once again it was emphasized that while they should not target only special populations, FQHCs would primarily be mobilized in medically under-served areas. Importantly, they must provide medical services to all residents in these designated catchment areas regardless of their ability to pay.[21]

Public Health

How we define public health, and, even more importantly, how we define the mandate and scope of public health in the COVID-19 pandemic climate, is the most hotly contested topic in this book and its main focus. Clearly, in order to describe solutions we must define the basic scaffolding of the problem.

Charles-Edward Amory Winslow, a preeminent bacteriologist and one of the "godfathers" of American public health, defined it as "the science and art of preventing disease, prolonging life, and promoting health through the organized efforts and informed choices of society, organizations, public and private communities, and individuals."[22] Put more simply, it is the science of protecting and improving the health of people and their communities (note the intersection with community health here, which will be fleshed out further in part III). The Centers for Disease Control and Prevention (CDC) describes this work as achieved by promoting healthy lifestyles, researching disease and injury prevention, and detecting, preventing, and responding to infectious diseases.[23] It defines its scope as primarily concerned with protecting the health of entire populations (note the intersection with population health) and not merely individuals, which is a straightforward way of distinguishing it from medicine. These populations can be as small as a local neighborhood or as big as an entire country or region of the world.

Public health experts analyze the effects on health due to genetics, personal choice, and the environment to develop interventions and policies that protect the health of families and communities, such as vaccination programs and education on the dangers of tobacco and alcohol. The American Public Health Association makes an important claim that "public health saves money, improves our quality of life, helps children thrive, and reduces human suffering."[23] While this can be debated (and is emerging), the five core historic disciplines of public health are as follows:

- Behavioral science / health education
- Biostatistics
- Environmental health
- Epidemiology
- Health services administration

Public health professionals focus on the prevention of disease and the promotion of wellness for populations, thereby strengthening communities through implementing educational programs, recommending policies, administering services, and conducting research. This can be contrasted with the general clinical fields, in which professionals (e.g., doctors and nurses) focus primarily on treating individuals after an illness or injury.

While the core academic disciplines of public health are generally agreed upon, the execution of public health varies greatly across the globe. Much of this variation is related to funding. Drawing upon the four financial models described above, the Beveridge model practiced in the United Kingdom and Cuba have robust public health clinical service delivery models that are tightly integrated with population and community health direct clinical services. This should be the global gold standard. In stark contrast, in the United States our public health systems have historically lacked those direct clinical services built into the public health systems, with the exception of certain more progressive states (e.g., California and New York) that provide services such as vaccines and testing and treatment for HIV/STD (actually, the correct term would be sexually transmitted "infections," which often do not lead to symptomatic disease).

If public health systems were well aligned with other health systems, the need for direct clinical services would be less important. This is not the case in the United States (or in much of the Global South), thereby generating serious fault lines that cause people to fall through the cracks during times of "population stress," classically precipitated by a public health emergency.

Population Health

So if public health is the science of protecting and improving the health of populations, what is population health? The Institute for Healthcare Improvement (IHI) defines it as the health outcomes of a group of individuals, including the distribution of such outcomes within the group.[24] These groups are often geographic populations (e.g., nations) but can also be other groups that share similar characteristics (e.g., employees, prisoners, racial / ethnic groups).[25] Since the advent of a more formalized definition in 2003, the practical focus of population health has been through the lens of the "Triple Aim," which identifies three linked objectives with the goal of

- improving the individual experience of care,
- reducing per capita cost of care, and
- improving the health of populations.[26]

The "Quadruple Aim" tacks on "improving medical provider satisfaction," a hot-button item given the degree of physician burnout throughout the nation (figure 1.2).[27]

The CDC views population health as "an interdisciplinary, customizable approach that allows health departments to connect practice to policy for change to happen locally."[28] So, again, how does this differ from *public health*? The CDC aims to distinguish population health from

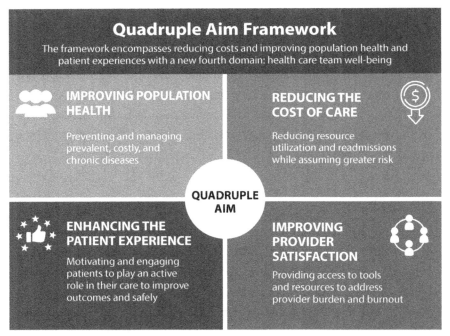

FIGURE 1.2. Quadruple Aim framework defining population health, which stems from quality improvement efforts in population health across the United States.
Source: Wellness Equity Alliance.

public health by emphasizing the latter's mission as aiming to protect and improve the health of populations through policy recommendations, health education and outreach, and research for disease detection and injury prevention. On the other hand, population health provides "an opportunity for healthcare systems, agencies and organizations to work together in order to improve the health outcomes of the communities they serve." In other words, public health is the nail, and population health is the hammer. Importantly, the direct application of public health policies to defined populations and the measurement of that change is the bridge that aligns the islands of public and community health, respectively.

For public health practitioners, improving population health involves understanding and optimizing the health of a population broadly defined by geography or discrete groups with common characteristics. Health reform encourages all sectors to think more broadly than the sum of the individual parts. This is certainly the case when it comes to the social determinants of health (SDoH, a concept described in more depth in chapter 2) and understanding how they influence access and, in turn, outcomes to population health measures. Ensuring population health goes well beyond the clinical care, support, and services provided by the health care system to include the government's public health policies, a corporation's wellness plans, and a school district's nutrition programs. A mosaic of systems and stakeholders are involved.

From a Triple and Quadruple Aim standpoint, many "population health" departments in hospitals have largely focused on cost-reduction components. While those are clearly important, the architects of the Triple Aim clearly describe their three goals as linked, so focusing on one measure while ignoring the others is a mistake. The term *population management* better encapsulates the predominant focus on cost reduction and, therefore, should be clearly distinguished from population health, for which a puritanical perspective would include analyzing and addressing the encompassing sociopolitical determinants of health. Applying practices to better address these SDoH is the term now coined *population health equity*.

An emerging term that may help to crystallize these concepts is *population medicine*. The IHI defines it as "the design, delivery, coordination, and payment of high-quality healthcare services to manage the Quadruple Aim for a population using the best resources we have available to us within the healthcare system."[29] Many examples of multisector multidimensional quality improvement applications can be found in this space, including patient registries, patient-centered medical homes, risk stratification, and ACOs. But for population medicine to be successful, it must focus on innovative clinical service delivery models, redesigned integrated data and information platforms, and a general shift to nontraditional health care workers (e.g., community health workers). Much of part III will take a deep dive into these concepts.

CHAPTER 2

Defining the Social (and Political)
Determinants of Health

Medicine is a social science, and politics is nothing but medicine on a large scale.
—RUDOLF VIRCHOW

Historically, a constellation of terms have attempted to describe the reality that health care workers—especially those in the social health space—are all too familiar with, but the *social determinants of health* (SDoH) appears to have become the gold standard. In fact, it's difficult to imagine folks engaged in the current health care workforce not encountering this term in any of the literature they have laid their eyes on since the COVID-19 pandemic emerged. There is no doubt that this salient paradigm shift was greatly needed, and if there is any silver lining to the COVID-19 pandemic, this undoubtedly tops the list. So what does it all mean, and how does it intersect with population and public health? Allow me to explain.

The theory of fundamental causes of health is rooted in Lieberson's concept of basic causes, which was first applied to the association between socioeconomic status (SES) and mortality by House and colleagues and developed primarily by Link and Phelan.[1,2,3] It was in my master of public health courses at Mailman School of Public Health at

Columbia University in the early 2000s, in a course taught by Bruce Link, where I first encountered this theory. Of course it made sense. From a nascent standpoint, poverty leads to higher rates of disease.

When I first went to South Africa in 2002, I clearly recall a fiery speech by the South African prime minister Thabo Mbeki at the XIII International AIDS Conference in Durban, where he famously denied the causality link between HIV and AIDS. His argument was multifactorial and largely wrong, to be clear. He did have an important message, however: that AIDS is the corollary of extreme poverty. He wasn't wrong with that statement.[4]

It got me thinking deeply about the link between poverty and disease. While interning with Doctors Without Borders (they prefer the French translation, Médecins sans Frontières) and assisting with the Essential Access (to Medications) Campaign in South Africa, my mind couldn't move beyond the sinister fact that >75% of HIV at the time was located in sub-Saharan Africa, the same place where access to treatment was impractical given the costs and poor infrastructure. These associations formed my thinking for years regarding intersections of the social sciences and medicine.

According to Link and Phelan, a fundamental social cause of health inequalities has four essential features. First, it influences multiple disease outcomes. Second, it affects these disease outcomes through multiple risk factors. Third, it involves access to resources that can be used to mitigate risks or to minimize the consequences of emergent disease. Finally, the association between a fundamental cause and health is reproduced over time via the replacement of intervening mechanisms. It is the persistent association of SES with overall health in the face of dramatic changes in mechanisms linking the two that led Link and Phelan to call SES a "fundamental" cause of health inequalities.[5]

Starting in the early 2000s, the World Health Organization (WHO) facilitated the work on the SDoH in a way that provided a deep understanding of health disparities from a more global perspective. Building on the Centers for Disease Control and Prevention's (CDC) definition of the SDoH, the WHO further describes the conditions in which people are born, grow, work, live, and age and the wider set of forces and systems shaping the conditions of daily life. These forces and systems include economic policies and systems, development agendas, social norms, social policies, racism, climate change, and political systems. They can be divided up into five domains, as follows:

- Economic stability
- Education access and quality
- Health care access and quality (health equity)
- Neighborhood and built environment
- Social and community context

To these I've added a sixth domain:

- Political determinants

Economic Stability

Economic stability is one of the most straightforward and compelling examples of the SDoH. Again, as described above in my exploratory and inquisitive mind of my 20s, the correlation between poverty (especially extreme poverty) and disease was axiomatic. Of course, science is never that simple, so it's best to unpack this core determinant into four subcomponents:[6]

- Employment
- Food insecurity
- Housing insecurity
- Poverty

Employment

Our labor force in the United States has been a moving target for decades, from the Industrial Revolution to an era of informationalism, and many communities have been unable to make the switch. The "Rust

Belt" (namely Buffalo, New York; Pittsburgh; Detroit; Cleveland) is a salient reminder of this poor transfer of relatable skill sets. Francis Fukuyama describes the period between 1970 and 2006 as a set of iterative intervals marked by a mass exodus and associated period of economic decline in areas around the Great Lakes.[7] He describes this decline as "readily measurable in statistics on crime, fatherless children, broken trust, reduced opportunities for and outcomes from education, and the like." Cleveland, Detroit, Buffalo, and Pittsburgh lost about 45% of their population, and median household incomes fell, with Cleveland and Detroit faring the worst.[8] Importantly, this employment insecurity has also been the targeted area of political campaigns—most notably, with the Trump administration) and will be described further below in the section on the political determinants of health.

High rates of unemployment lead to a dearth of reliable benefits (including insurance), as well as harmful workplace conditions, which ultimately impacts health care access and, in turn, outcomes. At the time of writing this chapter, I am the public health officer for the city of Vernon, California. This city is unique with >50,000 daily workers, many of whom are low-skilled workers and over half of whom are either uninsured or underinsured. They are employed by >1,800 businesses in this enclave of industrialism in south Los Angeles. During the COVID-19 pandemic, these folks were true heroes, coming in to work every day and contributing to the ongoing production of goods and services to keep the nation thriving. Unfortunately, and despite federal requirements, many businesses will not provide insurance to their workers through a wide array of manipulative tactics and loopholes, most of which are entirely legal. As a result, these daily workers lack the financial resources (and time) to access primary care and behavioral health services—areas in which many were particularly vulnerable during the pandemic. To protect this core workforce, my team at Wellness Equity Alliance (WEA) and the city of Vernon conducted a community health needs assessment and are now operationalizing these critical clinical services to provide necessary access to these essential workers. Sadly, this innovative partnership between public health and businesses is a unique delivery model.

Occupational health is a serious concern. In 2019 workers suffered 2.8 million nonfatal and 5,333 fatal injuries while on the job. Workers are particularly prone to injuries and illness if their job includes a lot of manual labor that places an undue level of stress on the musculo-skeletal system. Ironically, many people in these roles do not have ready access to structured physical fitness, causing even more severe delete-rious effects. Long-term exposure to harmful chemicals (e.g., pesticides, aerosols, and asbestos) or a noisy work environment can also have adverse consequences. In addition, highly demanding jobs and lack of control over day-to-day work activities are sources of psychosocial stress at work.

Other sources of workplace stress include high levels of interper-sonal conflict, evening shifts, working more than eight hours a day, and having multiple jobs. These stressors put people at risk for mortality and depression and may be correlated with increased parent-child con-flict and parental withdrawal."[9] People in highly stressful jobs may also exhibit unhealthy coping skills such as smoking or alcohol abuse. The prevalence of occupational health injuries is increasing. I recall moonlighting as an occupational health physician, typically in low-income communities. My day would be replete with a rapid increase in workplace injuries, as more Amazon warehouses were emerging and in-creasing the amount of productivity requirements. The combination of a lack of primary care medical offices, poor access to care facilities due to work schedules, a lack of meaning in their employment, a sense of collective disempowerment, and poor physical fitness leads to a com-posite of poor health outcomes, particularly for low-skilled workers with few other employment options.

Food Insecurity

Another correlate of economic instability is food insecurity, which leads to malnutrition. Most people assume that malnutrition is largely seen in iconic images of undernutrition, such as children with *kwashiorkor* (protein malnutrition) in nations like Ethiopia or Niger. This is deeply inaccurate.

Let's simply deconstruct the word. The prefix, which is all telling, *mal-* (meaning "poor") plus *nutrition*. That's all. This can mean either under- or overnutrition. The WHO notes that the levels of obesity have actually more than tripled since 1975, with >40% of the world marked as overweight and >15% as obese.[10] These rates are amplified in nations like the United States, with the CDC reporting >73% of the country as overweight and >41% as obese.[11]

Malnutrition is one of the world's most preventable causes of death and can have significant economic impact because of the costs of obtaining medical care or lost wages due to missing work. We are not even incorporating micronutrient (e.g., vitamins and minerals) deficiencies into this calculus, something that I've studied—especially among refugees.[12]

In South Sudan I was the only physician for >29,000 refugees and internally displaced people and was responsible for the care of a pediatric hospital for the malnourished and undernourished. I will expound on these experiences below, but all too often I held such extreme frailty in my arms that either did or could have led to their tragic demise—cases that fundamentally changed me as a doctor. In other settings, such as the Wind River "Indian" reservation managed by the Indian Health Service (IHS), where I served as community health director, I would frequently see adults with a body mass index (BMI) >50, the benchmark for extreme obesity. In fact, I once had an 11-year-old patient who weighed >400 lbs. We had trouble getting them through the door. While working in Harlem, I had a patient with a BMI >45 who collapsed after I had been examining him for only a few minutes because his knees buckled. He could not stay on his feet or get back up after he fell. The fire department had to come in with a gurney to raise him up. This is the reality we live in.

These narratives are largely driven by the SDoH, including poverty or economic instability, access to affordable health care, and low health literacy. Underserved communities are often considered "food deserts" because of the lack of access to supermarkets that provide affordable and nutritious foods. The US Department of Agriculture defines food deserts as places where "at least a third of the population lives greater than one mile away from a supermarket for urban areas, or greater than 10 miles for rural areas" (figure 2.1). I prefer the following: "low-income census tracts with a substantial number or share of residents with low levels of access to retail outlets selling healthy and affordable foods."[13] By this definition about 19 million people in America live in a food desert. Even in highly urbanized areas like New York City, a number of food deserts abound in low-income communities such as the South Bronx, where I used to work.

Clearly, other more obvious areas exist, such as tribal communities in *frontier medicine environments* (defined by the number of patients/physicians available) like the Wind River "reservation" (we don't favor this term as it assumes this land was somehow reserved for them; *territories* is the preferred term), where >30% of deaths are

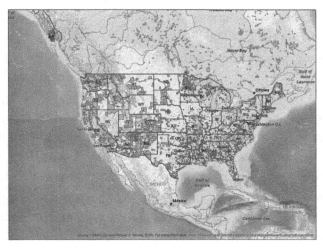

FIGURE 2.1. Food deserts and opportunity zones across the United States according to the *Food Access Research Atlas* of the US Department of Agriculture. *Source:* USDA Economic Research Service, October 20, 2022, https://www.ers.usda.gov/data-products/food-access-research-atlas/documentation.

attributable to diabetes.[14] Ironically, the same Indigenous communities that have historically prided themselves in their reliance on the land and intuitively nutritious fruits and vegetables often contemporaneously lay off of "commodified" foods provided by the US government, many of which are poorly nutritious processed foods.

Housing Instability

"Wow . . . homelessness in California is really bad." This is an all-too-common mantra chanted by out-of-towners as they visit our "left coast."

Let's unpack this statement. A state of communal anomie should not be described with a judgmental qualifier such as "bad." The homeless are not "bad," and homelessness is not necessarily "bad" either, despite the common myth. Is there an issue of homelessness in California? Indeed, there are over 170,000 unhoused Californians (that we are aware of), a number that has increased by over 30% in the last five years.[15]

Los Angeles has the largest homeless population in the United States, with Skid Row the epicenter of that epidemic. In 2018 the United Nations even wrote a scathing report regarding the state of homelessness in California in 2018, calling it "cruel and inhuman."[16] Let that settle in.

In greater Los Angeles County, the 2022 count by the Los Angeles Homeless Services Authority, or LAHSA, revealed approximately 70,000 unhoused people (an increase of 4.1% from 2020), with 41,980 unhoused people in the City of Los Angeles alone (up 1.7% from 2020).[17] Those estimates are likely low, as the RAND Corporation published an analysis of the methodology used by LAHSA showing dramatic increases in the population estimates that cannot be accounted for. This report found that on average, homeless populations in Los Angeles had actually increased by 18% from 2022 to 2023 in areas that had reported a decline.[18]

Let's zoom out further and explain how housing insecurity scales on a national and global level. In the United States, the Department of Housing and Urban Development reports that 1.5 million people a year are experiencing homelessness,[19] while other estimates find up to twice that number are housing insecure.[20] The United Nations Human Settlements Program estimates that 1.6 billion people worldwide live in inadequate housing, and the best data available suggest that >100 million have no housing at all.[21] Housing instability may also impact some populations more than others. Moving three or more times in a year has been associated with negative health outcomes in children. Households are considered cost burdened if they spend >30% of their income on housing and severely cost burdened if they spend >50%. Black, Indigenous, and people of color (BIPOC) households are almost twice as likely as white households to be cost burdened.[22]

So, yes, it's an issue, particularly in regard to the health implications for people experiencing homelessness (PEH). In general, homeless men are up to eight times more likely to die than the general population—a statistic informed by other factors, including suicide, opioid overdose, and sudden cardiac death.[23] Other important health-related issues are poorly controlled chronic diseases, a high prevalence of traumatic brain injury, disproportionate victimization, and high rates of tobacco use. The COVID-19 pandemic has further threatened the health of PEH.

Let us be clear: Being homeless is not the result of an obvious cause-and-effect relationship as is so popularly described. One does not simply wake up unhoused as the result of one poor decision, or even a string of them. Nor is it all about drugs. Much of this crisis is socially or politically determined—both in the United States and beyond. The upstream causes of poor health in the homeless population include extreme poverty, harsh living environments, trauma in childhood, and structural barriers to care. So uninformed efforts to cast blame on millions of folks is just not grounded in reality or science.

Homelessness is one of the most formidable issues when it comes to health care access in the United States and beyond. We can't begin to describe homelessness unless we have a broader definition of "housing insecurity": a lack of security in a residential setting resulting from high housing costs relative to income, poor housing quality, unstable neighborhoods, overcrowding, and, but may not include, homelessness.[24] Homelessness can take many forms, with people living on the streets, in encampments or shelters, in transitional housing programs, or "doubled up" with family and friends. Overcrowding—defined as more than two people living in the same bedroom or multiple families living in one residence—may affect mental health, stress levels, relationships, and sleep and may increase the risk of infectious disease.[22]

Homelessness is a complex issue, sitting at the intersection of public health, housing affordability, intimate partner violence (IPV), behavioral health (including mental health and substance use), urbanization, racial and gender discrimination, infrastructure, and unemployment. The connection between housing and homelessness is generally intuitive, but the strong link between health and homelessness is often overlooked, especially for physically demanding jobs such as construction and manufacturing. The loss of employment due to poor health then becomes a vicious cycle: Without funds to pay for health care, one cannot heal to work again, and if one remains ill, it is difficult to regain employment, and without income from employment, an injury or illness quickly becomes a housing problem. In these situations any available savings are quickly exhausted, and relying on friends and family for assistance to help maintain rent/mortgage payments, food, medical care, and other basic needs can be short-lived. Once these personal safety nets are exhausted, very few options are usually available to help with either health care or housing, let alone both.

My interest in homelessness started to develop when I moved back to California in 2016. While the intersections between homelessness and health care were well described in other areas of the world, I had not been as aware of them until moving back to California—coincidentally, my birthplace. Life had come full circle.

At the time I was working in the South Bronx seeing patients daily and was primarily focused on leading two programs: an HIV initiative to improve care for transgender women of color and the first integrated primary care/mental health program for refugees in New York City. I was heavily recruited to come out to interview and tour a prestigious HIV organization based in Hollywood—the AIDS Healthcare Foundation (AHF), which is in fact the largest community-based HIV organization in the United States

What a coincidence that this was World AIDS Day.[25] I was taken out on the streets during an HIV protest facilitated by the organization. I witnessed the passion of its members and the collective action of activists synchronizing their frustration at corporate America reaping profit off of the lives of those who suffer from chronic virological illnesses.[26] I was later wined and dined at a celebrity-led private concert with headliners from Harry Belafonte to Common. But it was the dedication at the grassroots level that had mesmerized me. As I grabbed a quick dinner with an old friend before I boarded the flight back to New York City, my mind was spinning from the events of the day and how my career might turn from there. My friend inquired about my facial expressions of deep consternation and what I had ultimately decided. After a long pause, I took a deep sigh and (somewhat) confidently responded, "I guess I'm moving back to LA."

In that job, as the medical director for the largest HIV clinic in the nation (as well as AHF's national director of infectious disease), homelessness and the substance use that is associated with it became an everyday reality looming over my patient care. More than a quarter of my patients (n > 2,000) were housing insecure, and approximately half were using drugs (mostly methamphetamine, some of which was injected daily). While an undeniable association existed between the two, my patients included plenty of housing-insecure folks who had previously been soccer moms who had merely fallen upon hard times. Now they were afflicted with methamphetamine dependence and infections like syphilis. The reality is that once the vicious cycle of housing insecurity is activated, it is an inescapable rabbit hole for most.

That job fundamentally changed my viewpoint on how I would perform clinical care. I prided myself on providing top-quality health care to all my patients, regardless of their ability to pay. I would often get teased about the long waits that patients had to endure (15–20 minutes, which is all that most Medicaid or Ryan White health plans afforded us to manage AIDS, schizophrenia, methamphetamine use, homelessness, and syphilis, just isn't enough time). But once they were in a room with me, I did my best to ensure they felt there was no other competing concern, and they had my undivided attention.

How naive I was. I recall one reckoning in which I ordered a Holter monitor for a Palestinian patient who had identified dysrhythmias, decompensated depression, and active methamphetamine use and, importantly, was living under a bridge. Of course, they don't teach you in medical school that without active sources of electricity, much of Western biomedicine's advancements have absolutely no applicability. It was reported that despite the patient's family trying to find him under this said bridge to bring him portable batteries, he ultimately ran away from them. That experience made me realize that, for many communities, the best care is simply meeting "them where they're at." Nowadays, this mantra is currently seared into the minds of nearly every community medicine medical resident, as well it should be. For me, another series of developments awaited that would further reify this expression.

As indicated in figure 2.2, the upstream causes of poor health in the homeless population include extreme poverty, harsh living environments, trauma, and structural barriers to care. The downstream causes range from staggeringly high rates of mental health issues and substance use disorder (SUD), including tobacco use, to a wide spectrum of cardiovascular, pulmonary, and hepatobiliary diseases and can be organized into the following domains of health concerns.[27]

- Mental health
- SUD
- Infectious diseases
- Chronic health conditions
- Musculoskeletal injuries and wounds

Prolonged conditions for PEH can increase mortality rates by two to eight times higher than the general population.[28] Put another way,

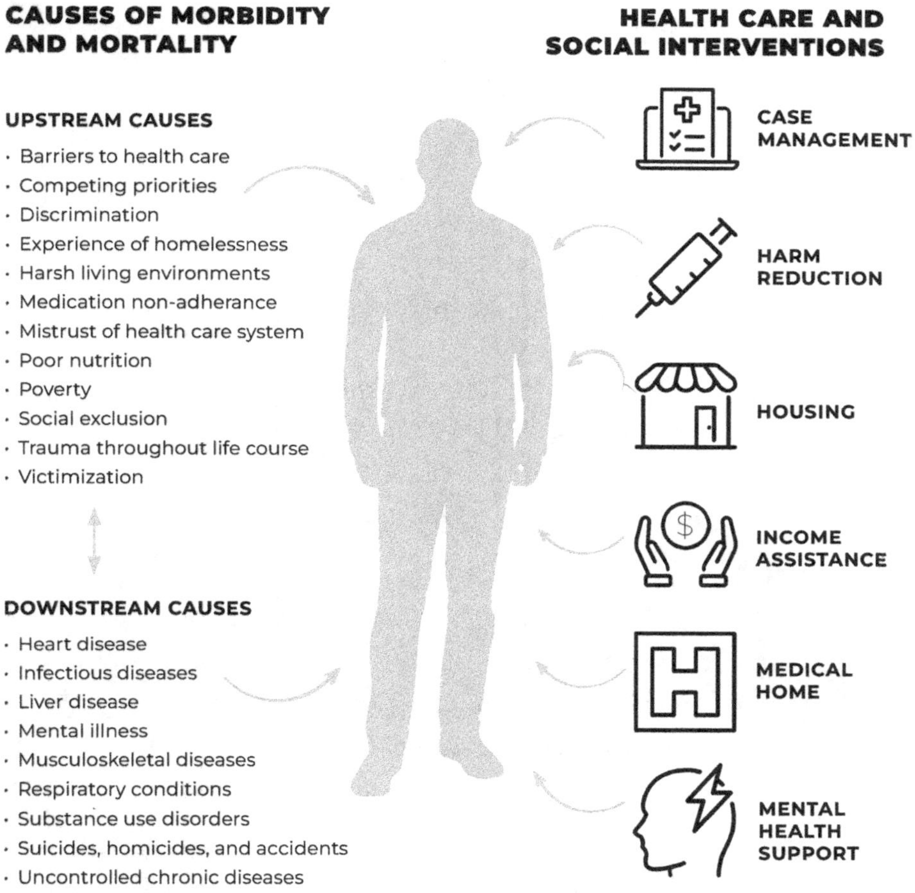

CAUSES OF MORBIDITY AND MORTALITY

HEALTH CARE AND SOCIAL INTERVENTIONS

UPSTREAM CAUSES

- Barriers to health care
- Competing priorities
- Discrimination
- Experience of homelessness
- Harsh living environments
- Medication non-adherance
- Mistrust of health care system
- Poor nutrition
- Poverty
- Social exclusion
- Trauma throughout life course
- Victimization

DOWNSTREAM CAUSES

- Heart disease
- Infectious diseases
- Liver disease
- Mental illness
- Musculoskeletal diseases
- Respiratory conditions
- Substance use disorders
- Suicides, homicides, and accidents
- Uncontrolled chronic diseases

CASE MANAGEMENT

HARM REDUCTION

HOUSING

INCOME ASSISTANCE

MEDICAL HOME

MENTAL HEALTH SUPPORT

FIGURE 2.2. Upstream and downstream causes of homelessness and the clinical interventions available for people experiencing it. *Source:* Graphic by author.

they die, on average, 12 years sooner than the general US population. When these conditions are further influenced by lifestyle factors as described by Maslow's hierarchy of needs (e.g., basic nutrient deficiencies, sleep hygiene; (figure 2.3), the health outcomes of PEH are further misguided.[29,30] The colliding intersectionality of this socially determined miasma of disease is well-known and understood by many who are housing insecure, but a collective sense of apathy or a lack of perceived agency influences either the will or self-determination to

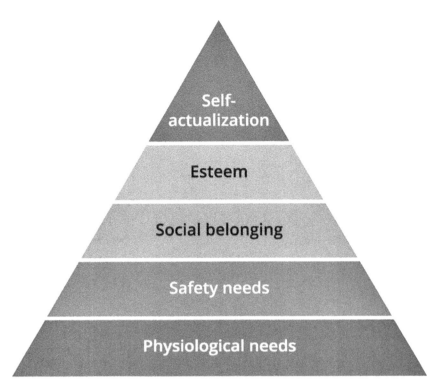

FIGURE 2.3. Maslow's hierarchy of needs. *Source:* Getty Images.

effectively manage their health care, or both. This sense of a lack of empowerment may be internalized as stress and somaticized to influence an effective immune response through a complex web of endocrine factors and immunomodulators.[31]

Homelessness creates new health problems and exacerbates existing ones. Living on the street or in crowded homeless shelters is extremely stressful and exacerbated by exposure to communicable disease (e.g., tuberculosis, HIV, COVID-19), violence, malnutrition, and harmful weather. Chronic health conditions such as high blood pressure, diabetes, and asthma worsen because there is no safe place to store medications properly. Behavioral health is particularly concerning. A recent study of newly homeless people in the New York City shelter system demonstrated that 35% and 53% experienced major depression and SUD, respectively.[22] These are all examples of syndemics, and we will delve more deeply into these in chapter 7.

Poverty

Imagine a space where the most elaborate decorations are junk-harvested aluminum cans adorned with colorful beads and a random assortment of dilapidated recliners and ripped-out car seats crowding the front porch. The home behind that porch is made of random building materials, most of which seem to be experiencing rapid decay, set within a constellation of apocalyptic-looking overhanging power lines. The home is populated by multiple humans—several generations in which health has manifestly not been a priority. They stare with expressionless faces at this white doctor approaching their home, all tied together by one unifier—poverty.

Allow me to paint another scenario with scattered makeshift homes emitting random plumes of smoke from indoor fires. Most of these homes appear to have been constructed in the matter of a week or less. People congregate in front of a few of these homes, in heavily soiled and tattered clothing with a common theme of poorly spelled American or European branding. Many do not have shoes; some wear flip-flops, mostly stitched together by duct tape (or some flailing and tenuous material). They, too, are staring, curious, albeit with flat affects chiseled by time and countless tragedies at this white doctor in a vest approaching in a Land Rover.

One of these scenarios was in South Sudan; the other on the Wind River Reservation in Wyoming. Can you guess which? It's unfortunate that we have this level of abject poverty in the United States of America, but that is the harsh reality. According to the 2010 US Census, 15.1% of Americans live below the federal poverty level.[32] Worse, according to UNICEF, the United States has the second-highest rate of childhood poverty among developed nations, second only to Romania.[33] Poverty is the universal influencer of health care access and probably the most formidable and compelling social and political determinant of health itself. Its causes are so multifactorial and intersect nearly every other determinant described in this chapter. This attention notwithstanding, it's important to devote an independent chapter to this determinant alone.

What does "poverty" even mean? We throw the term around so loosely that defining it is critical. Of course, the definition is relative to the environment in question. In its most atrocious form, *extreme poverty*, one cannot even obtain the basic needs for survival (i.e., food, potable water, and shelter). The World Bank has set the criterion for extreme poverty as anyone living on less than one dollar per day—a category that includes approximately 1.2 billion of our fellow human beings. (Barely better, 2.8 billion—1 out of every 4 people on Earth— have a daily income of less than two dollars.) These numbers have no doubt increased exponentially as a result of the COVID-19 pandemic.

Extreme poverty is not due to a lack of natural resources but results from human greed and oppression, frequently exacerbated by foreign exploitation. A country with homogenous poverty is tragic but morally digestible. It is far more horrific when a relative amount of wealth exists but is hoarded by a select few. As Mahatma Gandhi noted, "The world has enough for man's need . . . but not enough for man's greed."

An additional variant is relative poverty, defined by reference to the living standards of the majority in any given society. If the vast majority of a given society have access to particular resources, the minority who do not may be said to be living in relative poverty. If I am on the same aircraft with a man who is stretching out his legs and being served champagne and filet mignon while I am squeezed between two obese people with screaming children and consuming a vague approximation of tasteless chicken, the question may arise: Why is he being treated better than me?

Therefore, the real underlying driver of suffering is not absolute poverty but economic inequality. It is not the fact that one is lacking that is most unconscionable but the understanding that another is thriving at the expense of their less fortunate counterpart.

Historically, marginalized communities that are discriminated against because of race/ethnicity, geography, disabilities, or immigration status typically have much higher rates of poverty. The causal sequence is logical. The compositional features described above limit educational and employment opportunities, leading to poorer economic outcomes and associated agency. For example, those poorer communities will attract grocery markets with limited supplies of healthy and nutritious foods, as the residents generally lack the purchasing power to afford them, causing a concentration of food deserts as described above. The resulting poor nutrition leads to increased health issues, which worsen economic prospects and perpetuate the cycle.

In no other population is this argument more compelling than youth. Childhood poverty exists among a constellation of other issues described as "adverse childhood experiences" (ACEs) and is associated with developmental delays, toxic stress, chronic illness, and nutritional deficits. Moreover, the effect is cyclical, as individuals who experience childhood poverty are more likely to experience poverty into adulthood, affecting even their life expectancy. One study found that men in the top 1% of income were expected to live 14.6 years longer than those in the bottom 1% and women in that group 10.1 years longer.[34]

In short, massive and incessant human suffering need not exist amid the relative abundance of resources and technological proficiency that we possess in today's world. Yet it does. Jeffrey Sachs points out that the world's 200 richest people more than doubled their net worth between 1994 and 1998, to more than $1 trillion. The assets of the top 3 billionaires amount to more than the combined gross national product of all 43 least developed countries and their combined population of 600 million people. According to a recent World Inequality Report, 2020 actually marked the steepest increase in the global billionaires' share of wealth on record. Indeed, since 1995 the share of global wealth that billionaires possess has risen from 1% to over 3%.[35] Furthermore, the distance between the richest and poorest countries has expanded radically, from 3:1 in 1820 to 30:1 in 1960, 60:1 in 1990, and 74:1 at the turn of the century.[36]

Stated another way, approximately 20% of the world's population possesses 80% of the world's wealth, meaning that some people enjoy a high standard of living while others live in abject poverty and manifest misery. Human anguish is tragic at every level. From my observations, however, suffering is most acute when it materializes from inequality—namely, systematic oppression in which the "haves" maintain their privileged position at the direct expense of the "have nots."

Let's bring this back to health care in the United States, where structural access to that care is heavily influenced by poverty. In terms of funding health care access, the United States does provide insurance (Medicaid through the Centers for Medicare and Medicaid Services) for certain Americans falling below the federal poverty line. Sadly, it is still not enough for millions of Americans who fall just barely above that line and for whom the cost of purchasing insurance is out of reach. In an encouraging development, the Affordable Care Act (ACA; "Obamacare," a poorly contemplated term that would ultimately generate myriad political challenges) provided for the expansion of Medicaid, allowing many more Americans to obtain insurance who previously could not. Unfortunately, not all states adopted Medicaid expansion, resulting in even more inequality in the country—very much unnecessarily. As of 2021, about 27.5 million Americans—roughly 10.2% of the population—still lacked health coverage. In a bitter irony, many in that 10.2% have the greatest health care needs.

This discussion does not conclude our focus on poverty. In fact, poverty is one of the core drivers of health and is connected to nearly every other determinant, so it will remain a recurring topic throughout this book.

Education Access and Quality

While working with UNICEF in India in the early 2000s, my objective was to focus on the perception of HIV risk among adolescents in Tamil Nadu, a large province in southern India. Most of our research stemmed from interviews and focus groups at schools, many of which were rural in nature. What we found was a growing divergence of educational enrollment between boys and girls at or around age 11. More specifically, we identified that increasingly more girls would not attend classes because they lacked access to bathrooms. It embarrassed them to have to hold their toileting all day—especially once they started entering puberty. In many cases only one toilet (really a dug-out hole in the floor) served hundreds of aspiring young minds. Parents did not necessarily object to their young girls dropping out of school, as they often saw education as futile for girls who would be married off and have seemingly no purpose for it. This was more common in lower-resourced or more rural schools. So toilets literally determined the numbers of girls who would continue their education, which would further influence access to other resources for the rest of their lives. This cycle is a dominant theme throughout this book.

This group of social determinants is particularly important because it is a foundational building block that is largely deterministic of the ability to navigate through all other social determinants. While economics is highly correlated with education in what is commonly defined as socioeconomic status, education must be grouped and analyzed on its own. For purposes of clarity, the CDC breaks this group down into four subgroups.

Early Childhood Development and Education

The importance of early childhood development and education cannot be overstated. Early childhood (especially the first five years) impacts long-term social, cognitive, emotional, and physical development.[37] These developmental and educational opportunities are tenuous and deeply affected by various environmental and social factors, including socioeconomic status, relationships with parents and caregivers, access to early education programs, and above all, early life stress.[38] Other stressors such as physical abuse, family instability, unsafe neighborhoods, and poverty can cause children to experience inadequate coping skills, difficulty regulating emotions, and reduced social functioning compared to other children their age. Additionally, exposure to environmental hazards, such as lead in the home, can negatively affect a child's health and cause cognitive developmental delays.[39] Research shows that lead exposure disproportionally targets children from racial/ethnic minority and low-income households and can have an adverse impact on their readiness for school.[40,41]

The socioeconomic status of young children's families and communities also significantly determines their educational outcomes. Research shows that children from poorer communities are more likely to repeat grades and drop out of high school. Put simply, early childhood programs are a critical outlet for fostering the mental and physical development of young children to facilitate transitioning into thriving young adults.[38]

High School Graduation

Inequities in high school graduation rates are profound and continue to widen between race/ethnicity groups and states. The National Center for Education Statistics created an adjusted cohort graduation rate (ACGR) to help compare differences among students across the nation. The ACGR was 75% for American Indians/Alaskan Natives compared to 93% for Asian/Pacific Islanders and 90% for white students, respectively.[42] In terms of state differences, Washington, DC, had the lowest ACGR, followed by Arizona and New Mexico.[43] When we drill down the data further, we can see that these disparities are likely skewed by American Indians/Alaskan Natives living in the latter states.

I understood these communities very well, and some of my own lived experience is what brought me to work within the space I do and ultimately write these very words.

Dropping out of high school following a number of expulsions and having to care for my daughter was no easy decision. I ultimately decided to sit for a general equivalency diploma and enrolled in community college shortly thereafter. I had a second chance. I also had privilege. I was a white male living in the United States. Many others without that privilege would not have had that chance. Disparities in high school completion rates are highly correlated with race and ethnicity in the United States. Black and Brown communities have significantly higher rates of attrition for a number of reasons. According to data for the 2018–2019 school year, 93% of Asian / Pacific Islander, 89% of white, 82% of Hispanic, 80% of Black, and 74% of American Indian / Alaska Native students attending public high schools graduated within four years of beginning the ninth grade. This is multifactorial and several other factors contribute to the successful completion of high school, but race and ethnicity remain key.

These individual experiences ultimately brought me to South Sudan and New Mexico. An important area where health and education align is where we place these access points. School-based health centers (SBHCs) have increasingly become an innovative health equity tool focusing on the most at-risk youth communities.[44] SBHCs collaborate with the school nurse and augment the health care services to which a child may already have access. If a child lacks access to care, SBHCs, which are located in schools, can serve as a primary medical home. This greatly reduces factors such as transportation issues, parent availability, and missed appointments. WEA is currently building these out in Bernalillo County (including Albuquerque), New Mexico, focusing on substance use treatment and prevention, mental health, and sexual health. Our hope is to provide not only better health care outcomes but enhanced educational opportunities, as well (including high school graduation rates). Given the challenges encountered in New Mexico, this will be a highly welcomed program. There is more to come in part III.

Enrollment in Higher Education

The role of race and ethnicity in college and university enrollment rates is equally revealing. The college enrollment rate in 2020 was highest for 18- to 24-year-olds who were Asian (64%), followed by those who were white (41%), Hispanic (36%), Black (36%), or American Indian / Alaska

Native (22%).[45] How higher education determines access to health care is clear—most prominently through structural access with economic opportunity but just as compellingly through literacy levels, which will be described below.

That phenomenon is particularly true during pandemics. During the COVID-19 pandemic, the more education that workers had, the more likely they were to keep their jobs and work remotely, allowing them to avoid unnecessary exposure.[46] Other than health care workers, those considered "essential workers" were largely manual laborers in the food and agricultural sectors, many of whom did not have college or university degrees.

My perspective on this topic is highly influenced by my own experiences. At the time I was applying to universities, my father and grandparents had already passed away, and my mother was in failing health. I was alone to nurture my mother and care for my five-year-old brother. Obviously, my choices were limited in that it was essential for me to attend college within the Los Angeles area, so I submitted but one application—to the University of Southern California (USC).

One day I was called in to meet with the assistant to the dean of Admissions. As I was handed an acceptance packet, I could never explain the pride I felt as I watched my mother tear up. Two weeks prior to the beginning of my first semester at USC at the age of 21, my mother was hospitalized. My university dreams were shattered. Five months later, as my mature mind evolved within a 21-year-old body, I tragically and unexpectedly lost my mother to cancer and watched helplessly as the state placed my 6-year-old brother into adoption. My university dreams, it seemed, vanished.

My tenacity would not accept this. Following one of the most difficult years in my life, I was allowed readmittance and began my studies at USC. At the same time I was dealing with the financial fallout from my father's death, finding a home for my 6-year-old brother, and raising my 3-year-old daughter, all while taking physics, general chemistry, calculus, and Spanish in my first year at a university—with a mere 10th-grade education. Oh, and the Internet had also been born. . . .

Language and Literacy

Throughout my life I ended up learning six languages with variable levels of success—beyond my native English tongue, I picked up some Japanese, Korean, Thai, Hebrew, and Spanish. My wife would like me to add Arabic to this list (she is Egyptian), but I no longer have the neuroplasticity to engage, I'm afraid. While much of this linguistic mastery has atrophied, I was quite adamant about learning these languages in my 20s, as I traveled to >100 countries. As a doctor I enjoyed striking up conversations in my patient's native language and enjoyed being able to relate to folks in their native tongue. Even if it was just a few words, it gave them a great deal of comfort.

Let me explain further how this connects to health care access. Literacy has multiple components, including oral literacy (listening and speaking skills), print literacy (writing and reading skills), numeracy (the ability to understand and work with numbers), and cultural and conceptual knowledge.[47,48] Health literacy is the bridge between one's literacy skills and the degree to which individuals and organizations find, understand, and use health-related information or services. They are connected but certainly not the same. Research suggests that limited language skills and low literacy skills are associated with lower educational attainment and worse health outcomes and are a barrier to accessing health information, using medication properly, and utilizing preventive services.[49,50,51,52] Individuals with limited literacy face additional difficulties following medication instructions, communicating with health care providers, and attaining health information—all of which may adversely affect their health.

Because the average level of literacy in the United States is calibrated at a fifth-grade reading level, all governmental agencies (as well as organizations who receive considerable federal funding resources) must ensure their educational materials meet this mark. The fact that the largest economy in the world has an average reading level this low is obviously a formidable issue. In addition, several other countries (most in sub-Saharan Africa) have rates of illiteracy that exceed 50%—a disparity that predominantly afflicts women.

Institutional barriers such as a lack of well-trained interpreters and culturally competent health care providers adversely affect the health of individuals with low literacy and limited English proficiency. For migrants dealing with language and literacy challenges, cultural barriers and financial difficulties may create additional obstacles to accessing and comprehending health information.

When I was working with Doctors Without Borders in South Sudan, our primary mission was to build a pediatric malnutrition hospital, but of course, we would do everything possible to see any patient we could. Many of these were adults. Most had never seen a doctor before.

Empirically, we found that many of these patients were women. Headaches, abdominal pain, and "seizures" were the most common complaints, but even after reasonably extensive workups, we were not able to determine any actual source of disease for many of them. In fact, the reason I placed seizures in quotation marks is because we were quickly able to identify an interesting pattern of adult women presenting with convulsions. Someone who is having a true seizure essentially loses consciousness. We created a small team of observers who were able to discover nuggets of evidence of consciousness during these convulsions (e.g., eyes opening and peering around or intentional motor movements).

These presentations would then be classified as pseudoseizures and have very different motivating factors. The condition is complex, and we did not have the resources to study it, but we suspected that much of it was precipitated by stress and a large scope of mood disorders—primarily depression. In case conferences we were also able to uncover that many of these patients had undergone deeply traumatic experiences and simply needed to "check out." We suspected that a hospital visit would give them an escape from the grueling world they faced on a daily basis. The reality was that they lacked a structural way to say this, as the words "depression" and "stress" did not exist in the tribal languages they spoke, and they certainly could not express this to Western doctors. In an impoverished nation with one of the highest rates of illiteracy in the world, this would bleed into poor health literacy.

Health literacy, however, certainly cannot be chalked up to an "African problem," as the low reading level in the United States shows. I encountered this issue systematically throughout my career, almost everywhere I worked. During my medical educational training in a Harlem hospital, I would cringe when I heard medical residents or attending physicians speak to patients with unnecessarily complex words (e.g., oncological, hypertension), especially while delivering diagnoses with very sensitive courses of treatment. See table 2.1 for a cheat sheet for unnecessarily complex medical speak. They weren't speaking with the patients—they were speaking at them. As a result, when I worked in areas like the Wind River Reservation with American Indians or in the South Bronx with Dominicans, Puerto Ricans, or recently resettled

Table 2.1. Common terms used in medicine, "medical speak," that can confuse patients and put distance between physician and patient

Medical term	Layperson term
Acute	New, sudden, urgent
Benign	Without serious consequences
Diabetes	High blood sugar
Hypertension	High blood pressure
Intubate	Insert a breathing tube in the airway
Lipid	Fat
Morbidity	Complication or undesired result
Oncology	Study of tumors or cancer
Prenatal	Before birth
Renal	Related to the kidneys
Thrombus	Blood clot

refugees (we created a migrant health program), I would be very intentional about speaking in a language that people could understand and relate to. Using those few words in Urdu to my Pakistani patients or discussing the best Biryani with my South Indian patients meant something to them. It meant that I saw them and understood where they came from, and I tailored my recommendations and treatment courses in a way that made sense to them. Many times this required a medical interpreter, but I did my best to engage them in communication techniques that would help them feel heard and understood. Doing this during a public health emergency is slightly more complex and will be the subject of extensive discussion in chapter 7).

Health Care Access and Quality (Health Equity)

Access to Health Services

When I worked in rural Indian-controlled Kashmir, the volume of patients I saw was untenable—sometimes beyond 100 a day. I felt it was important, however, to always ask them a few relatable questions. One included the location of their village and how far they had walked in order to be seen that day. In the United States, patients complain if they need to travel over an hour. In Kashmir, it was several days.

The National Academies of Sciences, Engineering, and Medicine (NASEM) defines access to health care as the "timely use of personal health services to achieve the best possible health outcomes."[53] This sounds vague and ambiguous. What does timely actually mean? What are personal health services? The reality is that access to health services is one of the most seemingly complex concepts and cannot be distilled into one sentence. It comprises a wide array of mechanics and influences but can generally be divided into two buckets—one is real, material access, while the other is the perception of access. They are both equally important and should be evaluated separately.

Material Access

Material access to health care can be broken down into a number of smaller subsets, many of which are socially determined, including the following:

- **Access to primary care**: NASEM defines primary care as "the provision of integrated, accessible health care services by clinicians who are accountable for addressing a large majority of personal health care needs, developing a sustained partnership with patients, and practicing in the context of family and community."[54] A primary care provider (PCP) or general practitioner is usually an internist, family physician, pediatrician, or nonphysician advanced practice provider (e.g., family nurse practitioner, physician assistant).[55] The limitations can be further broken down into the following four causes:

  ○ **Limited number of PCPs in the area:** The United States suffers from a general shortage of PCPs, especially in low-resourced areas. The reasons are multifactorial, starting with the medical educational system and the lack of value that we place in clinical specialties involved with primary care. In addition, there are salient disparities in PCPs in areas of greatest need. As a result, the National Health Service Corps aims to recruit talented PCPs in areas of the United States with limited access to care, known as *health professional shortage areas.*[56] This only scratches the surface, I'm afraid.

  ○ **Limited transportation services to access those PCPs:** Transportation is one of the most formidable barriers to health care globally. Research showed that individuals from racial / ethnic minority groups who had an increased risk for severe illness from COVID-19 were more likely to lack transportation to health care services. Recall the story above in which the patients in rural Kashmir needed to walk for days to reach a doctor. It's important to note that this is not just an issue of deeply rural areas in the Global South, as a number of very troubling cases can also be seen in the United States. At WEA we have been working on the southern border of the United States in Texas for a few years now. In that region in unincorporated low-income areas known as the *colonias*, close to 2 million people are living in squalid conditions on what are difficult to describe as other than "slum ranches": scattered rural homesteads on inappropriately subdivided land, with substandard housing made of salvaged materials and lacking utilities and even basic services such as drinking water, sewage treatment, and paved roads. (Curiously, most are legally documented US citizens.)

○ **Limited cultural competence:** We know of an increasing number of communities whose youth no longer have the appetite to engage with a conventional exam room experience. They don't want to wait, they don't want to feel judged, and they often do not want to feel "sick." I've seen a great deal of this and would incorporate these wanted changes systematically into my operational practice when I was running health centers across the nation. Sexually transmitted infections (STIs) are what we describe in public health as "reportable" and therefore need to be traced, investigated, and then managed by public health agencies. Many agencies, however, do not have the bandwidth to provide direct clinical services, at least in a way that meets the needs of the communities they serve. The reality is that people with STIs (many of whom are active and healthy young adults) do not want to come into a "gray" government clinic and be asked to wait for hours. They want to be in and out in under 30 minutes and have as little contact as possible with a medical provider. As a result, I ran a network of STI clinics across the nation that we branded as "wellness centers." Wellness trends quite well for these communities because they prefer to avoid a space that suggests infirm or sick patients would attend (i.e., a "clinic").

- **Access to specialized care:** The United States is not generally lacking in medical specialists, an issue that leads to extreme excess in US health care spending, which is more than twice that of any other developed (or Organisation for Economic Co-operation and Development member) nation. As is the trend in this book, most of these specialists are concentrated in areas of wealth and heavy resources. For example, in the South Bronx we had access to dozens of tertiary medical centers within a 10-mile radius and a relative abundance of specialists in key fields such as rheumatology, dermatology, and even psychiatry, but it was seemingly impossible to access them simply because many would not accept Medicaid.
- **Access to health insurance:** People with lower incomes are often uninsured, especially in states that did not engage in Medicaid expansion as allowed by the ACA. Tragically, minority groups account for over half that group.[57] Individuals without health insurance may delay seeking care when they are ill or injured and are more likely to be hospitalized for chronic conditions. It's also important to note that this is not a binary concept, as many are not uninsured but "underinsured." In either case, inadequate health insurance coverage is one of the most formidable barriers to health care access, as the unequal distribution of coverage contributes to profound disparities.[58] In addition, out-of-pocket medical care costs may lead individuals to delay or forgo needed care and cause considerable medical debt to accumulate.

Let me share another story in order to help bite into these discussions. Between missions with Doctors Without Borders and the time that the ACA was passed, I was moonlighting as a doctor in emergency rooms and urgent care clinics—fortunately, in states where Obamacare was in effect, such as New York and Connecticut. All of a sudden, millions of Americans now had access to health care, seemingly overnight, but didn't know what to do with it. What was needed, especially in areas of concentrated poverty, were community health workers (CHWs) to help people navigate access. CHWs are a critical workforce due to the simple fact that they have the trust of key communities who historically distrust systems—especially the government. I had remarkable experiences working with CHWs in South Africa, where they would help get HIV medications to communities that struggled with access, particularly in deeply rural areas. Unfortunately, in the United States CHWs have no practical mechanism for reimbursement. In the US system, if you cannot bill for it, it doesn't exist. As a result, CHWs have been largely excluded from conventional health systems, especially in the areas they are needed the most. This needs to change, which I will discuss further in part III.

Interestingly, in the United States only five populations are guaranteed access to health care (of course, I'm simplifying): veterans, American Indians, people living with HIV and AIDS, older adults, and prisoners. How many still lack health coverage in the United States? The number of uninsured nonelderly individuals dropped from 46.5 million in 2010, prior to the ACA, to <26.7 million in 2016, then climbed to 28.9 million in 2019 before dropping again to 27.5 million (or 10.2%) in 2021.[59] Unfortunately, as irony would have it, that 10% often have the greatest health care needs. When the needs are so profound that they can no longer avoid consuming health care services, the costs are considerable. There was no greater example of this than the COVID-19 pandemic.

In much of the Global South, as described above, most health care must be covered through out-of-pocket expenses. At one point during the Ebola pandemic of 2014–2015, I was working in Sierra Leone, in the eastern province of Kono, which happened to be the poorest province in a country with one of the lowest average survival rates in the world. Kono was impacted heavily by Ebola, and the government hospital was largely abandoned. In December 2014, the WHO reported that over 11 days, "two teams buried 87 bodies, including a nurse, an ambulance driver, and a janitor drafted to remove such bodies. . . . One response team also discovered over 25 accumulated dead bodies in a cordoned area of the (government) hospital."[60] This was deep in the jungle on the border of Guinea and was fittingly the setting of the film *Blood Diamond*.

In Kono I would make rounds in the general medical wards in order to help teach some of the junior physicians and would commonly write up treatments that could be locally sourced—often fluids and antibiotics. I was deeply troubled when I discovered a number of patients had not made it through the night. When I investigated further, I discovered that many patients never received the treatment I ordered. This was not neglect on behalf of the clinical staff but a visceral and extreme example of an out-of-pocket insurance system in which patients would quite literally die if they (or their families) did not have the few dollars to cover their treatment. There was absolutely no safety net. The frustration experienced was extreme, and one evening I wrote this excerpt while working in these wards:

Patients are admitted with inaccurate diagnoses and management with very little follow up after such admissions (e.g., patients languish for weeks without being seen by a health care professional once admitted). . . . Blood transfusions are ordered as a perceived panacea (with frighteningly poor quality in screening and frequent fatal consequences) . . . and those requiring emergent care (including a number of patients in shock) are denied treatment unless they can buy the actual medications and supplies themselves (all treatment must be purchased before administration for all populations other than children under 5 years and pregnant women).

All of these egregious phenomena are not a fault of any one hospital, but rather the corollary of a system that is deeply fractured by corruption naturally feeding off of poverty that is contorted further by actors who regulate access to essential resources. Such valuable resources abound in this area, but the local actors entirely lack access to their benefits and are subjugated into a state where they remain vulnerable to adversarial forces—whether that be war or disease.

Perceived Access

Perceived access to health care is largely driven by health literacy. Of course, the universal trend here is that personal health literacy is associated with racial/ethnic minority status, age, poverty, health insurance coverage, educational attainment, language spoken before starting school, and self-reported health.[61] If one does not understand risk factors or value the importance of primary care including prevention, material access is meaningless. As a result, community health outreach and education are critical to inform communities of this importance—especially in high-risk communities. As discussed above, this outreach and education is most effectively delivered by CHWs, especially those of lived experience who remain relatable and accessible to the communities they serve.

Another important element to illuminate is the concept of digital literacy: the incorporation of technical and critical thinking skills to navigate through our increasingly digital world. We find that this literacy, unlike other types, is considerably influenced by age. There is a growing senescence of digital literacy through age but an equally important one driven by resources. As a result, we have a digital divide of people throughout the Global North, one that is increasingly impacting health care as we continue to digitize health care resources. As noted earlier, in one of the companies I was running during the COVID-19 pandemic (Curative Medical), those with preferential access to the lifesaving vaccine were the "triple Cs": Caucasians with cars and computers. Digital literacy has therefore become a highly deterministic element of whether people have access to lifesaving vaccines. This barrier notwithstanding, we may be able to flip this to help serve the needs of large populations through generative artificial intelligence (AI), and I am currently leading a group on this at *Open AI*. Part III will continue this discussion.

Health Equity

Addressing both material and perceived access is critical when approaching the subject of health equity. Many folks not in health care will falsely associate equality and equity, but they are actually quite different. If you google "health equity," you'll find a number of definitions attempting to define this word, which is a relatively fashionable term. I'll simplify it. It's doing more for communities at higher risk of poor population health outcomes in order to reduce disparities during both "blue skies" (chronic health) and "gray skies" (population and public health emergencies).

While this book predominantly focuses on the determinants of "gray sky" conditions, it's important to understand the connection of access during "blue sky" environments as well. Health equity is certainly not equality because the reality is that not every population should have the same access to health care. Put simply, those who are educated, health literate, younger, working in tech, and have insurance frankly do not need to work that hard to navigate access to their health care needs. We must work harder to optimize access for those in the South Bronx, in South Chicago, or in South Los Angeles. Once engaged we must optimize the quality of those services for those folks, focus on communication they understand, and provide the necessary resources they need in order to follow up on the recommendations their PCPs have provided. We need to do better. We must do better. My entire career has been dedicated to this fight. At the end of this book, you will better understand how you can contribute meaningfully.

Neighborhood and Built Environment

Access to Foods That Support Healthy Dietary Patterns

I stare at the man in front of me on the exam table. His left leg has been amputated above the knee. His fine touch of certain items is severely limited. He's on dialysis. He weighs over 500 lbs. He is disheveled. His sugar level is so high it's unreadable. His carrying bag contains extensive evidence of an array of artificial foods made in laboratories—including all the typical offenders, such as Cheetos, Oreos, and Pop

Tarts. He is unemployed, relying on disability coverage. He is in the South Bronx. Curiously, he is not here for any of these reasons. He is seeing me today because his eyesight is worsening (retinal damage is a common consequence of uncontrolled diabetes). He seems to have no insight as to the common denominator for all of these issues. He keeps eating—food that will kill him.

As described above in the section on food insecurity, food deserts are all too common throughout the world. What's curious is that they're not necessarily correlated with development, as the United States is notorious for having thousands of food deserts—over 6,500 to be exact. Interestingly, they are not necessarily correlated with rural environments either. In fact, we see them all too frequently in urban areas. Indeed, they compose the vast majority, 82%, of all such food deserts in the country.

An estimated 13.5 million people in the United States have low access to a supermarket or large grocery store.[62] In 2019, 10.5% of US households faced food insecurity, and this number has only worsened since then (see below). Much of this is socially determined, as the rate is the worst among households with incomes below the poverty line (34.9%) and single-mother households (28.7%). Latinx and Black households experienced food insecurity rates of 15.6% and 19.1%, respectively—disproportionately higher than white households (7.9%).[63]

We will discuss this further in chapter 5, but the COVID-19 pandemic amplified the shortcomings of food insecurity in the United States and beyond. The drastic rise in unemployment, lost access to school meals, and volatile food supply chains all contributed to food insecurity rates doubling among all households from February–May 2020. Even worse, food insecurity among households with children tripled in the same period. Communities historically lacking infrastructure also lacked a buffer to withstand some of the adverse impact of this pandemic, and their respective access to nutritious foods was disproportionately affected. We saw a significant rise in obesity (often lightly referred to as "COVID-19 fat"), a prime example of how stress highly influences malnutrition and how this term can refer to poor nourishment laden with highly caloric foods.

Crime and Violence

Growing up in areas of Los Angeles and New York City with high rates of criminality, I was immersed in gang and drug violence at the ripe age of 15, as my family no longer had the means to sustain a more privileged zip code. In the process I was also exposed to a mentality that saw the world differently than my previously privileged white experience. Trust was not a known commodity. Respect was not given—it was earned. People in these neighborhoods did not often think about long-term thriving, only survival. As a result, sustainable and quality-based health care was not often at the top of their priorities.

My education progressed, taking me into very different environments throughout my 20s and beyond. From favelas in Brazil to shantytowns in South Africa, I saw the harsh realities of survival in highly urbanized (and criminalized) societies. I asked myself: How could I possibly address meaningful health care access in these conditions?

Structural violence strongly impacts access to health care in a number of ways that are linked to historical inequities and the underlying causes of violence. In the *New Jim Crow*, Michelle Alexander discusses a number of connections between social conditions and higher rates of crime and violence. A prime example was the transition of US government spending in the 1990s from public housing to prison construction. Under President Bill Clinton's tenure, the United States slashed funding for public housing by US$17 billion (a reduction of more than 60%) and correspondingly boosted corrections by US$19 billion (an increase of more than 171%), effectively making the construction of prisons the nation's main housing program for the urban poor. Given this seemingly perennial threat for survival according to Maslow's hierarchy of needs (see figure 2.3), how can communities such as this possibly focus on quality of health or thriving when they need to eke out a basic living?

If we frame communal levels of violence as a public health concern (which we should), we can attribute the social etiology of patterns of mass violence to Link and Phelan's *fundamental causes model*. Once again, this theory stipulates that people will be "at (greater) risk of risks" if they live in more unequal societies and are located at the bottom of these respective social gradients. Therefore, we may speculate that a higher income inequality translates into a greater incidence of relative poverty. Economic prosperity almost invariably enhances the incidence of crime in the form of more goods and services to steal and internalize resentment over. Ironically, crime is least likely to be a serious problem in a society that is economically challenged. Cuba, with its relatively nonexistent crime rate, is a perfect example.

Neighborhood factors, such as higher rates of community violence, can also deeply affect health by influencing health behaviors and stress.[22] In criminology the broken windows theory states that visible signs of crime, antisocial behavior, and civil disorder create an urban environment that encourages further crime and disorder, including serious and violent criminal activity.[64,65,66,67,68] This is further internalized into poorer perceptions of self, which leads to an inevitable sense of hopelessness that can easily translate into higher rates of behavioral health outcomes, especially depression, anxiety, and substance use.

Hopelessness or despair is one of the most dangerous conditions in any community. In fact, that was largely the outcome of research I completed in the early 2000s around culturally supported suicides—namely, suicide attacks by Palestinians. Psychologists have often found connections between community pride, hopelessness, and suicide attacks, from Japanese kamikaze pilots to Hezbollah militants. We will further explore these concepts and how they intersect with the worsening of public health emergencies.

Environmental Conditions

Flint, Michigan, is an area known well by Americans for a number of reasons. One of the poorest small cities in the United States and the focus of a number of documentaries by Michael Moore, Flint's chronic issues were polarized further in 2014 due to a public health disaster. When Flint changed its municipal water supply source from Lake Huron, which supplied Detroit, to the Flint River, the switch caused water distribution pipes to corrode and leach lead and other contaminants into the drinking water. In 2016 a public health emergency was identified when the citizens of Flint were advised not to drink the tap water. While the issue of potable water access is all too familiar for communities in the Global South, Americans did not have a contingency plan to circumvent these issues. The unintended consequences were profound, with two-thirds of households in Flint reporting one or more adult members experiencing at least one behavioral health issue.

Five years later I set up COVID-19 vaccine clinics across the city. This municipality differed from many others. Folks seemed emotionally unmoved by the pandemic. They were neither fearful nor concerned. As a result, most of our "mega-clinics" were full of mothballs. When we did see the occasional straggler, they were busy and did not wish to speak. Where was the sense of community? Why did public health fail here?

The correlation between poor environmental health and poverty is clear. Buffalo, New York; Detroit; Cleveland; and Milwaukee were once some of the wealthiest cities in the United States, but because of the rapid transformation from an economy largely supported by manual labor to one driven by information, these cities lacked a strategic civil engineering plan and mostly atrophied. Given the cascading impact of prior industrial empires and the lack of resources to maintain sustained abatement programs, they also have some of the worst environmental conditions—including unsafe water, unregulated air emissions, and housing still rife with lead paint. As a result, many of these areas are now Superfund sites, flagged with sufficient hazardous waste that cleanup has become a federal responsibility.

While certain areas are categorically afflicted by environmental health concerns, other cities in the United States are deeply divided with respect to risk. Much of this inequality is the result of *red lining*, a term that originates in the New Deal homeownership initiatives of the 1930s. At the time, certain areas in the United States were designated as likely to depreciate in value, and therefore residents of those neighborhoods were systematically disqualified for home mortgages, further polarizing existing inequalities. Of course, many of these communities happened to be Black. Darryl Fears chronicles the historical origins of redlining, in which the federal Home Owners' Loan Corporation marked areas across the United States as "unworthy of loans" because of an "infiltration of foreign-born, Negro, or lower grade population" and shaded them in red starting in the 1930s.[69] This made it harder for home buyers of color to get mortgages; the corporation awarded A grades for solidly white areas and D's for largely non-white areas that lenders were advised to shun.[70] Throughout redlining's history, local zoning officials worked with businesses to place polluting operations such as industrial plants, major roadways, and shipping ports in and around these neighborhoods that the federal government marginalized.

Residential segregation is a major cause of differences in health status between African American and white people because it can determine the social and economic resources for not only individuals and families but also for communities.[71] Because many local public health resources are funded by local property taxes, most of these underresourced areas lacked robust public health prevention resources. In addition, city planning was designed so that large transportation arteries (e.g., highways, train tracks, etc.) bisected these neighborhoods, and air and noise pollution naturally followed suit.. In one study an association was found between redlining and poor mental health, a nondermatological cancer diagnosis, and a lack of health insurance. Another study found that small-for-gestational-age birth, prenatal mortality, and preterm birth have a higher prevalence in redlined neighborhoods than in other areas.

Basing credit-lending decisions on property location has created a legacy of urban areas experiencing chronic health inequities. A recent study of over 200 cities across the United States analyzed levels of nitrogen dioxide (an indicator of smog), and found strong correlations of redlining to air-pollution levels. A large body of research has already shown that redlined communities experience other environmental challenges, including excessive urban heat, sparse tree canopy, and few green spaces. The new analysis, according to the authors, is the first look nationwide at how redlining leads to disparities within different cities.

Some prime examples in some of the United States' largest cities are the Bronx, New York, and Boyle Heights, Los Angeles (figures 2.4 and 2.5). Without even knowing this background, while I was practicing at a community clinic in the South Bronx, I saw clearly that rates of asthma were much higher than I had seen in other parts of the city.

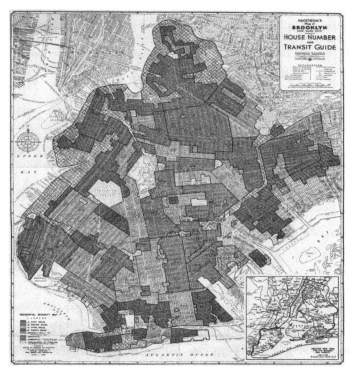

FIGURE 2.4. Residential security map of Brooklyn, New York, 1938. Redlining led to disparities in the city. *Source:* Mindy Thompson Fullilove, "Escaping the Catastrophic Logic of Separation," *Health Equity* 7, no. 1 (2023): 53–60, https://doi.org/10.1089/heq.2022.29021.mtf.

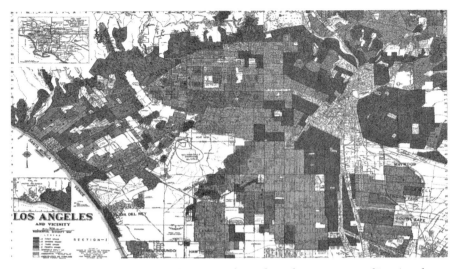

FIGURE 2.5. Homeowners Loan Corporation's residential security map of Los Angeles, California, 1938. Redlining led to disparities in Boyle Heights, Los Angeles.
Source: "Newly Released Maps Show How Housing Discrimination Happened," *National Geographic* (website), October 17, 2016, https://www.nationalgeographic.com/history/article /housing-discrimination-redlining-maps.

Poor children of color would innocently present for their inhaler refill not knowing that the racist policies implemented nearly a century before were largely the root cause of their inability to play a game of basketball without their lungs constricting. Years later I would become the public health officer for Vernon, California, a city with over 1,800 businesses surrounded by a number of other cities. Here, we are a few miles from the famed Los Angeles River, notorious for the levels of toxins it contains. Between the emissions of the factories of Vernon and the toxic sludge of the Los Angeles River, residents in adjacent communities like Boyle Heights—which were, of course, also redlined—are incarcerated in an inescapable prison of air pollution. They are scared, and I must address this socially produced fear. As I represent the government, my words are not likely to have an effect. Of course, the COVID-19 pandemic merely intensified these existential fears.

Quality of Housing

The intersection of housing and health is salient and has been repeatedly illustrated, including in one paper published in *Health Affairs*, which describes the pathways of that intersection in four segments.[72]

First, the "stability pathway" describes an emerging body of evidence demonstrating the impact on health outcomes from housing instability. People who are chronically homeless face substantially higher morbidity in terms of both physical and mental health and increased mortality.[73,74] Many people experience traumas on the streets or in shelters, which have long-standing adverse impacts on psychological well-being. These challenges can result in persistently high health care expenditures due to emergency department and inpatient hospital use. We discussed this above, especially as it related to adverse childhood experiences.[75,76]

The "safety and quality pathway" describes environmental factors within the homes of poorer communities. Substandard housing conditions such as water leaks, poor ventilation, dirty carpets, and pest infestation have been associated with poor health outcomes, most notably those related to asthma.[77] Additionally, exposure to high or low temperatures is correlated with adverse health outcomes, including cardiovascular events—particularly among the elderly.[78] Residential crowding has also been linked to both physical illness (e.g., respiratory diseases) and psychological distress.[79] We saw the risk of COVID-19 and SARS rise exponentially in smaller multigenerational homes across the world. We also often see the rates of indoor air pollutants rise significantly in homes that lack ventilation. This is widely demonstrated in cases of extreme poverty throughout the world, such as the South Sudanese refugee camps described above.

The "affordability pathway" describes the sheer cost of living and its impact on the affordability of other resources, such as health care. While the cost of living from a housing perspective is highest among Europeans, as they mostly follow either the Beveridge or Bismarck models, health care access is largely provided through other resources. In the United States (where we have some of the most expensive cities in the world), our spending on housing largely precludes spending on other necessary resources, such as health care. In fact, over 40 million Americans are considered "cost burdened" (spending >30% of their income on household expenses) and >20 million are "severely cost burdened" (spending >50% of their income).[80] This burden, of course, disproportionately affects renters, further eclipsing their agency and leaving them that much more vulnerable to pandemics. We saw this happen to far too many New Yorkers during the COVID-19 pandemic, when they would get sick and miss one or two rent cycles, precipitating acute housing crises for them. We would find them hotel rooms (during isolation or quarantine) but were then stuck in a predicament, as we could not discharge them without a responsible housing plan. This impacted thousands of our patients, which we will discuss further in chapter 5.

The final "neighborhood pathway" can be clearly understood by our "redlining" example given above (figures 2.4 and 2.5).

Social and Community Context

Civic Participation

Civic participation encompasses a wide range of formal and informal activities from volunteering to participating in group activities to community gardening.[81] Some are individual activities that benefit society (e.g., voting), while others are group activities that benefit either the group members (e.g., recreational soccer teams) or society (e.g., volunteer organizations). In addition to the direct benefit that civic participation provides to the community, it also produces secondary health benefits for participants.

Simply belonging to groups can improve both physical and mental health. Membership in formal groups (e.g., Boy Scouts, Rotary Club, Parent-Teacher Association) or informal ones (book clubs, bird-watching clubs) has been shown to increase social capital and decrease social isolation among members. Many such groups also engage in charitable activities that directly benefit health research (e.g., Ice Bucket Challenge, Susan G. Komen Race for the Cure).

Civic participation varies by generation and education. For example, one study found that while young people may be less likely to engage in mainstream media consumption, 90% of high school students surveyed had engaged in politics in general, and 40% had engaged in participatory politics. This civic engagement primarily occurs through social media. Individuals with higher education levels may have more opportunities for civic engagement, as college students become involved in community affairs through fraternities, sororities, or other student organizations, though male college students are less likely to engage in civic activities than female students. Other studies have found that BIPOC university students are more likely to intend to volunteer than their white peers.

Discrimination

Isabel Wilkerson describes global caste systems with three salient examples: Nazi Germany, India, and the United States. The impact of discrimination occurs at both structural and individual levels. Either can cause intentional or unintentional harm, whether or not it is perceived by the individual. Discrimination can be understood as a social stressor that has a physiological effect on individuals (e.g., irregular heartbeat, anxiety, heartburn) and can manifest as stress with very durable and measurable long-term negative health outcomes.[82]

Structural Discrimination

Structural discrimination (or "violence") refers to macrolevel conditions that limit the "opportunities, resources, and well-being" of less privileged groups. It is a systemic issue, not one of individual bigotry, though such bigotry—individually and collectively—may be the root cause. It is also a highly complex problem with multiple factors that reinforce each other in negative ways. For example, residential segregation is a form of structural discrimination in the housing market—redlining, as described above, being a very concrete example—which in turn leads to disparities in access to quality education. Most school districts generate their income locally through property taxes, so residential segregation by income translates into vastly different funding across school districts. Children who enroll in poor-quality schools with limited health resources, increased safety concerns, and low teacher support are more likely to have poorer physical and mental health, which has negative economic consequences, perpetuating the cycle of poverty.

Structural discrimination reflects a deep-seated, ingrained bias that disadvantages members of certain marginalized groups and is built into the infrastructure of a given society, independent of the personal feelings of its individual citizens.

Individual Discrimination

By contrast, individual discrimination refers to overt negative interactions between individuals in their institutional roles (e.g., health care provider and patient) or as public or private individuals (e.g., salesperson and customer) based on individual characteristics (e.g., race, gender, etc.).

Discrimination is a fairly common experience: 31% of US adults report at least one major discriminatory occurrence in their lifetime, and 63% report experiencing discrimination every day. While only 8% of all US adolescents report experience with racial / ethnic discrimination, there is significant variation between white (2%), non-Hispanic Black (17.1%), and Hispanic (11.0%) youths. A number of factors influence how individual discrimination comes about.[83] These events are often picked up in ACEs, when screened effectively.

Such discrimination occurs when people or groups are set apart from the group that defines itself as normative through "othering" and labeling on the basis of any number of characteristics including physical attributes, SES, sexual preferences and practices, religious beliefs, race, ethnicity, and association with disease.

Let us examine several of the key attributes that drive discrimination.

DISCRIMINATION BASED ON RACE

It is incontestable that the most manifest and insidious form of stigma, and therefore of discrimination, is on the basis of race (*racism*). We harbor a glaring contradiction between the conviction that a person's race is an irrelevancy and the reflexive social practice of attending assiduously to racial identity. We say people should be "judged by the content of their character and not the color of their skin," yet we routinely make decisions on the basis of the latter. I refer to this as our natural inclination to perceive the world as a *pigmentocracy*. The notion that we somehow are or should be "color blind" is an illusion.

As Wilkerson writes:

> In America, race is the primary tool and the visible decoy for caste. Race does the heavy lifting for a caste system that demands a means of human division. . . .
>
> Caste and race are neither synonymous nor mutually exclusive. They can and do coexist in the same culture and serve to reinforce each other. Race, in the US, is the visible agent of the unseen force of caste. Caste is the bones, race the skin. Race is what we can see, the physical traits that have been given arbitrary meaning and become shorthand for who a person is. Caste is the powerful infrastructure that holds each group in its place. Its very invisibility is what gives it power and longevity.[49]

Racism has been linked to a number of adverse health outcomes, including low birth weight, high blood pressure, and poor health status in general. For example, the infant mortality rate among the non-Hispanic Black population is 11.11 infant deaths out of 1,000 live births, while the overall rate in the US is only 5.96 infant deaths per 1,000. Further, the 2019 National Healthcare Disparities Report indicated that white patients receive better quality of care than 40.6% of Black patients, 40.5% of American Indian/Alaska Native patients, 34.5% of Hispanic patients, and 28.6% of Asian and Pacific Islander patients.[84]

In the Global South, racial discrimination has been inextricably linked to colonialism and is one of its most pernicious vestiges. As colonialism emerged, the world became substantially integrated and mixed—and the color of skin became the prime differentiator between the powerful and the powerless. It seems that humans, intrinsically, have great trouble accepting differences, resulting in stigma and discrimination. Man inherently fears what he doesn't understand, hates what he fears, and marginalizes what he hates. This power asymmetry led to persistent and profound oppression, or what sociologists refer to as *structural violence*, puppeteered by the dominant social class, which has traditionally been white, male, and wealthy relative to others.

In other words, social and economic status was largely based upon the color of one's skin—and the darker the skin, the poorer one was, with the least access to resources, increased violence over these miserable conditions, and increased disease, leading to further poverty, which concomitantly precipitated in the worst possible epidemics mankind has ever seen.

DISCRIMINATION BASED ON GENDER OR SEX

Experiences of discrimination based on gender or sex (*sexism*) have been shown to have adverse impacts for cisgender women. (Gender refers to "the cultural roles, behaviors, activities, and attributes expected of people based on their sex," while sex is "an individual's biological status as male, female, or something else assigned at birth.") One study found that after adjusting for other influences, levels of unhappiness, loneliness, and depression are about 30% higher for women who reported experiencing recent discrimination compared with those who did not.[85]

DISCRIMINATION BASED ON SEXUALITY ORIENTATION
AND GENDER IDENTITY (SOGI)

People who identify as LGBTQIA+ (lesbian, gay, bisexual, transgender, queer / questioning, intersex, and asexual / aromantic / agender) also endure frequent exposure to discrimination due to sexual orientation and gender identity (SOGI). Sexual orientation refers to "a person's sexual and emotional attraction to another person (i.e., lesbian, gay, bisexual, etc.)," while gender identity refers to an "individual's sense of themselves as man, woman, transgender, or something else." The two are very different, though many clinical institutions casually lump them together.

Evidence suggests that adolescents who identify as LGBTQIA+ are more likely than heterosexual adolescents to exhibit symptoms of emotional distress, including depressive symptoms, suicidal ideation, and self-harm, all related to the stress of having a stigmatized identity. Additionally, research has found that the increased risk of discrimination and violence for transgender individuals contributes to high rates of suicide attempts among this population—some of the highest of any marginalized group.

DISCRIMINATION TOWARD PEOPLE WITH ACCESS
AND FUNCTIONAL NEEDS (DISABILITIES)
People with access and functional needs (AFN) are particularly vulnerable to experiences of discrimination (*ableism*) if they fall into any of the following groups of physical, developmental, or intellectual characteristics:

- Suffer chronic conditions or injuries
- Have limited English proficiency
- Are older adults
- Are children
- Are low income, homeless, or transportation disadvantaged
- Are childbearing patients
- Have intellectual / developmental disorders

This number is substantial, with well over 25% of US citizens having at least one disability or AFN. A history of discrimination and institutionalization for people with disabilities has caused grave health inequalities in this population. Adults with disabilities are more likely to report their health to be fair or poor than people without disabilities: specifically, 50.8% of adults with a complex activity limitation (e.g., a work or self-care limitation) and 31.5% with a basic actions difficulty (e.g., a movement difficulty, cognitive difficulty, seeing or hearing difficulty), compared to 3.4% of adults with no disability.[83] In addition, adults with disabilities are 2.5 times more likely to report skipping or delaying health care because of cost. They also often experience a number of secondary adverse outcomes, including consistently higher rates of obesity, a lack of physical activity, and higher rates of cigarette smoking: all disparities in health that are likely socially determined.

DISCRIMINATION BASED ON AGE

The health vulnerabilities of older adults may amplify the health effects of discrimination, something I have often seen play out in my work as a gerontologist. The United States does not demonstrate the filial piety that we see in Asia. In fact, in the United States discrimination based on age is the most common type of discrimination. One study found that experiences of discrimination are frequent among older Americans, with 63% and 31% of older adults reporting everyday discrimination and major discriminatory events, respectively.[83] After controlling for general stress, everyday discrimination still had effects on emotional health, such as depressive symptoms and self-reported health in older adults.

INTERSECTIONALITY WITHIN DISCRIMINATION

Although categories such as race or gender alone may influence how individuals experience discrimination, it is equally important to understand how being a part of several affected groups simultaneously can impact experiences of discrimination. To that end, according to the Center for Intersectional Justice, intersectionality is defined as the ways that systems of inequality based on gender, race, ethnicity, SOGI, disability, class, and other forms of discrimination "intersect" (or synergize) in order to amplify the effects of each category of identity.[86] For example, as members of two marginalized groups, Black women are differentially situated economically, socially, and politically—and may experience discrimination differently—than other women or Black men, which may also affect health outcomes. Specifically, racial discrimination as a psychosocial stressor may increase the risk of preterm and low-birth-weight deliveries for Black women. We see this commonly playing out in public health outcomes.

Incarceration

I'm staring into the eyes of inmates at Rikers Island. They are full of angst and determination and seem to follow a script of toughness as they parade around the waiting area to see the doctor. Once they step into my exam room, I can sense a prescriptive agenda. After I begin to engage in an attempt to disarm them, I see an entirely different person. I see vulnerability and pain. I give them the space to be themselves. I connect with them because I used to be them, incarcerated.[87]

My adversity throughout my youth precipitated a period where I was left with almost nothing. The hurt and loss I felt when my family passed away in rapid succession were overwhelming, and I acted out in an effort to mollify the pain, even as I was trying to raise my own daughters. This led to a series of juvenile incarcerations. I felt the need to become quickly hardened and emotionally numb to the stressors I was suddenly immersed in. In these jails corralling the spirits of tough Angelenos and New Yorkers, I felt like I connected with these other youth who were also merely reacting (mostly) to adverse childhood experiences. The difference was my privilege. I was ultimately surgically excised from these sociologically sordid environments because I had "such potential." This mostly translated to a young white American male with a precocious intellect and reasonable grade point average. I was given the chance (with a scrubbed and sealed record) that young children of color are rarely afforded. I took that chance seriously. I was in medical school a decade later.

Tales of systematic oppression can be traced back thousands of years. A fairly linear trend can be traced between colonialism (which killed off >90% of the Indigenous populations), slavery, and our contemporary practice of mass incarceration across the Global North. Michelle

Alexander writes that the birth of mass incarceration was rooted in the US quest to replace race as legitimate and legal grounds for systematic oppression. The "war on drugs" in the United States was initiated by President Richard Nixon, raised through President Ronald Reagan, and optimized under Clinton. Reagan mastered the "excision of the language of race from conservative public discourse" and thus built on the success of earlier conservatives who developed a strategy of exploiting racial hostility or resentment for political gain without making explicit reference to race. In October 1982, President Reagan officially announced his administration's war on drugs.

Between 1980 and 1984, US Federal Bureau of Investigation (FBI) antidrug funding increased from $8 million to $95 million. The Department of Defense's antidrug allocations increased from $33 million to $1,042 million in the decade from 1981 to 1991. During that same period, US Drug Enforcement Agency antidrug spending grew from $86 to $1,026 million, and FBI antidrug allocations grew from $38 to $181 million. By contrast, funding for agencies responsible for drug treatment, prevention, and education was dramatically reduced. The budget of the National Institute on Drug Abuse, for example, was reduced from $274 million to $57 million from 1981 to 1984, and antidrug funds allocated to the Department of Education were cut from $14 million to $3 million.

Determined to ensure that the "new Republican majority" would continue to support the extraordinary expansion of the federal government's law enforcement activities and that Congress would continue to fund it, the Reagan administration launched a media offensive to justify the war on drugs. Central to the media campaign was an effort to sensationalize the emergence of crack cocaine in inner-city neighborhoods—communities devastated by deindustrialization and skyrocketing unemployment. The media frenzy the campaign inspired simply could not have come at a worse time for urban Black communities. In the early 1980s, just as the drug war was kicking off, inner-city communities were suffering from economic collapse. As described above, the blue-collar factory jobs that had been plentiful in urban areas in the 1950s and 1960s (especially in the Great Lakes areas) had suddenly disappeared—seemingly overnight.

Once elected, Clinton endorsed the idea of a federal "three strikes" law, which he advocated in his 1994 State of the Union address to enthusiastic bipartisan applause. The $30 billion crime bill sent to the White House in August 1994 was hailed as a victory for the Democrats, who "were able to wrest the crime issue from the Republicans and make it their own." The bill created dozens of new federal capital crimes, mandated life sentences for some three-time offenders, and authorized more than $16 billion for state prison grants and expansion of state and local police forces. Far from resisting the emergence of the new caste system, Clinton escalated the drug war beyond what conservatives had imagined possible a decade earlier. As the Justice Policy Institute has observed, "The Clinton Administration's 'tough on crime' policies resulted in the largest increases in federal and state prison inmates of any president in American history."

While the United States has both the highest number of people incarcerated/imprisoned and the highest percentage of incarcerated/imprisoned per capita, other nations are known to follow a similar pattern of criminal justice—namely China, Brazil, Russia, India, Mexico, Iran, El Salvador, Turkmenistan, and Cuba (notably, all nations with very questionable human rights records). We must examine this issue of health care from a global lens.

As the US now is incentivized by racial domination in addition to salient financial incentives, with nearly 10% of current inmates/prisoners housed in private, for-profit facilities, it's critical to understand the determinants of health care inequities. While access is reasonable within jails and prisons, referrals and follow-up upon release is less than ideal. The stressors placed on individuals released from or at risk of incarceration are severe (primarily for people of color), making their engagement in meaningful health care options very challenging, especially when it comes to behavioral health for the trauma they certainly must process. Alas, these needs remain largely unmet. We have some promising opportunities that we will discuss more in chapter 7.

Social Cohesion

Before I spent time in Israel, never before had I witnessed such impressive examples of solidarity and social cohesion.[88] Anti-Semitism has pervaded the globe for millennia. Only in the past 60 years have the Jewish diaspora found one place to call home. Due to this oppression, they have had to maintain strong ties of kinship. We may reflect upon the Durkheimian concept of social anomie here. It simply does not materialize in Jewish society. In fact, Jews have some of the lowest suicide rates in the world, largely because they keep in place such strong support networks. As a nation pieced together with individuals from all over the world, this solidarity has manifested in unprecedented ways. Constantly assuming they will not be welcomed or accepted, they have created a strong and unique sense of communal self-reliance. While certainly a complex web of confounding and interacting factors, Israel also has some of the best and equitable (for Jewish citizens) health care access in the world.

When examining the social cohesion of a place like Israel, it's helpful to describe a place that directly contrasts with it and exemplifies the quintessence of the aforementioned social anomie, as described by Durkheim. I choose Indigenous communities in the United States to provide that contrast and will share some thoughts I wrote back in 2014 regarding my perception of this community obsessing over obituaries, as I called it at the time (figure 2.6):

As I skimmed through the local Wyoming newspapers (*Wind River News, The Lander Journal, The Ranger*), my attention was frozen by their disproportionate focus on one particular section—the obituaries. While I scanned these melancholy narratives for possible casual mention of any of my patients, my mind would seemingly sediment over one inescapably common discovery—"They are all so young."

As a physician and epidemiologist, my mind was trained to recognize patterns. While working in developing contexts throughout the world, I have found that death is often evaded, as people often accept the inevitably truncated ends of their struggling existence. It is something that people prefer

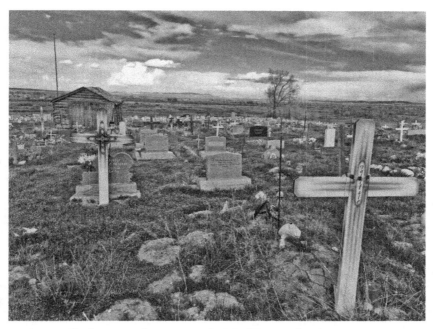

FIGURE 2.6. The Sacajawea Cemetery on the Wind River Indian Reservation in Fort Washakie, Wyoming. *Source:* "Guest Commentary: Native Americans' Obsession with the Obituaries," *Denver Post*, updated April 22, 2016, https://www.denverpost.com/2015/07/10/guest-commentary-native-americans-obsession-with-the-obituaries/.

to remain reticent about. As my travels took me to an area within the borders of my own birthplace and native country, however, I began to notice the approach to death take a salient turn.

With a combined mean age of mortality of 51.7 years, the Northern Arapaho and Eastern Shoshone have some of the worst health indicators in the nation. With a combined population exceeding 12,000 and living on more than 2.2 million acres of the Wind River Reservation, these communities are isolated and burdened by the historically traumatic events that have cast a harrowing shadow over their ability to pursue the almighty "American Dream."

So how did they cope while drowning in such pervasive trauma? Much like other American Indian societies, ceremonies remain a prominent and proud reminder of their cultural identity. These rites were historically focused on life transitions—namely marriage and childhood honor feasts. In a more contemporaneous context, with premature mortality dominating their daily lives, funerals (ironically) represented one of their most common forms of social interaction. It was on such days that clinical traffic at the Indian Health Service (IHS) Arapahoe and Fort Washakie Health Centers reached a distinct nadir.

Deference to death had always played an integral part in their lives, but the practices took on morphological changes as their lifestyles gravitated toward sedentary conscription. Prior to reservation lifestyle, death was followed by burial within the same day—usually limited to the immediate family. With increasingly "Western" influence, however, such funerals took on a more elaborate and fanciful character, often involving the entire community. What were the reasons that precipitated this paradigm shift to involve such large numbers, I asked myself?

Many of the Indian reservations in the United States are distinguished by their isolation from the more progressive areas of the nation. Despite the existence of the national / international media, many members of the community adopt a more insular perspective, preferring to focus on their tribal identity and cultural cohorts. As a New Yorker, my media prism was relatively global. There- fore, it was the very preoccupation with (truly) local news in Northwestern Wyoming that initially captured my attention. I found it odd that there were three local periodicals covering a combined area of less than 30,000 and with a keen interest on the obituaries in particular.

It was striking how many people discussed the obituaries on a daily basis. From patients and staff at my clinic to community-dwelling residents, the reservation seemed to be connected through this one very common portal— death. When I investigated further, I was informed that such obituary surveil- lance was a connective interface between them and the rest of the tribe. One IHS psychologist speculated "it was a way to reconnect and reaffirm the family system after all of the historical disruptions that underlie everything." One tribal patient mentioned it was a mechanism for them "to validate their grievance and resentment toward the white man's oppression." Another patient noted "it made (me) feel needed at a time where (my) friends were dying too damn fast and too damn young." In other words, it made them feel relevant in a society that was deteriorating at an alarming rate.

This somber occurrence gave me considerable pause and led me to ponder the underlying symbolism of such an "obsession." Could it be that such demonstrable preoccupation with community deaths is a proxy for their own collective fatalism? Is it possible that scanning these death pages was somehow creating an introspective portal to view their own imminent destinies? Would such frequent reminders of their historical trauma cause them to choose a different path, or would they passively accept their perceived destiny instead?

It is an ignoble blemish on humanity to allow such premature epitaphs to be written, and it is high time that such proverbial slates are wiped clean. This is anomie.

Political Determinants

Public health is arguably one of the most politicized professionalized fields, as it touches upon core issues such as choice and access. This has not always been the case. In fact, we have never seen the impact of politics so strongly as with COVID-19 vaccinations. I would argue that outside the core political diversities of division in this nation—abortion, guns, and religion—I have never seen public health play so strongly into politics. It should not. We must depoliticize public health, as the foundations that we build impact communities from all walks of life in the United States. These foundational services are intended to be accessible to all and should support a healthy, functional, and productive society.

Daniel Dawes describes the political determinants of health as "more than merely separate and distinct from the SDoH: they serve as the instigators of the SDoH with which many people are already well acquainted.[89] They involve the systematic process of structuring relationships, distributing resources, and administering power, operating simultaneously in ways that mutually reinforce or influence one another to shape opportunities that either advance health equity or exacerbate health inequities." Dawes describes those political determinants as the core foundational stage in a theatrical production of health outcomes that are largely driven by the social actors on the stage. They are inextricably linked. Government, of course, is a key political determinant.

Let's begin with examining the political influences of vaccine hesitancy around the globe. In a paper for the *New England Journal of*

Medicine (NEJM), Larson et al. describe vaccine hesitancy as an attitude or sentiment, whereas vaccination is an action measured to determine vaccine coverage.[90] The period of hesitancy and indecision is a time of vulnerability, as well as opportunity.

As vaccine hesitancy became increasingly recognized as a global challenge and global immunization rates plateaued and even started to decline in some areas, the WHO Strategic Advisory Group of Experts on Immunization "noted with concern the impact of reluctance to accept immunization on the uptake of vaccines reported from both developed and developing countries." In 2019 (notably prior to the emergence of the COVID-19 pandemic), the WHO named vaccine hesitancy as one of the top 10 threats to global health.[91]

A framework developed from research done in the Global North, the 5C model of the drivers of vaccine hesitancy, provides five main individual person–level determinants for vaccine hesitancy: confidence, complacency, convenience (or constraints), risk calculation, and collective responsibility.[92] I would argue that distrust of systems is largely one of the most common deterministic elements of vaccine hesitancy in the United States and beyond. I would also argue that while these rates have been polarized for a number of reasons, largely through the increasing potency of social media channels worldwide, the core issues can be understood as a basic distrust, much of which is politically determined.

Although many observers point to the 1998 *Lancet* article by Wakefield et al. (retracted in 2010) as the source of parental fears that the measles, mumps, and rubella vaccination might cause autism, the search for the cause of the seeming increase in autism was already brewing (figure 2.7).[93] This was a systematic distrust, one that the COVID-19 vaccine took to a new level. In the United States, the lowest rates of COVID-19 vaccine uptake were among African Americans and non–college-educated whites.

In 2020–2021, the percentage of US citizens who voted for Trump was strongly and inversely related to the percentage vaccinated (figure 2.8). Most significantly, political views were not only strongly

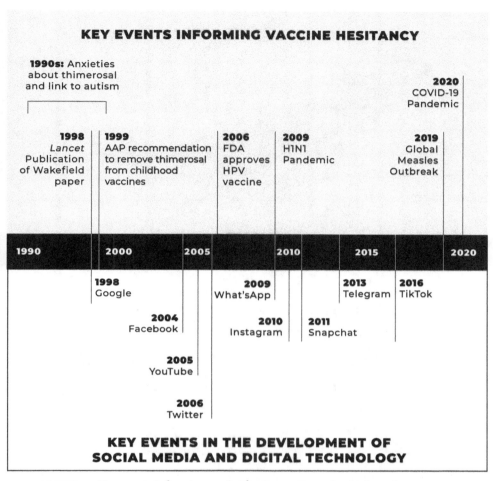

FIGURE 2.7. Key events informing vaccine hesitancy. *Source:* Graphic by author.

related to vaccination rates but also heavily implicated in COVID-19 cases and deaths. Counties with a high proportion of Trump voters had more per capita cases and deaths from COVID-19 than counties with fewer Trump voters.[94] In counties where Trump received less than 25% of the vote, death rates per 100,000 were less than half as high as in counties where Trump received 75% or more of the vote in 2021.

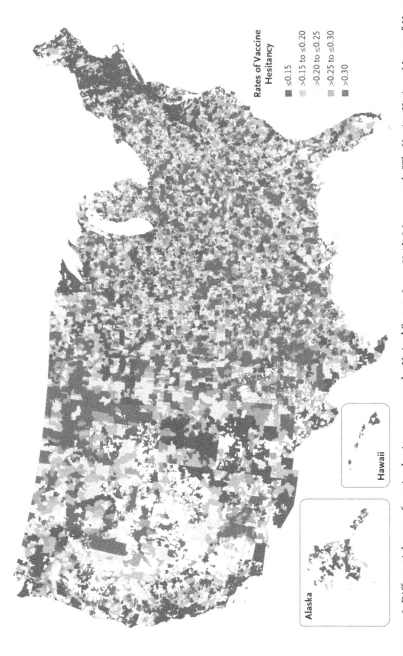

FIGURE 2.8. Differential rates of vaccine hesitancy across the United States. *Source:* Heidi J. Larson et al., "The Vaccine-Hesitant Moment," *New England Journal of Medicine* 387, no. 1 (2022): 58–65, https://doi.org/10.1056/nejmra2106441.

Rates of Vaccine
Hesitancy

≤0.15
>0.15 to ≤0.20
>0.20 to ≤0.25
>0.25 to ≤0.30
>0.30

Alaska

Hawaii

When the COVID-19 Johnson & Johnson vaccine came out, Christian church leaders around the nation publicly condemned it because of the use of stem cells in the research and production of the vaccines. In a few days, Black leaders from across the nation were in collective protest against the use of this COVID-19 vaccine, which only served to propagate hesitancy further among this community that had expressed the highest rate of hesitancy to begin with (and, ironically, was one of the most at risk of adverse consequences of those infections).

Studies around vaccine hesitancy exploded during the COVID-19 pandemic (my group in California also conducted one). While we understood the issue to be multifactorial and likely linked to the rise of a reliance on social media, we understood that the pockets of hesitancy were diffuse and not necessarily correlated with the historical levels of vaccine hesitancy among certain (socially determined) communities. If we were to distill a common understanding of the reasons for hesitancy, we could break them down into three buckets:[95]

1. Poor information: not necessarily too little or too much but simply the wrong information provided by the wrong messengers
2. Social media and digitization of information: a force multiplier for poor information
3. A core distrust of certain systems and institutions

While politics clearly contributed to this unfortunate public reception, the communities impacted often had little in common with one another. As a case in point, Black communities (largely Democrat voters) and registered Republicans expressed the highest rates of hesitancy during the COVID-19 pandemic.[96] While we could see a clear correlation between vaccine confidence and partisan politics, we understood that we needed our community leaders (including our interfaith and spiritual) to stand up and do what was right for their communities. So who should they have listened to?

In *NEJM* (one of the most trusted and prestigious journals in science),[97] Larson et al. wrote a review article on vaccine hesitancy and found that physicians and other health care providers are still among the most trusted persons when it comes to healthcare advice. The Wellcome Global Monitor surveyed people in 140 countries and found that 73% of the respondents said that they would trust a doctor or a nurse more than others; the percentage was 90% in the higher-income countries.[98] Vaccine acceptance can increase,[99] but healthcare providers need to offer support and encouragement and listen to what matters from the patient's perspective. Equipping physicians with information on the nature and scope of circulating concerns in their communities may help them address such concerns in the clinic, while also informing appropriate interventions at the community level.

Vaccine hesitancy (or confidence) is merely a proxy for public health confidence. From the beginning, Democrats were much more likely than Republicans to take the threat of the virus seriously and to support efforts to control it.[100,101] Subsequently, research found that counties with a higher share of Republican voters tended to have lower perceptions of the dangers of COVID-19, and these perceptions led to riskier behavior.[102] States with more Republican voters were more resistant to stay-at-home orders.[103] In more religious states, which tend to be heavily Republican, people were found to be more mobile during the pandemic despite recommendations to stay home.[104] Perry et al. found that Christian nationalism, which has strong ties to the Republican Party, was related to many of the far-right responses to COVID-19, including unfounded conspiracy theories.[105,106]

This experience was not unique to the United States. A number of studies have demonstrated these political determinants worldwide. One analysis looked at seven studies in low-income countries (Burkina Faso, Mozambique, Rwanda, Sierra Leone, and Uganda), five studies in lower-middle-income countries (India, Nepal, Nigeria, and Pakistan), and one study in an upper-middle-income country (Colombia).[107] Overall, it found that the average acceptance rate across the full set of studies in the Global South was 80.3%, with the lowest acceptance in Burkina Faso (66.5%) and Pakistan (66.5%), a nation with serious discrepancies over immunizations as a result of the state-sponsored assassination of Osama Bin Laden. (His location, in a compound in Abbottabad, was ultimately discovered through a sham polio vaccination campaign.)

Moreover, the acceptance rate in every sample from low- and middle-income countries (LMICs) was higher than that of samples from the United States (64.6%) and Russia (30.4%), which had the lowest.[108] The data show that vaccine acceptance is explained mainly by an interest in personal protection against COVID-19, whereas concerns about side effects are the most common reasons for hesitancy. Again, we know that trust in the government and science also largely determine engagement and acceptance of public health systems. A classic example were the rampant attacks on health care workers in the Democratic Republic of the Congo in 2018–2019 during the height of the Ebola epidemic. People naturally assumed that the state sponsored these public health systems in an attempt to wipe out certain populations, as they would see many members of their respective communities entering Ebola treatment units and never coming back out. Of course, this was not based on some government plot but resulted from case fatality rates often exceeding 25%.

Another survey was conducted by the African CDC, in partnership with the London School of Hygiene and Tropical Medicine in late 2020, in 15 African countries. Again, it was found that the majority of respondents in Africa (79%) would be vaccinated against COVID-19 if it were deemed safe and effective.[109] Perhaps it may be that lived experience in LMICs, where many vaccine-preventable infectious diseases still cause thousands of deaths annually, results in a higher perceived need for or value of vaccines. Alternatively, people in the Global North feel relatively protected and privileged.

Vaccine hesitancy is also currently prevalent in certain key European nations, including Eastern European ones such as Bosnia and Herzegovina, Georgia, Romania, Serbia, and Ukraine, as well as in several prominent Western European countries, including France, Germany, and Italy. Moreover, while vaccine hesitancy is an important factor, it is not the only one. For example, Ukrainians significantly mistrust government authority, but reports abound of corruption, lack of government commitment, and a weakened health system due to the ongoing conflict with Russia. In France, vaccine confidence has eroded partly due to a lack of government trust following the H1N1 influenza pandemic of 2009, when people felt that the health impact of the flu was less than conveyed by government authorities.[110]

The WHO defines hurtful messages that have precipitated issues such as vaccine hesitancy as infodemics.[111] In other words, too much information (including false or misleading information in digital and physical environments) come out during a disease outbreak, which causes confusion and risk-taking behaviors that can worsen the public's health. In addition, infodemics lead to a toxic mistrust in health authorities, thereby undermining the public health response. An infodemic can intensify or lengthen outbreaks when people are unsure what they need to do to protect their health and that of the people around them. With growing digitization—an expansion of social media and Internet use—information can spread more rapidly. In fact, the correlation of the spread of social media and the viral antiscientific perspectives that are infecting the world is curious. This is a double-edged sword and can aim to amplify helpful, as well as harmful, messages.

Vaccine hesitancy certainly does not exist on an island in terms of the political determinants of public health. Abortion has been historically tied to these political correlates. In the United States, the landmark *Roe v. Wade* Supreme Court decision protected access to abortion care for nearly 50 years. In 2022 that protection was largely overturned by the court's decision in *Dobbs v. Jackson Women's Health Organization*. This is a quintessential political determinant of health, as this de facto "abortion ban" has primarily been exploited by conservative states. A recent trend of political influences on health care access has now entered the transgender health care space, where gender-affirming care has been systematically banned in a number of conservative states that largely mirror areas that have applied the state ban on abortion. To say that these political influences on evidence-based areas of medicine are dangerous is an understatement of the highest order.

CHAPTER 3

Population Stress

In such a world of conflict, a world of victims and executioners, it is the job of thinking people, not to be on the side of the executioners.

—ALBERT CAMUS

Now that the reader is acquainted with the social determinants of health (SDoH), this chapter will tackle more substantive examples to illustrate how the SDoH operate in the real world, beginning with population stress.

As the cycle of poverty and disease continues, population stress can be not only a precedent to outbreaks but also the consequence of such. Countless previous examples demonstrate the association between population stress and infectious diseases such as leishmaniasis, cholera, typhus, trench fever, anthrax, and tuberculosis. Some cases are particularly compelling. HIV/AIDS and its rapid emergence in South Africa in 1999–2002 is one. While the origin is famously associated with a number of variable causal factors, the sociopolitical violence and associative population stress experienced during the latter stages of apartheid have been widely cited as significant contributing factors to the South African epidemic.[1]

Ebola has a similar tale. The outbreak of 2014–2015 was particularly telling, with over 14,000 infections and nearly 4,000 deaths.[2] The cumulative mortality for all previous outbreaks on record (starting in 1976) was fewer than 2,000.[3] So how did it emerge de novo in an area without any prior outbreaks on record? What exactly led to the outbreak in West Africa? What leads to such variable case fatality rates in divergent areas?

Sierra Leone has suffered from decades of war, foreign intervention, a highly precarious sociopolitical system, and an anemic infrastructure. It has one of the lowest recorded life expectancies in the world (at 45 years).[4] Moreover, as quality of health is inextricably connected with access to resources and highly correlated with general quality of life, it is no surprise that Sierra Leone is ranked sixth lowest on the Multidimensional Poverty Index and 183 out of 187 nations analyzed on the Human Development Index (often colloquially referred to as the "happiness index").[5,6]

As is often the case in impoverished settings, those systems that are most vulnerable will be attacked, whether as a result of some perverted irony or a manifestation of the very poverty-precipitating conditions that favor disease and warfare, combined with the lack of foundational strength to withstand disaster, either natural or anthropogenic. The association between violence and epidemics is particularly striking. It is likely that fractured health systems worsened by episodic social disruption place inordinate stress on societies and disproportionately impact the most vulnerable in those respective societies. Given such woefully inadequate health care systems unequipped to manage the needs of their citizens, coupled with latent microbes dormant for decades awaiting perfectly opportunistic moments, we can speculate that stark inequalities may be one of the strongest precipitants of infectious disease outbreaks.

These dynamics are not limited to the Global South. In New York City, months of government-facilitated isolation, quarantine, and separation for COVID-19; disproportionate adverse health consequences; and further economic distress on populations predisposed to adversity likely activated frustration already simmering due to decades of systematic oppression and violence. Social norms and civic boundaries dissolved, and it is plausible that populations felt more emboldened to express their sense of lived injustice. In New York City (as in cities across the world), the situation was aggravated by gross inequities that caused residents to take to the streets and demand justice. It caused thousands to break down the months of progress that social distancing had made on the incidence of COVID-19 in New York City. This, in conjunction with the anger and emotional exhaustion associated with the unjust killing of George Floyd, likely led to a widespread compromise of the immune systems of thousands, placing them at higher risk of infection and poor disease progression.[7] It was not surprising that COVID-19 case rates spiked after these events.

These provide just a few examples of how cracks in sociopolitical systems lead to chronic access barriers to health, which are amplified during public health emergencies. Historically marginalized communities become acutely polarized as the impact of these emergent conditions on other related factors (housing, food, jobs, education) cascades and leads to a pressure cooker of population stress. These stressful conditions, often fertile grounds for viruses, bacteria, fungi, and parasites, are compounded by impacts on immunology (stress) and amplified care barriers, leading to the unprecedented loss of health and life (morbidity and mortality, respectively). This population stress is a critical ingredient for pandemic stew. It is a core sociopolitical determinant and a recurrent thesis of this book.

CHAPTER 4

Selected Vulnerable Populations Around the World

The world is a dangerous place to live; not because of the people who are evil, but because of the people who don't do anything about it.
  —ALBERT EINSTEIN

This chapter applies the foundational principles of chapter 3 and provides concrete examples by zooming in on select historically marginalized communities that have known health care access barriers with salient infectious disease risk correlates. Some known communities have universal thematic elements around the globe that make them collectively at higher risk for certain infectious diseases (interchangeably referred to as "vulnerable," "key," or "priority"). I will also provide regional examples of some of these historically marginalized populations and how the SDoH impact their health outcomes.

Poverty

While sitting in morning rounds in eastern Sierra Leone, the charge nurse would report how many children had passed away overnight. The fact that it was invariably more than zero was disturbing, as so many of these conditions were treatable or avoidable. The fact that it was occasionally in the double digits was unconscionable. Students / medical residents would often inquire why sickness among certain pediatric populations would recur or fail to abate. When I pointed out that these communities could often not afford a lifestyle that could either treat or prevent recurrent episodes of malaria—in a part of West Africa where malaria infections are as prevalent as the common cold—it was refreshing to see reactionary "light bulbs" illuminate. The reality is that certain fundamental structural population prevention measures must be implemented in certain high-risk communities. If the government cannot provide those measures, the individuals will remain vulnerable. They cannot afford bed nets. They cannot afford bug spray. They cannot afford to stay indoors during the most dangerous time of day for bites from the mosquito vector that carries malaria in that region. And in many situations, they certainly cannot afford treatment.

Thabo Mbeki was the second president in postapartheid South Africa, following in the footsteps of Nelson Mandela. In a 1995 report to the World Health Organization, Mbeki claimed that extreme poverty, not HIV, was the primary cause of AIDS—a claim I heard him repeat in person in 2002. While this position on "HIV denialism" precipitated feelings of deep consternation from HIV/AIDS activists around the world, and despite the salient implausibility of his scientific claim, his sociopolitical claim was not wrong. Poverty is the prime influencer of health care access across the world. As poverty is so inextricably linked with so many other elements that lead to a higher risk of infectious disease corollaries (e.g., sanitation, nutrition, living conditions, occupational risk), it is no surprise that higher incidence rates (this means the number of new infections in a given population) and higher prevalence ratios (the number of infected people / the number of the defined population at risk) of infectious disease naturally ensue.

Infections have always had a predilection for areas of poverty and inadequate access. Rudolf Virchow, a well-known German microbiologist, famously wrote: "As disease is so often associated with poverty, physicians are the natural attorneys of the poor"—a mantra that resonates with many social justice–driven infectious disease special-ists. Vulnerable populations across the world (including New York City) are at the highest risk of adverse health consequences based on the woefully inadequate resources provided for people living in poverty.

COVID-19 seems to be the gold standard of this amplification of health inequities, but nearly every infectious disease outbreak of global significance follows a similar narrative. The lack of access to basic san-itation, hygiene, vaccinations, and nutrition as well as to the principles of isolation, the distrust of the very governments empowered to fa-cilitate these isolations, and the decades of preceding sociopolitical violence create perfect storms of infectious disease outbreaks and associative violence.

Poorer populations across the world had significantly higher rates of COVID-19 infection and associated rates of death (mortality), with salient examples in England, France, India, Mexico, Peru, Sweden, Bra-zil, and the United States Within those nations, the case rates were sig-nificantly higher in poorer areas. As a case in point, New York City had the highest rates of infection in 2020 in the poorest and more ethnically diverse zip codes—with Corona, Queens (ironically), having the highest prevalence.[1] Another compelling example was Brazil, where analysis of income inequality rates across the nation showed an association be-tween COVID-19 and the Gini coefficient (a measure of the distribution of income in a population): Neighborhoods with greater income inequality had higher COVID-19 incidence and mortality. The patterns are unmistakable, and we will discuss them in more detail in part II.

Neighborhoods

Low-Income Housing Communities

The cascading impact of poverty and housing creates a very compel-ling case for a higher risk of infectious disease transmission. Congre-gate facilities are one of the most obvious cases, where shared utilities and common spaces naturally increase the risk of transmitting communicable diseases spread through the air or respiratory droplets. The scope of congregate facilities is immense and can range from housing shelters to carceral (i.e., jail or prison) settings to social support programs to single-room apartments to facilities for those with intellectual and developmental needs to skilled nursing facilities.

During the COVID-19 pandemic, I helped lead an initiative that focused on categorizing and analyzing congregate care facilities across New York City. We would look at a number of principles that would help categorize the level of risk at each facility and then implement a number of safeguards at each. If the facility was determined to be too dangerous for sheltering in place, we would decant or de-densify those facilities and transport the residents to other more suitable ones (decanting differs from de-densifying in stratifying by risk profile and only transferring the lowest-risk patients to hotel sites). You can imagine the reluctance and fear in these communities as the city forcibly relocated them. Certainly, this would trigger trauma for many who had had similar adverse experiences in the past, especially if dealing with behavioral health or intellectual or developmental disabilities. It was an ongoing challenge that placed an additional assault on communities that were already historically displaced.

Outside of congregate care facilities, crowded housing—typically representing multigenerational homes—is an independent risk factor for infectious disease transmission. This was certainly the case both with SARS-CoV-1 (popularly known as the 2002–2004 SARS outbreak) and -CoV-2 (COVID-19). A study of counties in the United States showed that each 5% increase in the percentage of households with poor housing conditions led to a 50% higher risk of COVID-19 incidence and a 42% higher risk of COVID-19 death.[2] Crowded multigenerational households, which are partly culturally defined, also had elevated risks. A cross-sectional analysis of deaths in England found that relative mortality from COVID-19 was five times higher in households consisting of nine or more members.[3]

As 1 billion people worldwide live in slums, crowding can be categorized as one of five indicators of deprivation. Studies of influenza in slums in Delhi, India, indicate that a slum resident has 50% more contact with other individuals than a nonslum resident, leading to higher rates of disease infection and transmission.[4] In a study in Chennai, India, SARS-CoV-2 infection rates were much higher in higher-density areas.[5] In Medellin, Colombia, residents of slums and informal settlements had higher mortality rates due to COVID-19 than those of other areas in the city.[7]

In nations with some of the greatest inequalities, these conditions can manifest in extreme ways. In parts of Brazil, urban slums known as favelas create conditions with high demographic density and very poor resources. The conditions described in the "broken windows" theory would certainly apply, as most people there live on less than two dollars a day amid staggering crime rates and poor access to the most basic public services, such as health care, education, and space for recreation. This results in a significantly high incidence of malnutrition, diarrhea, pneumonia, leptospirosis, skin diseases, rotavirus, hepatitis, gastroenteritis, hypertension, heart disease, and strokes, as well as infant mortality rates (IMRs) that are often 5–10 times the rate of those in wealthier neighborhoods.

As a medical student, I worked in the favelas with HIV/AIDS physicians and would consistently encounter the same issues with respect to health behavior, including a sense of anomie when it came to the importance of health prevention and maintenance. This was during the early 2000s, when the communities most heavily impacted by HIV/AIDS did not have access to health care. Brazil was an exception, as it defied the World Trade Organization and started to produce its own HIV medication despite the fact that it was still under international patent. Therefore, people actually had access to the medication. This privilege notwithstanding, the people I worked with generally had minimal interest in taking their lifesaving medication. While the reasons behind this behavior are certainly multifactorial, it seemed reasonable to me that the poverty and violence (both micro and macro) these communities experienced on a daily basis was internalized and impacted their will to control their health.

Moving to a different southern continent, over half of Africa's population live in overcrowded informal settlements. In the Cape Town metropolitan area of South Africa, residents in two areas with a high concentration of informal settlements, Khayelitsha (where I spent considerable time as a student and intern) and Klipfontein, live in abject poverty, and their rates of health indicators are often consistent with this. During the COVID-19 pandemic, 2,000 cases occurred per 100,000 residents in these areas, while the rate was 1,639 in the rest of Cape Town (this proxy was very much consistent with the HIV and TB rates I saw decades prior when interning with Doctors Without Borders).[6]

Geography is often described as a compelling SDoH, as it concentrates many of the other determinants into hot spots or clusters of access barriers. Early in the COVID-19 pandemic, we found much higher cases in areas with historic patterns of poverty. Of course, many of these areas were placed at risk because of governmental machinations to systematically exclude people of color, not unlike the redlining examples noted earlier. Consequently, we saw the majority of infections taking place among Black, Indigenous, and people of color (BIPOC) communities in certain areas with chronically poor health care access and outcomes.

In South Chicago, for example, >60% of COVID-19–related deaths were found among African Americans despite the fact that they represent only 12% of the US population.[7] Why were they so disproportionately infected? Why was the mortality so much higher? It was largely due to the conditions described above, with many individuals living in either low-income housing complexes or multigenerational homes where the probability of the risk of transmission (based on the sheer density of populations) was significantly increased. Once infected they would also experience far worse health outcomes because they chronically suffered from factors (e.g., obesity, high blood pressure) that put them at higher risk of COVID-19 death.

But this case is not specific to South Chicago. In fact, we could see similar scenarios playing out in the South Bronx, in South Los Angeles, in South Boston, and in the southern United States (as well as South

Africa). I often make the argument that some of the worst social and health indicators seem to have a common predilection for "southern" areas. This is not arbitrary. Much of the redlining we discussed historically took place in these areas. Why southern sectors of these cities were targeted is beyond the scope of this book.

The Bronx has the worst health outcomes of any county in New York, with the South (again) Bronx, where I worked for years, mostly seeing HIV+ patients, bearing the brunt. Though the manifest conditions are difficult to describe, I will try my best.

There is a humming feeling of vivacious activity in poor, dirty corners of the city. The sounds of trains (of all kinds) are ubiquitous and overwhelming. On a sunny summer day, you will see bustling human activity rising out of industrial poverty. None of the traffic lights seem synchronized, and the clustered traffic just adds to the cacophony of urban tones, with a percussion section of cars crossing nearby bridges competing with the effervescent vocals of "Hey Mamis" emerging from the construction labor. Everyone appears busy with the exception of the smattering of older adults resting their varicosed legs on their sunny two-by-four stoop outside their homes.

The reality of the residents' health and social status, however, is diametrically different. They have the highest rates of nearly chronic and acute health issues in New York City. As an infectious disease doctor, I was very keen to the fact that the rates of sexually transmitted infections (STIs) were also some of the highest in the country. The curious irony is that this is not the result of inadequate health care facilities: In fact, the Bronx has nine hospitals, in addition to several others less than five miles away in Manhattan, plus multiple health centers like the one I ran. Unfortunately, when it comes to the SDoH, the problems exist on so many levels that they impact communities' perception of access and the importance of health care, especially prevention. This, in addition to other social determinants such as transportation and childcare, makes it nearly impossible to access the resources that they do feel are important.

While slums may classically exist in more urban areas throughout the world, the influence of geography may manifest in a number of settings. At the regional level in the United States, poverty is disproportionately concentrated in the rural South (again). In 2014–2018 the South had an average rural poverty rate that was 20.5% higher than any urban area in the United States, where the average urban poverty rate is just above 15%. Mississippi is the poorest state, with most other southern states placing in the top 10.[8]

How does this impact infectious disease? The South now experiences the greatest burden of HIV and deaths of any US region and lags behind in providing quality HIV prevention services and care. Clearly, a host of historically racist policies precipitate disparities such as these—many of them going back to Jim Crow laws. In science, however, we often cannot prove causality and frequently allude to associations as a means to explain the impact on one or another. In the next part, we will do a deeper dive and demonstrate how and why these associations exist.

Southern states today account for an estimated 51% of new HIV cases annually.[9] In 2017 the South also had a greater proportion of new HIV diagnoses (52%) than all other regions combined.[12] Diagnosis rates for people in the South are also higher than for Americans overall, with 8 of the 10 states with the highest rates of new HIV diagnoses located in the South. The impact of HIV in the South also varies by race. African Americans are disproportionately impacted in every risk group, accounting for 53% of new HIV diagnoses in the region in 2017.[10] Black men who have sex with men account for 6 out of every 10 new HIV diagnoses among African Americans in the South. To complicate factors, access for treatment is significantly impacted in these regions. For example, 80% of southern counties do not have an HIV medical provider who has followed more than 10 patients for three years.[11] In addition to a dearth of trained providers, the current workforce does not begin to match the demographic characteristics of the populations most impacted by HIV; in particular, greater numbers of BIPOC providers are needed, as well as medical providers across the spectrum of sexual orientation / gender identity (SOGI), to engender patient trust and retention in care.

Another rural example can be drawn from the colonias, where Wellness Equity Alliance (WEA) continues to work, whose residents have almost no access to health care and struggle every day just to get by. In conversations with the residents of these communities are two salient findings. One is that there is a serious distrust of all angles of government. The second is that they seem to have no knowledge or agency when it comes to their eligibility for certain services or resources. Their checks are often received by their landlords, and they are given a certain net amount and "told" what to live on. They also lack access to information that could help them remedy the situation because the Internet is often spotty or completely inaccessible. The most unsettling fact is that this is entirely legal.

Finally, it is important to note that not all people living in geographic areas of risk are people of color. Several areas are populated by poor rural whites whose socially determined limited access to health care places them at higher risk of public health emergencies. Appalachia is a prime example, as a region that touches 13 different states on the East Coast and is heavily afflicted with poverty. Importantly, it also has one of the highest IMRs and drug overdose rates in the nation.[12] The COVID-19 pandemic further worsened these disparities in the area as people often had to travel hundreds of miles to the nearest community hospital. During times of population stress, this is an unreasonable cost for these communities.

People Experiencing Homelessness

The Organisation for Economic Co-Operation and Development (OECD)—the wealthy nations' club—estimates that nearly 2 million people are currently experiencing homelessness in 35 OECD countries.[13] The global homeless population is growing rapidly, owing to increasing urbanization, austerity, income inequality, and natural disasters. Moreover, people experiencing homelessness, or PEH, are becoming more diverse and increasingly include populations not previously considered at risk, including youths, women, families, seniors, refugees, Indigenous, and LGBTQIA+ (lesbian, gay, bisexual, transgender, queer / questioning, intersex, and asexual / aromantic / agender). The SDoH are critical in understanding why this is such a pervasive and growing issue, part of which was addressed in our section on housing.

How does homelessness impact health care, particularly infectious diseases? Population stress weakens the immunological response of certain frail and vulnerable communities. PEH are a quintessential example of such an immunocompromised population.

Another salient example is the rise of congenital syphilis—especially among unhoused mothers. While the reasons are clearly multifactorial, a profound rise in injecting drug users—especially methamphetamine use—is likely one of the most formidable contributors. Meth, the molecular prefix and common abbreviation, is a unique drug that, unlike other drugs, actually leads to hypersexuality with more profound disinhibition. These risky behaviors (e.g., multiple sexual partners, inconsistent condom use, sex work) lead to inordinately higher rates of STIs in general but, given the epidemiological propensity of sexual networks, selectively increase STIs among certain communities more often than others.[14] For a number of reasons, syphilis has a predilection for women who have sex with men and inject drugs. From 2013 to 2017, the percentage of women with primary and secondary (P&S) syphilis who reported meth use and sex with a person who had injected drugs within the past 12 months more than doubled, and conversely, the percentage of women with P&S syphilis reporting meth use increased nearly threefold, from 6.2% to 16.6%.[15] Given the SDoH and the risk of homelessness among people who inject drugs, the rate of congenital syphilis is significantly higher among the unsheltered homeless.

As discussed in chapter 2, the prevalence of communicable disease is often higher in PEH, partly because of congregate settings, which are exacerbated by this population stress, causing them not only to be at higher risk of disease transmission but to have worse outcomes of those infections as well.[16] Classically, this is seen in high rates of TB, HIV, and viral hepatitis. Infectious respiratory diseases are no exception, and disproportionate rates of COVID-19 have been demonstrated among PEH, who are also at higher risk of contracting SARS-CoV-2 and developing severe disease.[17] Homeless shelters facilitate transmission owing to crowded living quarters and high population turnover, and common health problems in this population (respiratory conditions, heart disease, and tobacco use) are risk factors for severe COVID-19 disease.[18]

Studies of the seroprevalence of COVID-19 among homeless people in France showed that these populations are more exposed to COVID-19 than the general population.[19] In Belgium the hospitalization rate of homeless people for COVID-19 was three times that of the general population.[20] The risk of disease transmission is further complicated by structural access barriers to care when an outbreak takes place—for example, in a street encampment—where the risk of a delayed (or entirely missed) response is high. The cascading impact of these multiple risk factors makes it extremely important to implement additional protections during public health emergencies.

So what do we do about it? We'll exploring such opportunities further in part III, but one concept to plant here is that of *HIV street medicine*—an area that WEA is leading in Southern California.

Minority Race / Ethnicity

We've discussed the pigmentocracy association of race and disease: in other words, the darker you are, the higher your risk of disease. While I am clearly oversimplifying, this correlation is salient and ubiquitous— especially in the context of risk of infectious disease. Regarding COVID-19, systematic reviews comprising almost 19 million patients in 26 studies showed higher rates of infection and mortality in historically marginalized racial and ethnic communities. In the United Kingdom and United States, the risk ratios for infection were twice as high for Black people and 1.5 times as high for Asian people than for white people. In yet another systematic review of studies in England and

Brazil, historically marginalized communities were also found to have more severe outcomes (e.g., respiratory difficulties, kidney failure).[21]

Indigenous Communities

While a granular sociomedical analysis on all minority races/ethnicities is beyond the scope of this book, a focus on Indigenous communities can offer our readers a tangible and powerful example of how color and disease collide. Colonialism is well-known to have decimated Indigenous populations through a number of ways—infectious disease, albeit accidental, having been one of the most effective. The tragic irony is that this level of vulnerability still continues today. Indigenous people number 476 million around the world (about 5% of the global population) and are spread across more than 90 countries, representing more than 5,000 different Indigenous groups and speaking more than 4,000 languages. Over two-thirds live in Asia.[22]

Indigenous communities make up 15% of the world's extreme poor.[23] Globally, they also suffer higher rates of landlessness, malnutrition, and internal displacement than other groups and often face explicit discrimination in countries' legal systems, leaving them even more vulnerable to violence and abuse. Let's be honest: The main element that precipitates this overt discrimination is the clear cultural differences that distinguish those Indigenous communities from the dominant social structures around them.

Indigenous communities' unique historic, social, and political experiences yield distinctive SDoH such as self-determination, settler-colonialism, migration, globalization, cultural continuity and attachment, relationships with land and nonhuman relatives, social support, capital, cohesion, racism and social exclusion, and justice systems. The colonial process manifested in a diminished self-determination and anemic influence in drafting policies to protect the rights of the Indigenous. Consequently, all communities suffered a systemic loss of land, language, and the essential resources to thrive. Forced assimilation through salient examples such as residential schools can help the reader begin to understand how difficult it was for these communities to sustain the agency needed to develop healthy lifestyles. This has led to historical trauma, which is the cumulative, multigenerational, collective experience of emotional and psychological injury in communities and in descendants.

Indigenous health is an emerging field of research but is seriously limited by a lack of reliable and accurate data in all but a few regions of the world—namely, Canada, Australia, the United States, and New Zealand. In the United States, health indicators among American Indians (the general term preferred by most Indigenous communities) are the worst in the nation in many ways and often reflect those of low- and middle-income nations. Relative to the general US population, American Indians are 770% more likely to die from alcoholism, 650% more likely to die from TB, 420% more likely to die from diabetes mellitus, 280% more likely to die from unintentional injuries, and 52% more likely to die from respiratory illnesses (pre–COVID-19) than the rest of the general US population.[24] As a result of these increased mortality rates, American Indians have a life expectancy that is 5 years less than the rest of the US population.[25] At the Wind River Reservation where I worked in 2015–2016, we found the average life span to be 53 years of age, a shockingly low number comparable to that of many Central African nations.

Historically, pandemics tend to have a predilection for Indigenous communities. Alaska Natives represented 80% of the state's death toll from the 1918 Spanish flu. Their mortality rate from the 2009 H1N1 influenza was four times higher than the general population.[26] Despite over one hundred years of progress, the epidemiological data from COVID-19 was hardly different. According to the Centers for Disease Control and Prevention (CDC), American Indians and Alaska Natives were 3.5 times more likely to be diagnosed with the disease than non-Hispanic whites, with a mortality rate that was 2.8 times as high. Of course, this is not merely limited to English-speaking nations.[27] In Brazil, nationwide serological studies demonstrated that the prevalence of COVID-19 in Indigenous patients was more than 4 times higher than in their white counterparts.[28] Moreover, inequitable COVID-19 outcomes were reported for Indigenous people in several other communities all throughout North America. Specifically, people who spoke an Indigenous language were more likely to be hospitalized and die as a result of COVID-19 than those who did not.

Romani People

The Romani, colloquially known as the Roma (and widely known by the pejorative exonym Gypsies, or Gipsies) are a traditionally nomadic Indo-Aryan ethnic group. They live predominantly in Europe and Anatolia but have a well-known diaspora with significant concentrations in the Americas. The recent admission of several central European countries to the European Union has caused an increased migration of the Roma population to Western European countries. While immigration rates of Roma vary from country to country, those countries encounter similar problems in housing and supporting this population.

Several studies have addressed the important health inequities between Roma and the general population, with most findings indicating that Roma have a significantly shorter life expectancy and higher IMR and are more at risk for a wide variety of diseases, findings recently confirmed in a report published by the European Commission.[29] From an infectious disease standpoint, viral hepatitis has been found in unusually high proportions among this socially vulnerable community. A study in Spain found a seroprevalence of hepatitis A virus (HAV) antibodies of 82% in deprived Roma children compared to 9.3% in more affluent non-Roma children.[30] In another Spanish study, the overall seroprevalence was 63% among the Roma, 46% in the orphanage group, and 23% among the controls.[31] Overcrowding seemed to be a factor, as did poverty and sanitary practices. An excess in the seroprevalence of hepatitis B in pregnant Roma women has also been described.[32] Hepatitis C may also be more prevalent among Roma, especially those in carceral settings. Finally, evidence points to an excess of hepatitis E morbidity among the Roma, with a study in Bohemia showing their seroprevalence of hepatitis E antibodies to be double that of non-Roma STI clinic attendees.[33]

Bedouin

The Bedouin are nomadic Arab tribes that have historically inhabited the desert regions in the Arabian Peninsula, in North Africa, in the Levant, and in Mesopotamia. The Bedouin originated in the Syrian and Arabian Deserts but spread across the rest of the Arab world after the coming of Islam.[34] The Bedu (the English word "bedouin" comes from the Arabic *badawī*, which means "desert dweller") are traditionally divided into tribes, or clans, and historically share a common culture of herding camels and goats. The vast majority of Bedouins adhere to Islam, although a small number are Christian Bedouins.

The Bedouin have been subjected to decades of expulsion, internal transfer, land confiscation, and invariable policies of forced sedentarization. This is particularly the case in Israel, where approximately 200,000 Bedu live. While this book is intended to depoliticize several public health and associated social drivers, it is important to describe some key objective findings, some of which I directly witnessed and documented.

Many Bedouins (>60%) live in the state of Israel's "unrecognized villages," which are not dissimilar from the colonias or American Indian reservations described above.[35] The systematic application of nonrecognition and neglect accompanied by concentrating the population in urban settlements leads to a number of downstream health issues.

When I was working with the Bedouin while in medical school in the 2000s (figures 4.1a–d), I kept some journal entries, which can be helpful to our readers.

Picture a large power plant with dozens of high-voltage power lines that traverse the adjacent village. The hazards involved are irrefutable: electromagnetic radiation, electrocution, chronic noise pollution, and polluting emissions well beyond the acceptable national standards.

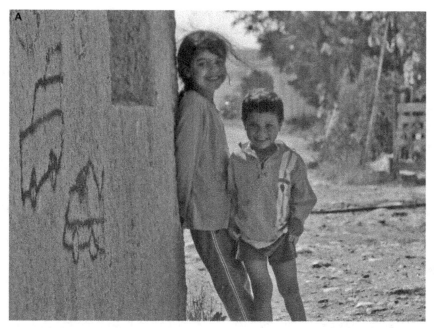

FIGURES 4.1. A–D Assortment of personal photographs of the bedouin, Negev, Israel, 2009. A: children in Umm Batin; B: Hebron stream running through Um Barin; C: diesel-operated generator to power CPAP device; D: Zenzun's home (Wadi El Na'am, Negev, Israel). *Source:* Photos by author.

It is here that Zenzun and his family reside. He is unemployed. He and his family were relocated to this site by the State of Israel some 30 years ago. This power plant was built in 1982. Toxic gasses are released into the open air daily—including nitric oxides, sulfuric oxides, and hydrogen combustion gasses. Despite this risk, ironically, Zenzun and his family do not have access to electricity.

Studies of prolonged, daily exposure to noise show physiological symptoms ranging from loss of hearing to heart disease. Others manifest intellectual and developmental disorders, affected rational judgment, and increased interpersonal and community conflicts.[36] Wadi el Na'am residents continue to suffer from unbearable noise originating in the power plant—loud to the point that conversations amongst villagers were simply inaudible, albeit even several kilometers away from the power plant.

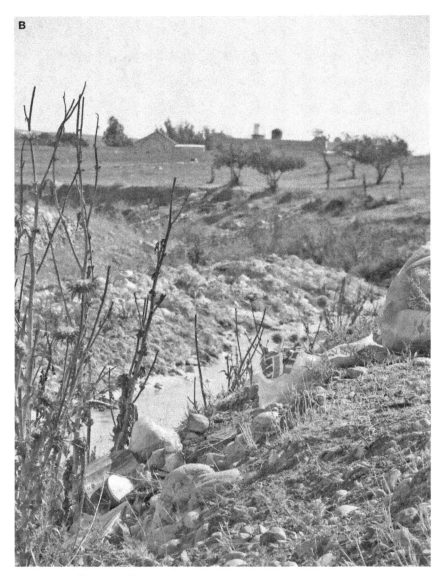

FIGURES 4.1. (Continued)

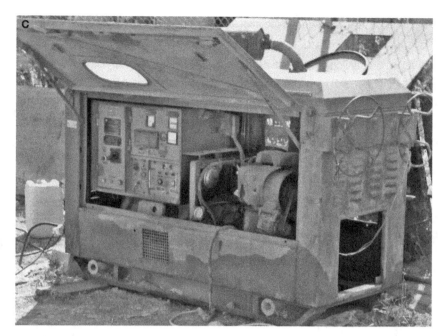

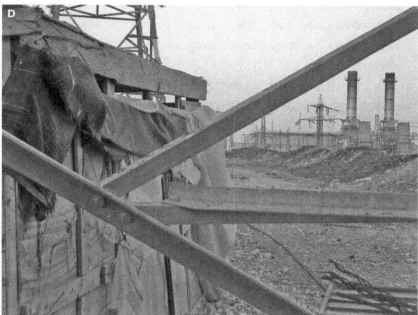

FIGURES 4.1. (Continued)

Finally, electromagnetic radiation here (although unproven as of yet) has the most profound impacts on the health of these residents. It is difficult to garner valid epidemiological data on a population that "doesn't exist." Zenzun, his wife, two children, and several other villagers are frequently ill—mostly with chronic illnesses. Symptoms range from difficulty breathing and weight loss to dizziness, fainting, and vomiting—most of which can be attributed to nerve-related disorders.

Imagine this cacophony of buzzing electric lines as a backdrop with Zenzun required to shout above the suffocating sounds with a look of despair: "My whole family is sick. . . . The doctors say we are sick because of the power and chemical plants nearby. They tell us to leave the area—but we have nowhere to go. We would prefer to struggle than lose our land. We have nowhere to go. We are not recognized."

Unrecognized villages are in violation of the provisions of international conventions defining the state's responsibility toward its citizens—conventions that have been signed and ratified by Israel. The social needs and actual services in these villages and the situation in the neighboring Jewish communities prove the extent to which the condition of the residents of the unrecognized villages in the Negev desert is inconsistent with the basic obligation to avoid discrimination.

This "lack of recognition" results in the absence of basic infrastructures and services such as connections to the electric and water grids, running water, sewage and refuse disposal, proper access roads to the villages, and the providing of decent health, education, and social services. The residents of these villages are also subjected on a regular basis to land confiscations, house demolitions, fines for "illegal" construction, destruction of agricultural fields and trees, and systematic harassment and persecution by the Open Areas Inspection Unit (or the "Green Patrol"). Furthermore, the Israeli government's policy of settling Bedouins into 7 "recognized" settlements has caused high levels of unemployment and loss of livelihood.[37]

This dilemma also bleeds into other complexities, such as inhibited access to shops and banking services. Moreover, the villages do not appear on the official and accepted maps of the State of Israel—creating significant problems in terms of access to health care, particularly emergency relief. A typical Bedouin village has no road sign directing traffic from the nearest paved road, and no sign bearing its name. A dirt road leads to the main clusters of homes. Most of the villages have only a mosque and local grocery store, albeit with limited supplies.[38]

This absence of infrastructure and basic utilities form some of the core sociopolitical determinants that place these communities at severe risk of disease—particularly for their most vulnerable members, in this case women and children.[39]

Minority Sexual Orientation / Gender Identity

LGBTQIA+

LGBTQIA+ is a broad term that includes multiple SOGI minorities. The sexual orientation bucket covers lesbian, gay, bisexual, and queer identities, which describes humans who are often attracted to the same sex / gender or a plurality of orientations. Many folks find these terms restrictive and prefer more fluid identity references, which partially explains why they are constantly evolving and why this alphabet soup continues to expand. A more recent preferred term among some is pansexual (a human sexually attracted to others of any sex / gender). In medicine we refer to gay men as men who have sex with men, as it simply defines the act and the associated risk of STIs but does not reference the presumed identity.

Transgender represents the gender identity bucket and describes humans who are assigned one particular gender at birth but experience a degree of gender incongruence and identify with another or do not identify with either binary gender identity (e.g., gender nonconforming or gender fluidity). Intersex is a completely different bucket and describes multiple (generally two) sets of genitalia. It is a term often used to describe individuals who develop atypically in regard to some or all aspects of their biological sex (chromosomal, hormonal, gonadal, or genital). Intersex conditions, of which there are many types, are anatomical, enzyme related, or neurological. Gender identity issues can arise but do not themselves form part of the intersex condition. Most intersex conditions are not readily visible. Asexual (no known sexual attraction) or, recently, "allies" (supporters of the LGBTQIA+ but not necessarily identifying within this spectrum) represents the final letter, and the plus sign simply flags that this list is incomplete.

This large bucket can intersect with a number of other identities, which may lead to cascading impacts in terms of the risk of given health outcomes. While the group is vast, if treated as a monolith from an epidemiological standpoint, we know that certain factors place members of this group at an increased risk of physical or sexual abuse, intimate partner violence (IPV, which is a broader definition than domestic violence), depression, post-traumatic stress disorder (PTSD), substance use disorder (SUD), and self-destructive behaviors. They are also particularly vulnerable to suicidal behaviors, with LGBTQIA+ youths representing up to 40% of all young PEH. STIs, particularly HIV, are also a common health outcome—especially among adolescents and young adults.[40]

The group consistently at highest risk for HIV is African American gay men, who are at six-times greater risk than white gay men, thereby representing the critical intersection of sexual orientation and racial disparities.[41] Poverty, discrimination, stigma, inequality, xenophobia, and other social conditions facilitate HIV transmission by influencing community prevalence. These conditions are greater in the southern United States, where the majority of new infections take place.[42]

Working with these communities has been an absolute privilege. The amount of delightful stories I have heard over the years are far too numerous to list, but I will do my best to share a few compelling ones.

At one point, as described earlier, I was the medical director for the largest HIV clinic ($n > 2,000$ patients) in the largest chain of community-based HIV clinics in the United States. As we were chronically understaffed, I would often have to manage a few dozen patients per day, which is a high number for a single physician. The complexities of these appointments are difficult to describe, as we would often be responsible for handling multiple (if not dozens) of health and colliding social issues in the span of 15–20 minutes per patient. In other words, we would be managing someone's HIV in addition to their poorly controlled diabetes, their schizophrenia, their high blood pressure, their rectal gonorrhea, their insatiable methamphetamine use (and associated behavioral outcomes), and often their housing insecurities to boot.

It was stressful but also exhilarating and enjoyable. When people asked me "what kind of doctor" I was, I would often coyly respond that I managed meth and syphilis all day (this wasn't far from the truth). One time a patient walked in out of breath. Eventually, he was able to share that he had just had sex with more than five men (separately) at a local bathhouse and was so high on meth that he needed to sit on the floor (we later gave him intravenous fluids, as it seemed he had been up for days).

Fortunately, his HIV was controlled and was the least of his issues. As my nurse, my social worker, and I sat next to him, providing a comforting look and reassuring pat on the back, I asked him to evaluate his life choices. This triggered a disarming chuckle from him, and we were able to jump into some meaningful interventions. The point was that we didn't judge: We provided a harm-reduction approach. This means supplying health care that meets the patient's needs in the place where they are at the moment. We do not preach about poor health-related behaviors because the reality is that our multipolar world is too complex for some "magic" Western biomedicine approach to be effective. Who am I to judge this person's actions? I can simply ask him / her / them to reflect on the current outcome of some of those choices, point to likely health outcomes if the behavior continues, and ask if they wish to make any changes. The LGBTQIA+ (like so many other communities we're describing) have had so many colliding factors that influence the course of their lives, many of them socially determined, that as effective leaders it is critical that we simply meet them "where they're at." I certainly tried with this patient. Over time our efforts were met with success.

Many transgender (TG) people live with the constant threat of violence. International research documented a total of over 2,000 murders of TG humans between January 2008 and April 2016.[43] (These findings are likely greatly underreported.) Even more widespread is nonlethal violence against TG communities. A national US study indicated that 35% of TG/nonbinary (NB) youths between the ages of 5 and 18 (roughly) fell victim to physical violence and 12% to sexual violence.[44] In the same study, 6–7% had been either physically or sexually assaulted at work.

The sum total of this violence and discrimination naturally affects behavioral health. Of the participants in the US study noted above, 41% reported attempting suicide (compared with 1.6% of the general population). In addition, a national Australian study found that over 50% and 38% of TG humans had been diagnosed with depression and anxiety, respectively, at some point in their lives, which is four times the rate for the general population. Even worse, TG/NB youths are disproportionately burdened by poor mental health outcomes. These disparities are likely due to high levels of social rejection during the formative development years, such as a lack of support from parents and bullying.[45]

Outside of poor mental health and SUD outcomes, multiple factors stemming from stigma and discrimination likely also contribute to high rates of infectious disease—namely HIV. In a large multinational study, the overall standardized HIV prevalence was nearly 20.0% and 2.56% for TG women and men, respectively. Just to add more clarity, TG women's odds of being infected with HIV were a staggering 66-times higher compared with rates in the general population (the rate was 6.8 times higher for TG men).[46] Breaking this down regionally is also helpful to allow us to better contextualize how risk translates for TG communities. In sub-Saharan Africa, the infection rate odds were 30% for a sample of 1,192 individuals, which was 21.5-times higher than for the general population.[47] In Latin America the prevalence was 25.9%, which was 95.6 times higher than for the general population. In

Asia the prevalence was 13.5%, which was 68 times higher than for the general population. Last, Australia, Europe, and North America demonstrated a prevalence of 17.1% with an odds ratio of 48.4 (compared to the general population).[48] Hopefully, these stark comparisons can begin to tell a story. I have a few. . . .

While finishing up my residency training, I was moonlighting as an HIV doctor in Buffalo, New York. I was so excited to complete my seemingly endless training (17 years in total) and be "unleashed" on the medical world to make my own autonomous clinical decisions. A few months in, my boss, the medical director, dropped a manual on my desk and sternly asked me to learn it by the next day. The manual was on gender-affirming care for TG communities. I was shocked. Was he serious? I wasn't trained for this. No one really was at the time. So I did what I was told, as any upstanding medical resident would, and spent several hours assimilating this information. I was about to have the health of a human being transferred into my care with a "disease" I was completely unfamiliar with yet stood the chance to learn so much and help this person. Learn, I did.

This physician-patient relationship became one of my most memorable. The TG female (or male / female) patient ended up becoming one of my favorites, and I devoured anything I could on the subject. She was trying hormone therapy for the first time (surgeries were far from being approved by major insurance payers at the time), and I was helping her navigate the complexities of transition within the social milieu that she lived in. While my understanding was still nascent in this space, I did know a fair bit about generally counseling patients about socially driven grief and anxiety. As it turns out, there were few differences between the two, and even the notion that she suffered from a "disease" (often classified as gender identity disorder so that insurance companies would pay for the encounter) was wrong. This ultimately became a highly contentious discussion throughout the nation.

Another remarkable patient who came under my care years later in East Hollywood was a TG person with some of the most complex health issues I had ever seen in an outpatient clinic. In addition to having HIV (well controlled), she was schizophrenic, diabetic, and deaf, with recurrent STIs, hepatitis C, meth use, and end-stage renal disease, on dialysis, and to top it all off, she was homeless. She also had one of the most challenging "no show" rates (for many of the reasons noted above) and likely could have made more effective choices, but we knew that if we could help her with housing, stability would follow. We were right.

We were able to get her a single-room occupancy unit (with a common bathroom), and after a few months, she was adherent with her insulin, on hepatitis C medication, and quickly en route to a cure, as treatment nowadays can take place as early as two months. One day when I went to visit her at her apartment, one of the case managers told me that she was generally doing well but that he was frustrated because she consistently defecated in the corner of her room. I couldn't help but chuckle and simply assured the case manager that this was yet another scenario where we must not impose our standards on certain communities who live differently and simply "meet them where they're at." The problem is that most of the health care world does not see it that clearly.

Religious Minorities

The plight of religious minorities is well described and nearly ubiquitous—most notoriously in the last century, with the horrific events of the Holocaust. Sadly, religion continues to have a formidable impact on health care access and outcomes throughout the world.

The reasons are multifactorial. In the Global North, we often do not have the cultural competence to provide adequate care to religious minorities, leading to systematic delays that can determine the difference between life and death. Then, of course, there is implicit bias. This type of bias (unconscious though it may be) is the process of associating stereotypes or attitudes with categories of people without conscious awareness, resulting in actions and decisions at odds with one's conscious beliefs about fairness and equality. Sadly, there are far too many examples of these injustices. I will merely present a few salient contemporary examples I have personally seen throughout the world.

One example is Israel. For Palestinian populations there is no doubt that implicit bias and systematic barriers have led to much poorer access and outcomes with regard to health care. As a medical student, I would often volunteer in the Palestinian territories nearly every weekend (typically with Physicians for Human Rights), working among both Jewish and Arab Israeli physicians and nurses. Because of the systematic distrust in both communities, as well as the procedural barriers for certain communities to gain access, health care was significantly compromised. In addition, while Arabs (mostly Muslims) would have access to health care institutions once they crossed the security checkpoints, there was likely implicit bias among the medical providers once they did so. Too often we saw people with medical emergencies (including a number of pregnancies) stuck in their villages without access to structured medical care. We were all they had.

This section is even all the more germane given the current war with over 1,000 casualties on the Israeli side and over 30,000 (and counting) on the Palestinian side (the average casualty ratio between both sides since 1948 is 100:1 Palestinian / Israeli). Anyone with media access is all too familiar with the problem benignly dubbed "the Israeli-Palestinian conflict." At the same time, however, many of us fail to fully understand the intricacies of this energy-consuming nightmare. I was one. Here are some thoughts I jotted down in my late 20s upon arriving to the famed "Holy Land." . . .

Upon arriving in Israel at the age of 29 to commence my graduate medical studies, I quickly began absorbing everything around me. Yet my baseline ignorance was soon supplanted by the unknowns and curiosities that emerge due to erudite knowledge. I decided I needed more. In an attempt to reify all the abstract statistics and historical narratives with irreplaceable reality. I soon entered that "bomb-ridden, terrorist-proliferating" forbidden land that us Westerners only read about in our suspense novels or Hollywood blockbuster films. I was on my way to the occupied Palestinian Territories. . . .

In this geographical area smaller than Los Angeles County, I expected to encounter sheer unequivocal hell, even worse than some of the conditions I had encountered in sub-Saharan Africa, Latin America, and South Asia. What I was met with was something very different. I was immediately welcomed by stunning geography, lush vegetation, a paucity of superficial infections and diseases, and well-fed stomachs. Where was the pervasive trauma that the media would flood our media digests with?

Over the course of my repeated excursions into the West Bank, I began noticing something completely different from my experiences in other developing nations: populations seemingly void of emotion. This was new to me. One of the heartwarming aspects of working in least-developed countries was the prevalence of warmth, gratitude, and appreciation targeted towards the outsider, despite the disproportional poverty, famine, presence of triadic pandemics, desperate acts of violence, and sociopolitical volatility.

Was it possible that the Palestinian people were inherently cold and apathetic? After traveling to and researching several other parts of the Arabic world, it became inordinately clear that this was a cultural impossibility. Instead, I came to realize that they were suffering from a pain undetectable by the conventional differential diagnosis. Palestinian suffering was not rooted in the traditional forms of poverty and disease. Instead, it was the direct result of the daily oppression enforced upon them by the Israeli occupation. The proliferation of unplanned checkpoints, the repeated taunting by their Jewish settler neighbors, their inability to lead reliable and fulfilling existences all converge upon a suffering that is not experienced in most other parts of the globe.

Of course, the world is overrun by brutal sociopolitical and structural violence, but three significant components caused a very different experience in the near East. First, the majority of other forms of government or insurgency-led oppression are facilitated by members of the same or similar national, ethnic, religious, or racial group. The more features that differentiate the oppressors and their subjugated prey, the more their shared ideologies will rupture, the more resistant the marginalized group shall be, the more detrimental too shall be their consequences.

Second, most other domination manifests either in subtle, undetectable, and persistent forms (i.e., structural violence) or random and transient varieties. Therefore, the seemingly infinite formalized and structured oppression of the Palestinian is internalized differently—as a barrier to hope, dreams, and a realistic future. A university education cannot be properly sought after, a family cannot be appropriately planned for, a life cannot be organized if hope is an abstract concept.

If these restrictions on natural liberties do not seem to fade with time; if the strong Arabic pride is denigrated by children watching their mothers bear children or sisters die of acute trauma at military checkpoints; if nothing positive ever seems to materialize no matter how much resistance and infighting persists—human beings are gradually drained of the life that causes the human condition to subsist.

These two factors mentioned so far resonate well with the conditions observed under the apartheid regime in South Africa. But why? Why attempt to whip the nonconformist into absolute docility? The inclination to create such human dynamics emanates from a general culture of fear that we all live in. Aung San Suu Kyi stated that "it is not power that corrupts but fear. Fear of losing power corrupts those who wield it and fear of the scourge of power corrupts those who are subject to it." Curiously enough, prolific infectious disease and relative poverty still abound in South Africa, yet the element of human suffering has inarguably declined since 1994 and the dissolution of the oppressive apartheid state. This is quite a different experience from the Palestinian, who continues to be at higher risk of infectious disease and overall poor health.

A denial of physical freedom naturally impacts multiple dimensions of health care outcomes—especially behavioral health, which in turn, leads to a higher risk of infectious disease. George K. Anderson accurately coined this peculiar and illogical condition by stating "What man has done to man is the saddest chapter in the history of the world. The story of the peoples of the earth is in large measure the tale of how the world whipped the nonconformist with its displeasure and visited upon him dishonor and ignominy, torture and death." It is high time we wipe the tears of anthropogenic human suffering by drawing from lessons in the past and applying them to solutions in the future.

Rohingya Muslims

Another unlikely community to experience human rights abuses based on religious standing are the Rohingya Muslims of Myanmar (Burma). As this is a Buddhist nation led at one time by a Nobel Peace Prize laureate, one would assume this translated into a culture of tolerance. Unfortunately, quite the opposite materialized in 2016 when the Rohingya (who mainly reside in Myanmar's Rakhine region state and are not recognized as a legitimate minority by the state) fled to escape violent persecution by the Burmese army. A review published by *The Lancet* reported that the persecution of this population has led to killings, the destruction of their neighborhoods, and limits on their reproductive freedoms and movement.[49] Rohingya who violate Myanmar's restrictions are subject to imprisonment, torture, forced labor, and sexual violence. The shocking situation has caused over 300,000 Rohingya to flee to surrounding countries in Southeast Asia—namely Bangladesh, where they also face discrimination from that government.

This displacement significantly impacted health care access, making the health status in and outside Myanmar far worse than the majority population for several indicators. Childhood mortality (under five years) is two to three times higher than the general population; acute malnutrition is 14% higher; and pediatric diarrheal disease is five times greater than the general (Buddhist) population.[49] Moreover, in Bangladesh nearly 20% of Rohingya children are severely malnourished and 60% are stunted, rates that are both 50% or higher than in the rest of the Bangladesh population.[50] The situation facing the Rohingya stems from their statelessness. As the historian Joseph Reese Strayer noted: "A man can lead a reasonably full life without a family, a fixed local residence, or a religious affiliation, but if he is stateless, he is nothing. He has no rights, no security, and little opportunity." This was caused by religious differences.

Uyghurs

Another Muslim minority group suffering from systematic discrimination is the Uyghurs in China. About 12 million Uyghurs live mostly in Xinjiang (Northwest China). They speak their own language (similar to Turkish) and see themselves as culturally and ethnically close to central Asian nations. They make up less than half of the Xinjiang population, where the majority are Han Chinese. Recent decades have seen a mass migration of Han into Xinjiang, allegedly orchestrated by the state to dilute the minority population there.[131] China has also been accused of targeting Muslim religious figures and banning religious practices in the region, as well as destroying mosques and tombs.

Over the last decade, China has created a large system of arbitrary detention and enforced disappearance. Approximately 1 million Uyghurs (nearly 10% of the entire ethnic population) are currently imprisoned, for reasons as simple as practicing their religion, having international contacts or communications, or attending a Western university.[51] The Chinese government has defended the camps as "vocational training centers" aimed at combating violent extremism. But leaked government documents reveal that the state is in fact targeting people based on religious observance, such as praying or growing a beard, as well as family background.

Independent researchers have reported that individuals in the camps are often subjected to ill-treatment and indoctrination. Uyghurs who have been detained report being forced to renounce their religion and to sing songs and make statements swearing allegiance to the Communist Party. Some have reported experiencing torture and sexual violence. Those who are detained are often unable to communicate with or receive visits from their families. Children whose parents are detained are placed in government-run adoption centers, sometimes far from their homes and families. While some Uyghurs are charged with crimes through the formal criminal process, the majority of detentions occur without charges ever being brought. In these situations, family members, particularly those living abroad, are often unable to get information about their missing loved ones or even confirm that they have been detained, causing further trauma and fear within the community.

In terms of health care concerns, the Office of the High Commissioner for Human Rights (UNHCR) describes specific medical concerns about the treatment of Uyghurs in Xinjiang, especially between 2017 and 2019.[52] Testimonies were gathered that pointed to blood tests, injections, and medications being forced on Uyghurs without their consent, as well as rape, "invasive gynecological examinations," and sexual violence and humiliation. Investigations revealed that psychological torture produced mental suffering by creating an atmosphere of fear, stress, and anxiety. The report also expressed concerns about widespread violations of the right to the highest attainable standard of health—a lack of freedom to refuse nonconsensual medical treatment and a lack of access to clean water, sanitation, and food. Reproductive rights were also allegedly violated. Sterilizations rose sharply in 2017 and 2018—around eight times the amount in China overall—and this as well as the forced placement of intrauterine devices and forced abortions may have contributed to a rapid fall in the Uyghur birth rate in Xinjiang. Quality and neutral medical access is entirely absent, with a high risk of infectious disease outbreaks.

Low-Income Labor

The markets and industries in which people work often determine their risk of health access and associated outcomes. In several nations where the Bismarck model is employed (including the United States), full-time employment translates to health care coverage. The association is complex, with education and literacy further influencing the engagement of care. The recent COVID-19 pandemic also demonstrated the polarization of risk when it came to mostly white college-educated communities working safely at home in virtual meetings while their Black and Brown (non–college educated, mostly) neighbors worked in certain "essential" industries where they continued to be at risk. This is a common theme that we will highlight in part II. Below are two extreme examples.

Economic Migrants

The world is currently witnessing the highest-ever recorded number of international migrants, at over 300 million, though the percentage of the world's migrant population has remained fairly constant over the past several decades, at about 3%.[53]

Migrants endure several experiences that ultimately affect their health—particularly in settings where they face a constellation of legal, cultural, economic, social, communications, and behavioral barriers. We will delve into the plight of (political) migrants below, but in the context of migrant labor, health vulnerabilities can occur throughout the migration cycle. Economic migrants are those who voluntarily migrated to pursue economic development opportunities and were not necessarily forced from their homes (though many situations are a matrix of many reasons). The conditions in which they travel, restricted access to health services upon arriving to their destination country, exploitation, poor living and working conditions, discrimination, and the geographical distance from their families and support system are some aspects of the migration process that can impact the health of labor migrants and lead to the deterioration of their health status.

Many migrant workers are employed in high-risk and hazardous sectors such as mining, agriculture, and construction. These kinds of jobs usually involve long hours and hard physical labor, which can result in increased occupational accidents. Those in an irregular migration status, especially, endure dangerous working conditions and fear drawing attention to themselves and losing their jobs or being deported. Furthermore, migrant workers are often not allowed to form and join trade unions, which may be an additional obstacle to raising concerns about their health and safety in the workplace.

In addition, sexual exploitation has been widely reported in the context of female labor migrants working in informal sectors, such as domestic work. Unfortunately, much like the multiple vulnerable communities described above, migrant laborers were highly impacted by the COVID-19 pandemic. This was especially the case in California. When I was the COVID-19 vaccine czar in Marin County and one of the incident commanders for the entire Bay Area, we had a set of criteria created by the CDC Advisory Committee on Immunization Practice (ACIP, Advisory Council on Immunization Practices, composed of the most elite vaccine scientists at the center, who have the final say on all vaccine policy) for priority groups to receive the COVID-19 vaccine at a time when it was in exceedingly short supply. After age (the universal risk factor), essential workers were prioritized, starting with health care workers and moving to food and agriculture workers (many of whom were Latinx migrant workers). They were not enjoying the comfort of their homes on Zoom calls and wearing shorts; they were out working. As a result, Latinx communities in certain areas were at highest risk of COVID-19 in the early stages of the vaccine rollout. A recent study detailed farmworkers' fears of COVID-19 transmission at work, compounded by a lack of access to health care and social services, and their need to work in order to survive economically.[54]

Sex Workers

The common adage is that sex work is the oldest profession known to history (though some may argue that another profession needed to precede it in order to produce the currency to purchase the sex). For our definition, sex workers are adults (not those under 18 regardless of the country's laws) who receive money or goods for sexual services, either regularly or occasionally. This can include cis female or male and TG sex workers. We prefer the term *sex work* to other slightly more derogatory terms, as it provides more agency and less objectification to their profession (which may be volitional for many).

The genesis and ongoing influence for sex workers is highly variable—especially based on their country of residence. Some enjoy their work and see it as a way to express their sexuality. Others like the income and flexibility. Others view sex work as their best available option to earn an income. Yet, whoever sex workers are and whatever they do, they deserve the same protections as everyone else. This includes the right to health care, to safety, and to their wages.

Sex work provides a classic example of intersectional discrimination, as we discussed above. Stigma against sex workers leads to extreme barriers to health care. Sex workers often hide their involvement in sex work due to fear of being judged and treated poorly. When they disclose their occupation, they often experience stigmatizing behavior from medical staff. Many health workers have limited training on sex work (again, implicit bias likely plays a role) and do not know how to deal with sex-related issues in general. Sex workers often face structural barriers to accessing health care such as long waits, restrictive hours, unwelcoming spaces, fear of arrest, legal status requirements, inconvenient locations, lack of transportation, inability to pay, lack of confidentiality, and no access to culturally competent social workers.

Stigma is a particular concern and with its associated criminalization places sex workers in vulnerable positions. Access barriers to health care in addition to a number of other SDoH help explain why sex workers are over 30 times more likely to be HIV+ than the general population.[55] Research notes that despite likely popular opinion, these significantly higher rates are not attributable to irresponsible behavior. Conversely, they are often the result of systematic discrimination leading to high rates of violence (including sexual assault) that place these women or men at high risk. As a case in point, in Haiti UNAIDS found that 36.6% of women who engage in sex work report physical violence, and 27.1% report sexual violence.[56] It should also be noted that these results are likely highly underreported because of the concern for reprisals. In places where sex work is criminalized, police have used condoms as evidence of sex work. To avoid arrest, some sex workers engage in unprotected sex with clients, thereby increasing their risk of HIV infection.

COVID-19 lockdowns and restrictions have made in-person sex work more difficult, if not effectively impossible.[57] This in turn has made sex workers more dependent on the clients they do have, decreasing sex workers' agency and leading to higher rates of abuse. The COVID-19 pandemic has been particularly difficult for people whose only income is sex work, based on multiple reports from journalist and organization-led investigations, impacting sex workers in a number of formidable and unique ways.

Immigration Status of Political Migrants

Imagine a young boy orphaned by a mother eviscerated by AIDS and a father whirled away by conventional trends of abandonment. The local priests look after this boy until one day a tragic fate unfolds when all men of the cloth are systematically gunned down with antiquated Kalashnikovs. The locals seeking refuge there are not even offered the luxury of a bullet but instead meet their end by means of elongated machetes. The boy is spared . . . for he can be of use one day . . . to propagate their violence.

He is forced to rape, maim, and slaughter the very people he was taught to respect. He is caught in an ethical quandary and no longer feels he can operate as a vessel of war. He escapes his doom and, after various transnational peregrinations, procures a spot on a makeshift boat that can accommodate his passage to a land of proverbial promise. Sadly, he is intercepted 20 miles off the coast of his final destination by the local authorities.

He lacks any proper documentation—and is (importantly) from a least-developed nation. The question remains—which trajectory will this young boy follow? Such a query, though ostensibly axiomatic, posits a long-standing uncertainty in international law. Shall he be defined as a (political) refugee or a (economic) migrant? While the question appears to be one of insignificant nuance, the consequences of this decision may potentially determine the systematic survival of thousands (figure 4.2).

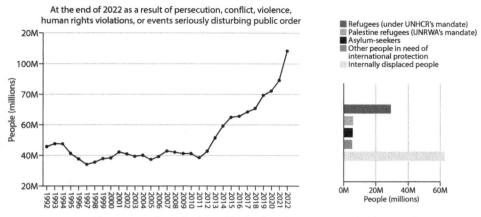

FIGURE 4.2. The temporal trend of forcibly displaced persons worldwide according to the UNHCR, 1992–2022. *Source: Procurement in UNHCR*, United Nations High Commissioner for Refugees, July 2024, https://www.unhcr.org/sites/default/files/legacy-pdf/54aeb4f39.pdf.

At least 108.4 million people around the world have been forced to flee their homes.[58] Among them are nearly 35.3 million refugees, around 41% of whom are under the age of 18; 5.5 million are asylum seekers. While the plight of refugees or asylum seekers can never be overstated, the opportunities for internally displaced persons (IDPs) are often far bleaker, as they sometimes lack the agency of the humanitarian clusters funded to generally help humans only after they cross borders. There are over 63 million IDPs. These are important distinctions. We have not even discussed victims of human trafficking (figures 4.3 and 4.4).[59]

The personal history of a refugee is often marked by physical and emotional trauma. Although refugees hail from a wide latitude of cultures and climates, their shared pattern of experiences allows some generalizations to be made about their health care needs and challenges.

So many terms are thrown around, but how precisely do we define a refugee? Today, the United Nations defines a refugee as anyone who, "owing to a well-founded fear of being persecuted for reasons of race, religion, nationality, membership of a particular social group or political opinion, is outside the country of his nationality and is unable or,

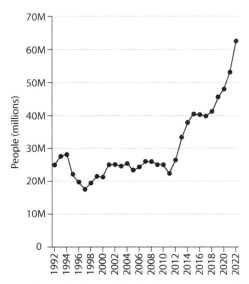

FIGURE 4.3. The temporal trend of internally displaced persons worldwide according to the UNHCR, 1992–2022. *Source: Procurement in UNHCR*, United Nations High Commissioner for Refugees, July 2024, https://www.unhcr.org/sites/default/files/legacy-pdf/54aeb4f39.pdf.

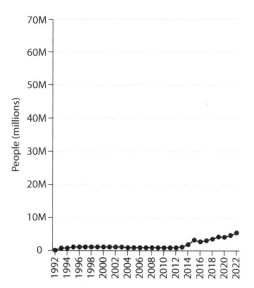

FIGURE 4.4. The temporal trend of asylum seekers worldwide according to the UNHCR, 1992–2022. *Source: Procurement in UNHCR*, United Nations High Commissioner for Refugees, July 2024, https://www.unhcr.org/sites/default/files/legacy-pdf/54aeb4f39.pdf.

owing to such fear, is unwilling to avail himself of the protection of that country."[60]

Over half of all forcibly displaced people (who have successfully crossed a border) came from just three countries (i.e., Syria, Ukraine, or Afghanistan). This certainly does not include the 4.6 million Palestinian refugees who are under the tutelage of the United Nations Relief and Works Agency (UNHCR, 2011). IDPs contribute the largest burden of displacement, but humanitarian resources are limited to address these populations based on international humanitarian law. Ten countries—Syria, Afghanistan, the Democratic Republic of the Congo (DRC), Ukraine, Colombia, Ethiopia, Yemen, Nigeria, Somalia, and Sudan—are home to nearly three-quarters of those who live in displacement. Several of them remained displaced because of unresolved conflicts.

Sadly, the numbers are going up dramatically. As of the time of writing (late 2023), there were 17 million displacements inside Ukraine, 8 million in Pakistan, and 16.5 million in sub-Saharan Africa, with the DRC, South Sudan, and Ethiopia seeing the most displacement on the African continent. I have experience working in all three countries.

Again, in 2013 I was the only doctor working in an IDP camp in South Sudan (figures 4.5a–f). The catchment area served approximately 29,000 IDPs. I was there on an emergency mission during a time of intensive fighting. In fact, I arrived less than a few weeks after a horrific attack on a hospital in nearby Malakal <60 miles away (figure 4.6), where dozens of health care workers and patients were murdered. I'll share an excerpt from my journal that I kept at the time, which I believe is telling. (This entry was made shortly after the referendum that created a division between Sudan and South Sudan, which is easiest to understand as the "newest country in the world.")

We have established a biweekly mobile clinic here . . . treating topical ambulatory conditions . . . but mostly focusing on our malnutrition cases here. Mostly, however, our presence is a proxy for the MSF commitment to neutrality. Their needs are minimal . . . and their numbers are far fewer than the nearby Dinka IDPs

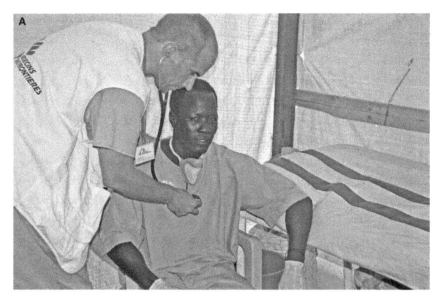

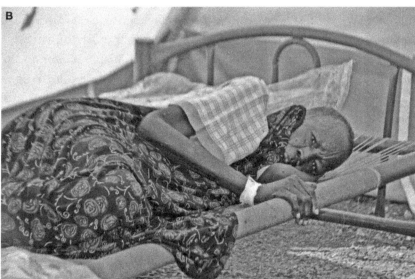

FIGURES 4.5. A–F Assortment of personal photographs taken while working at a pediatric malnutrition hospital run by Doctors Without Borders / Médecins sans Frontières in Mellut, South Sudan, 2013. A: Tyler examining patient in outpatient ward; B: patient in TB ward; C: Tyler and interpreter triaging patients during general pediatric clinic; D: makeshift MSF clinic at UNMISS IDP (refugee) camp; E: Tyler in MSF truck heading to UNMISS (UN Mission in South Sudan) camp where they housed n >1,100 IDPs; F: MSF pediatric malnutrition hospital. *Source:* Photos by author.

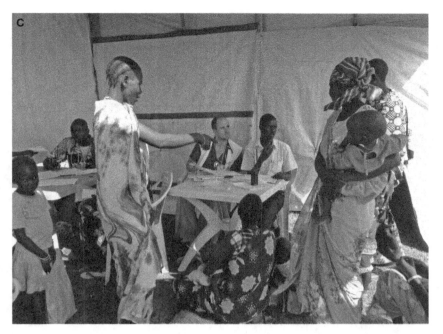

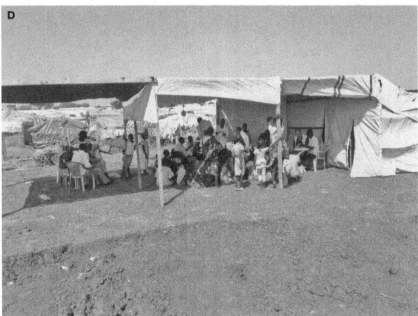

FIGURES 4.5. (Continued)

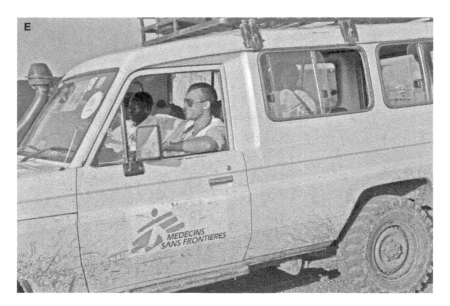

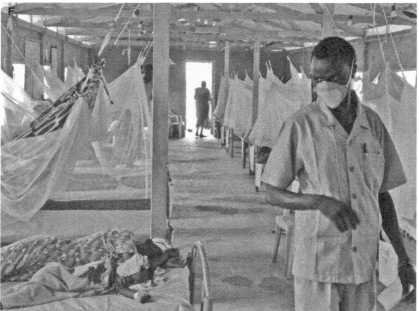

FIGURES 4.5. (Continued)

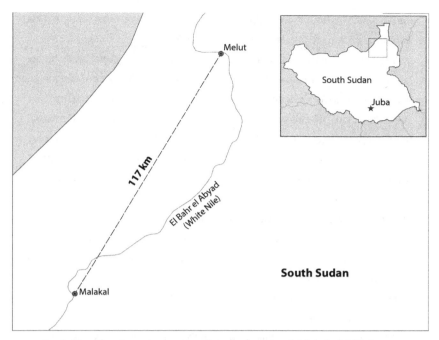

FIGURE 4.6. Map showing comparative distance between Malakal and Melut.
Source: "Map: Who Controls Upper Nile State?," Radio Tamazuj, October 14, 2014, https://radiotamazuj.org/en/news/article/map-who-controls-upper-nile-state.

(1,100 vs. 23,000), but the hope was to create an empiric surveillance system to identify truly ill patients and refer them to the appropriate locations. Sadly, that has not been the case....

I have never seen people (collectively) so paralyzed by fear. While the fear is the corollary of a rational source ... its practice is entirely irrational. These people will not move beyond the gates of this compound that is no more than a square kilometer. Over 1,100 people living on top of one another ... in shelters adorned by humanitarian aid. To define their existence as substandard would be a profound understatement. Latrines (built by Oxfam) now destroyed and overflowing with feces. Multiple children bathing in tin buckets. What is the purpose of survival for these people who will not leave this compound? We, arrogant westerners, philosophize about the meaning of life ... and all of its metaphysical permutations ... in our world of free-roaming movement and ideas. But these people are imprisoned ... or are they?

The camp is divided into two ... as there was a murder immediately before my arrival between two key members of the society ... and, as can be imagined, a man was killed. The offender moved approximately 60 people from his immediate clan. They claim we do not service their needs (an inappropriate request considering our demands elsewhere and the impossibility of making great strides to treat less than 100). In fact, even the main camp often complains to the Danish Refugee Committee that our "medications do not work." Love the entitlement. The reason why this may be is that most of them are placebos ... Tylenol ... multivitamins ... simply to placate their sense of entitlement. That word sounds harsh in this context, but this, sadly, is one of the consequences of a humanitarian presence. Those displaced often feel "entitled" to something. Anything. The underlying issues are far greater—deep-seated mental health pathologies caused by decades of intergenerational violence and trauma.

The problem is that they will not accept these referrals ... adamantly refuse. This absolute recalcitrance to accept transfers compromises everything I am doing for them. Four notable cases to date better elucidate these issues. The first two were severely malnourished. The skin hanging off their bodies as pudding accumulates on a spoon ... their eyes entirely sunken in ... large glass prisms waiting to be nourished ... but refused. One of the mothers finally relented to my pleas to be transferred to our facilities. UNMISS provided transportation. The problem was at the time that we closed at 5 p.m. This potentiated the fear of frequent transit back and forth. On the 3rd day, she did not show.... Two weeks later, her 9-month old infant was dead.

My time in the eastern DRC in 2018 was equally challenging, but our resources and the timing of our exploratory mission were substantively different from my time in South Sudan. As a board member of a small medical humanitarian nongovernmental organization, I was there leading a needs assessment on how we could help survivors of sexual and gender-based violence (SGBV). Below are some notes that I wrote on the plane returning home in 2018.

Congo: the very name that evokes the deepest realm of the imagination, conjuring up mystery and intrigue, but most of all, a sense of fear and "darkness"—a term often used to describe colonial Africa. This source of sensationalized sentiment has influenced literary minds for generations—from Conrad's *Heart of Darkness* to Coppola's *Apocalypse Now* to Crichton's *Congo*, yet none have even scratched the proverbial surface when it comes to actually describing the systematic suffering and dehumanization of the second-largest nation in Africa.

Such feelings of dismal discomfort could not be better demonstrated than by women affected by SGBV, which describes an act committed against an individual that is based on gender norms and unequal power relationships.[61]

A recent study demonstrated that 39.7 percent and 23.6 percent of women and men, respectively, reported sexual violence alone.[62] While these statistics are impressive, personal narratives are more effective at describing such atrocities. One woman described her harrowing experience:[63]

> The soldiers came in. They wanted to kill my husband. They had machete.
> They butchered him, like a slaughterhouse. I had to pick up all the pieces.
> I had to lie down on his body parts. I wept and they started raping me. There
> were 12 of them. And then my two daughters in the next room. After six
> months . . . my daughters were pregnant. They said it was my fault that my
> husband is dead. When my grandchildren ask me now about that scar, I can't
> tell them. It was their fathers who did it.

The DRC has been torn apart by wars since 1996. The neighboring Rwandan genocide garnered worldwide attention, but when the conflict between the Tutsis and Hutus ended in Rwanda, it spilled immediately into the DRC. At one point, it involved nine African nations—aptly referred to as the "First African World War"—often described as the deadliest conflict since World War II and continues today.

Reports vary, but it is estimated that as many as 6 million people have been killed since 1988.[64] Such widespread humanitarian complexities have precipitated the largest and most expensive United Nations peacekeeping operation in history.

In a society of lawlessness, poor infrastructure, and destructive leadership; all fueled by the greed created by one of the largest mining industries in the world, men and boys are insidiously drawn into conflict to seek identity, respect, and purpose.

Respect for human life (widely known to have been stripped of value starting with the oppressive colonization of King Leopold II) is further eviscerated within these caustic environments, thereby legitimizing murder and desensitizing rape. Militarized groups often use rapes as an instrument of terror—where gang rapes are reported by 33.4 percent of women.[65]

Yet little of the world is aware of this epidemic. In a contemporary era now acutely aware of gender-based discrimination (#MeToo), how are such women forgotten?

Such pervasive acts infect communities and provoke a constant state of fear and an internalized sense of weakness and hopelessness. This culture of violence bleeds into a feeling of collective inadequacy and humiliation among men (exacerbated by a lack of economic security), leading to a drive to procure a sense of power and domination.

Such inner turmoil and rage precipitate a familial destructive environment, which often includes SGBV. A recent study reported that 41.6 percent of women reported IPV.[66] It is not just women who are affected; 30.7 percent of men also reported IPV—an occurrence that is often overlooked. This culture of violence clearly causes a wide cascade of adverse effects on health, in particular, mental health. In the same study cited above, 40.5 percent and 50.1 percent of adults met criteria for major depressive disorder and PTSD, respectively. Even worse, 16.0 percent attempted suicide.

While the traumatic effects in the DRC are certainly not representative of the global South, mental health is generally not prioritized by global health and development organizations. In fact, countries in sub-Saharan Africa (SSA), on average, spend less than 1 percent of their total health expenditures on mental health (compared to approximately 20% on HIV/AIDS).[67] Even the WHO does not specifically address mental health in their Millennium Development Goals, recommending an expenditure of less than $0.25/person annually in low-income nations.[68]

African primary care physicians (PCPs) are not well trained to detect or manage mental health, and specialists are a relative rarity. (For example, there are only 4 in South Kivu, a province with a population of more than 6 million). Consequently, most mild and moderate mental health conditions are overlooked, and more severe conditions are dismissed as "foolish" or even "witchcraft." Public health and sociopolitical environments are closely related.

Countless examples demonstrate the efficacy of community empowerment to resist the caustic forces of corrupt and inept governments. If communities are ravaged by unresolved state-sponsored trauma, however, they will continue to remain powerless victims in a complex web of social injustice.

The tools needed to build resilience are necessary to empower communities. Such tools are a basic provision of care built into robust systems that support mental health care. Sub-Saharan Africa (particularly the DRC) is wholly lacking such systems, and it is time for these changes (figures 4.7a–f). It is within the scope of care of Congolese PCPs to manage mental health. Until they do, the health care system will continue to remain saturated by the more topical physical conditions with underlying mental health correlates, and a nation of such vibrancy and strength will never reach its full potential.

Zooming out on the issue globally, in terms of resettlement destinations, 76% of political migrants are housed in lower-middle-income countries, with Turkey, Iran, and Colombia hosting the most refugees (note this comment is fluid) while Germany has by far the greatest number of asylum cases—especially in Europe.[69] More than 2 million refugees have been resettled in the United States since 1975.[70] The three leading states of resettlement are California, Texas, and New York. If we factor in Cuban and Haitian entrants (a different class), Florida is also a top recipient of political migrants, and Washington state has started to recently accept a sizable number of refugees. While the United States used to be among the developed nations resettling the most refugees, the Trump administration slashed refugee admissions by more than 85%, setting record low-admission caps nearly every year: 30,000 for 2019, 18,000 for 2020, and just 15,000 for 2021.[70] These

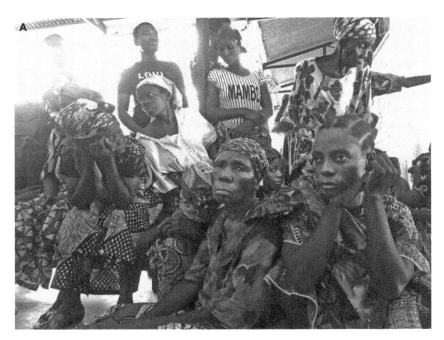

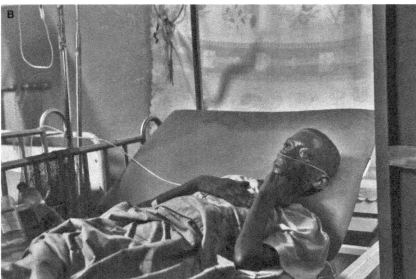

FIGURES 4.7. A–F Assortment of personal photographs from Nundu Deaconess Hospital, Nundu, Democratic Republic of the Congo, 2019. A: collection of women awaiting the workshop on sexual and gender-based violence; B: patient in the HIV ward; C: pediatric malnutrition ward; D: a survivor of sexual and gender-based violence; E: woman prostrated after receiving difficult news at the general outpatient ward; F: Tyler examining a psychiatric patient in the outpatient ward. *Source:* Photos by author.

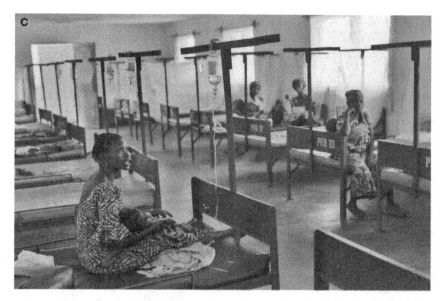

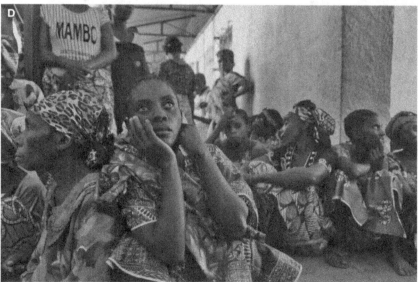

FIGURES 4.7. (Continued)

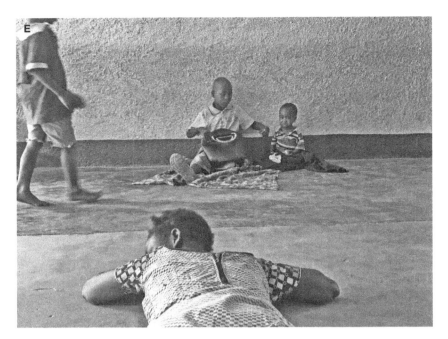

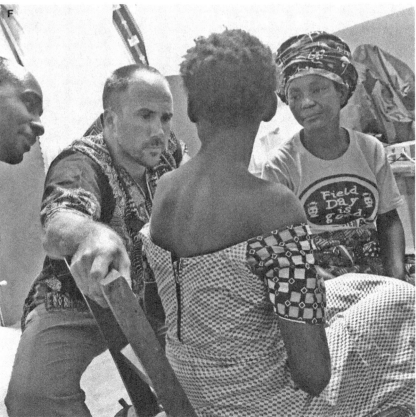

FIGURES 4.7. (Continued)

numbers represented a stark decline from the average annual admissions cap of 95,000 under both Republican and Democratic administrations since the program was founded.

In terms of health care access for political migrants, many barriers may be ascribed to culture and assimilation. First, the general Western notions of body, health, and illness are often incongruent from those of other cultures. Second, language and communication remain formidable challenges. Such barriers have major implications for informed consent and treatment cooperation, as well as comprehensive health education / health promotion. Third, even beyond the issue of communication is the very literacy level of health care, irrespective of language. It is typically quite low. For example, adherence to medication is problematic. The conceptual understanding of certain topics like medication refills is anathema with their backgrounds. Alternatively, they assume that the treatment is complete. Moreover, they often do not understand the distinction between primary care and other subspecialties, making an "arsenal" of physicians appear rather unnatural to them.

Fourth is the issue relating to the American emphasis on punctuality and efficiency—one that is often incongruent with their relative notions of importance. As a case in point, it is challenging for them to initially schedule appointments, as many have been exposed to previous systems that encouraged walk-in hours. Studies demonstrate that once appointments are made, however, they rarely miss them.

Fifth, a conceptual understanding of the US health insurance process creates an additional obstacle for them as utilizers. For example, in the United States, the Medicaid biannual reapplication process causes many to have repeated lapses in coverage secondary to missed deadlines. Finally, such acculturative stress is beginning to reflect the issues of their respective host nations of secondary asylum, where self-abusive behaviors (i.e., alcohol and drug abuse) are employed for coping.

Initial concerns for refugee health while still overseas essentially reflect the public health concerns for most developing nations, whereby infectious disease and heavy metal toxicity are underscored. Of course,

TB is of paramount concern. In fact, in one California study researchers found that 27.5% of refugees' initial visits with health care providers were related to TB.[71]

STIs (including HIV) are another main concern. Refugees are considered to be at higher risk for contracting STIs due to a basic lack of access to protection and / or treatment, as well as circumstances of war and flight, thereby making them subject to higher incidences of rape and sexual abuse. Hepatitis B is endemic to SSA, Southeast Asia, East Asia, northern Asia, and most of the Pacific Islands. The rate of chronic infection among those immigrating to the United States is between 5% and 15%.[72]

Parasitic infections are also known to be a profound public health issue among refugees—namely ascaris, *Entamoeba histolytica*, *Trichuris*, schistosoma, and *Hymenolepsis nana*. In fact, GI helminth infections alone are found in 19–36% of screened refugees overseas.[73] Of most considerable public health importance is malaria, a disease estimated to have a worldwide prevalence of 300–500 million. The CDC recommends that those planning on US immigration from sub-Saharan Africa or Southeast Asia undergo presumptive treatment with albendazole (or antiplasmodials for malaria).[74]

Finally, while less of a communicable concern, anemia and other blood-related disorders are a widely prevalent issue affecting nearly 2 billion globally. Acquired causes often seen among refugees include iron deficiency, malaria, parasitic infection, HIV, TB, and anemia of chronic diseases. Hereditary cases include α- and β-thalassemia, hemoglobin E, sickle cell disease, hemoglobin C, G6PD deficiency, and red blood cell membrane defects (e.g., spherocytosis).

Although many physicians associate infectious diseases with refugees, they actually account for less international spread than international travelers and other migrant populations. This is thought to be a result of such a tightly controlled population. Other diagnoses, such as musculoskeletal pain and mental health issues, are actually more prevalent. In fact, refugees have begun to mirror the same chronic conditions as their Western counterparts—including diabetes mellitus, hypertension, hyperlipidemia, and asthma.

Musculoskeletal pain can repeatedly be seen in the data as a primary factor for primary care visits—mostly neck and lower-back pain. Although this is comparable to the general American public, refugees seem to have different risk factors—including past physical trauma, current employment in jobs involving physical labor (e.g., housekeeping, factory work), and difficult living conditions (e.g., sleeping on hardwood floors, etc.). It turns out that the source of this pain may not be entirely organic.

Chronic headaches are another common pain presentation, as is ill-defined "whole body pain." Pain in the abdomen and pelvis is more common in women. Organic etiologies for such anatomical sources of pain are often difficult to identify. A higher prevalence of vague somatic complaints is reported in the literature on refugees seeking health care. We see this frequently, and it often seems to be attributable to underlying decompensated mental health issues. This is exacerbated by the fact that mental health often has no space for expression, and the number of medical providers often pales in comparison to the actual needs. (As mentioned in my notes on the eastern DRC, in that case there was but one public health psychiatrist in a province with >6 million people, >16% of whom had attempted suicide.)

Most studies reveal high rates of PTSD, combat stress reaction, anxiety, depression, and somatization among newly arrived refugees. Variations reported in the prevalence of PTSD and depression may be ascribed to a number of factors, including a lack of appropriate processing time and resources available after the trauma(s) to deal with such experiences.

Conflict precludes ample opportunities to deal with anxiety, and most autocratic regimes do not permit a meaningful expression of feelings. Living as an asylum seeker further contributes to a culture of precarious uncertainty. In secondary asylum, stressors such as social isolation, financial constraints, generational acculturation differences, culture shock, disability issues, and housing concerns also adversely affect refugees' mental and physical health.

Women are a highly vulnerable population primarily because of traditional cultural roles and perspectives that place them in subservient positions. They are extremely vulnerable to SGBV (particularly from soldiers and paramilitaries in refugee camps). Malnourishment is another significant concern, as their "inferior" status often prevents them from receiving prioritization in food rations. Female genital mutilation is another paramount concern among refugees that transcends the scope of this book. Multiple barriers preclude women from seeking help for mental health issues—including gaps in knowledge, worries about the stigma that is associated with depression, an unwillingness to share personal issues with an ill-defined "outsider," and an existential fear that their "instability" could be misconstrued as an indicator of poor parenthood, thus placing their custodial rights in jeopardy.

Studies among female survivors of SGBV in the DRC indicate that they suffer tremendous adverse health sequelae—particularly psychological, as well as familial / societal. In a study by Johnson et al., 39.7% of women were affected by SGBV in the DRC ($n = 997$), and >40% and >50% were suffering from depression and PTSD, respectively.[75] In addition to receiving <1% of total health care funds, insufficient training on mental health within medical education has led to a dearth of trained mental health providers in the DRC. This translates to a severely inadequate capacity for treatment in a region with high rates of traumatic experience.

In a different vein, reproductive health is a considerable concern. Refugee women tend to have greater parity, delayed prenatal care, obstetric complications, and low-birth-weight infants relative to their Western counterparts. As a case in point, in a group of refugees studied in California, only 11% had ever received a gynecological exam prior to resettlement.[76] Many operative factors may present, including cultural values that preclude the utilization of ob-gyn exams by Western practitioners (particularly men). Others may simply rely on traditional models of healing and treating illness and may distrust the very foundation of Western medicine.

Finally, populations affected by emergencies, including humanitarian emergencies and conflict, and migrants—in particular forced migrants—have higher risks of infection and severity from pandemics. Such was certainly the case with COVID-19. The International Organization for Migration has estimated that immigrants account for a high percentage of the population (at least 3.7%) in 14 of the 20 countries with the most COVID-19 cases.[77] Early outbreaks in Singapore were concentrated in migrant worker housing. A study in Kuwait showed that the odds ratios for admission to an intensive care unit for COVID-19 and death were two to three times higher for migrants than for Kuwaitis.[78]

One of the most formidable political determinants of health is the weaponization of public health policy against certain populations. We saw this taking place globally during the COVID-19 pandemic, with particularly challenging examples taking place in the United States with Title 42. Title 42 expulsion policy effectively closed the US border to nearly all asylum seekers based on the misapplication of an obscure, 75-year-old public health law (the Public Health Service Act of 1944). Responding to a cholera epidemic, Congress passed a law in 1893 that later became Title 42, giving the president authority to exclude people from certain countries during public health emergencies. According to Title 42, whenever the US director of the CDC determines there is a communicable disease in another country, health officials have the authority, with the approval of the president, to prohibit "the introduction of persons and property from such countries or places" for as long as health officials determine necessary. That authority was held by the US surgeon general until it was transferred to the CDC director in 1966.

Prior to 2020, Title 42 had never been used, and the law that became Title 42 had only been used once—in 1929 to keep ships from China and the Philippines from entering US ports during a meningitis outbreak. Quarantine authority was never meant to be used to determine which noncitizens could or couldn't be expelled or removed from the

United States. In March 2020, the Trump administration activated Title 42, which gave the US Border Patrol the power to turn away people seeking asylum. The administration claimed it was using Title 42 to help stop the spread of COVID-19 in immigrant detention centers, where many migrants and asylum seekers are placed when they arrive at the United States–Mexico border. Many believe that the real intent was to keep asylum seekers out of the country and to end asylum full stop, which was part of the Trump administration's overall anti-immigrant agenda and policies. Before that, migrants could cross illegally and ask for and be allowed entry into the United States. They were then screened and often released to wait out their immigration cases. Under Title 42, migrants were returned over the border and denied the right to seek asylum. US officials turned away migrants more than 2.8 million times.

What many US citizens did not understand was that this really did not prevent infections from entering the United States at all. We had infection prevention and control measures in place so we could easily screen and even vaccinate these communities. In fact, WEA was on the southern border of Texas doing this for the small minority that did make it through.[79] What Title 42 really did was prevent millions of folks with legitimate sociopolitical justifications for forced displacement from entering a nation that could give them a chance. These were not economic migrants. As a democratic nation whose history is based on flight from persecution, we could have done much better. This use of Title 42 was criticized by many civil and human rights organizations, who argued that it violated US and international immigration law. Unfortunately, it was not reversed even after a presidential administration change.

People with Mental Health and Substance Use Disorders

This is such a massive category with so many highly variable expressions around the globe that it is difficult to pigeonhole into one section. We described some of this impact on SGBV survivors in the DRC above. If we are to navigate back to the United States and just take the case of HIV, it may be easier to digest some of the complexities of this spectrum.

The health of people with SUDs is inextricably bound to their social environment. Drug-taking and risky drug-use behaviors are affected by social processes, and the health of drug users is a product of both behaviors and social determinants. The SDoH can directly shape health risk behaviors. Homeless drug users, for example, are more likely to engage in high-risk sexual activity. Inadequate housing increases the likelihood of infectious disease transmission, social relationships offer protective financial and emotional resources, and more cohesive neighborhoods have a greater likelihood of providing appropriate care. Moreover, a history of incarceration has a long-lasting impact on the ability of people with SUD who are in recovery to find employment, which is essential to reentry into family and society. The role of the SDoH is particularly relevant to the health of BIPOC drug users. BIPOC communities report levels of drug use similar to or lower than their white counterparts, but they experience a disproportionate number of health consequences from SUD. HIV is a classic example, where people who inject drugs (PWID) are one of the highest risk groups—especially among Black and Brown communities.[80]

PWID and PEH or unstable housing were routinely marginalized and stigmatized long before the beginning of the HIV epidemic. They currently have some of the worst outcomes of HIV infections in the United States—often leading to AIDS in approximately half of untreated domestic cases. Moreover, HIV prevention efforts among PWID have been woefully insufficient. For example, in one study only 2% of PWID in California were offered HIV preexposure prophylaxis (PrEP; this can be thought of as the birth control pill) despite nearly 60% indicating a willingness to initiate PrEP.[81,82]

Many nations criminalize drug use, as the United States did with the "war on drugs," which only exacerbated the issues. The reality is that it is a chronic, relapsing brain disease marked by physiological changes that have been documented by brain imaging. These changes drive compulsive drug seeking and use despite the harmful consequences to the users and those around them. Despite these high incarceration rates, the criminalization of SUD has been shown to have little impact on SUD rates. Instead, incarceration is linked with increased morbidity from viral hepatitis and increased mortality from overdose. Within the first two weeks after release, individuals with SUD are 129 times more likely to die of a drug overdose than the general population. Just let that sink in. People in carceral settings (jail / prison) have a high prevalence of hepatitis C, between 12% and 35% in US prisons, compared with 1.3% in the general population, with the risk of further spread through sex, tattoos, and continued drug use while incarcerated.[80]

On the same spectrum, people with mental health conditions have an increased risk of acquiring HIV, and in a case of the chicken versus the egg, people with HIV (PWH) are at higher risk of developing mental health conditions. In addition to affecting quality of life, mental health conditions can negatively affect HIV treatment adherence and treatment response. One US multisite study found that 36% of PWH had major depressive disorder and 15.8% had generalized anxiety disorder compared with rates of 6.7% and 2.1%, respectively, in the general population.[83]

Conversely, those experiencing serious mental illness (SMI) demonstrate HIV prevalence between 2% and 6% compared with 0.5% in the general population. Similar to the benefit of integrating care for SUD and infectious diseases into primary care, models that focus on integrated behavioral health care hold considerable promise for PWH and people at risk for HIV. This is another one of our models in California at WEA. As the need and demand for mental health services have increased during the COVID-19 pandemic, disparities in access to mental health care have become more pressing and are, in part, reflected in the overwhelming surge in preventable overdose deaths: more than 70,000 in 2020.[84]

Justice-Impacted Communities

I experienced many of the ingredients in my youth that should have led to a different outcome. They probably would have—had I been Black or Brown. As a white American in Los Angeles and New York, I grew up with privilege. As we have seen, however, privilege is relative. . . .

After a childhood spent among elitist "Hollywood" circles, my life took a very acute directional change. My father was laid off from his 20-year career as a pilot for Pan Am. Unfortunately, my parents lacked the foresight of investment and savings. Very quickly, I was cast out as a pariah among my peers. I was repeatedly ridiculed and ostracized from most "worthy" social circles. Similarly, my mother hopelessly strived to "be accepted," but because social status in Los Angeles was defined by the prestige of one's address, make of one's automobile, and size of one's swimming pool and silicone implants, she never had a chance.

It's often said that the first indication of alcoholism is denial. If so—insinuated by the massive stockpiles of vodka bottles both empty and full in her closet—my childhood intuition would inform us that the second sign must naturally be driving shit-faced with a small child in the passenger seat while dodging road construction signs at 2:00 a.m. Following this empirical pattern, allow me to predict the third step on the trajectory toward alcoholic self-degradation: stumbling around all hours of every night reciting slanderous mantras toward your loved ones. A night in my preadolescent home would not have been complete without my mother's drunken, vociferous assaults on my dad.

Upon reaching pubescent age, I was to be next. On late nights my friends would often inquire about the disturbing racket in the background as we conversed over the telephone. I would put them at a false sense of ease by dismissing these fits of chemically laced rage as my mother merely "singing" at my door. The reality was that she would embark on a seemingly endless loop commenting on how worthless and disappointing I was to her. Days later, they would find my door in shambles—beaten down by a baseball bat—and displaced cotton balls scattered throughout my room (I used these to filter out the screaming).

I share my own adverse childhood experiences (ACEs) because they allowed me to be vulnerable and open to empathizing with the plight of discriminatory factors that communities face across the world and that often leads to adverse social outcomes—as it did in my own life, leading me to repeated events of juvenile incarceration. I knew what it felt to be an "other." I knew what it felt like to not belong. I also knew what it felt like to be relatively hardened. I needed to create a protective shell around my emotions and engage with a crowd that would toughen me up. I did that and it led me into a number of challenging circumstances. As my family began to precipitously expire, I was clearly faced with a Frostian binary path. I chose the higher road and that made all the difference. I have no illusion about the critical importance that privilege played in helping me charter that course.

The United States has the largest carceral population in the world (followed by China, with a population four times greater than ours) and the sixth highest proportional rate of incarceration, rivaled only by far smaller nations that have recently experienced war or genocide. What does that say about Americans and our values regarding social cohesion? In 2016 over 6 million people were impacted by the justice system—including 2.16 million people incarcerated in state or federal prisons and local jails.[85] There is no argument that people of color are highly overrepresented in US carceral data. This basic class war has effectively thrown young Black and Brown communities (especially men) into intractably precarious situations. The data for incarcerated women shows similar racial/ethnic disparities. One study found the imprisonment rate to be over 48 per 100,000 for white women, 63 per 100,000 for Latina women, and 83 per 100,000 for Black women.[86]

Once youth have touched this "system," their ability to regain entry in a meaningful way is seriously impacted. They will continue to be treated as second-class citizens and flagged as social deviants when it comes to basic mechanisms to achieve economic security, such as education and employment. In fact, the US Department of Education does not allow US citizens with drug-related charges to receive financial aid. In other words, if an 18-year-old Black man is incarcerated for a marijuana joint and comes from a poor family, it is quite possible that that young man will never be able to achieve a college education.

Here is a little more background on how jails and prisons are run in the United States. People often use the terms interchangeably, but they are considerably different from one another. Local jails hold people sentenced to less than one year; people who violate parole or probation; and those awaiting trial, sentencing, or transfer to prison. State and federal prisons hold people sentenced to more than one year of incarceration.[87] Between 1980 and 2014, the US incarceration rate increased by 220%, which can be linked to state and federal policy changes that enacted harsher sentencing rules—including mandatory minimum sentences and the infamous "three strikes law."[88] As stated above, Michelle Alexander argues that this is not a partisan initiative, and in fact, there were more incarcerations under Clinton's administration than those of his predecessors. Much of this can be attributed to the "war on drugs" and its disproportionate impact on Black and Brown communities—whether deliberate or accidental.

Do we even know what the objective of our criminal systems is? Removal of the most violent offenders from open society? That seems fair. Punishment for an act that society (codified by our legal statues) deems incorrect? Okay, fine. But "whose" society? As stated above, HIV and its associated acts of risk, including sodomy, sex work, and drug use are illegal in a number of states. We have become so divisive in our society that it does not seem right to impose the values of one dominant caste on another. Finally, reform is often cited as an objective of incarceration. While this is certainly a laudable one, the evidence just doesn't support it.

Recidivism rates in the United States are quite dismal, with approximately 75% of those released rearrested in <5 years and 75% of them being jailed again.[89] While some folks may chalk this up to these individuals simply being "bad apples," if we are purely data driven about this decision, it's pretty clear that the current US justice system is broken. I am not here to argue how the root causes in society have led to these highly variable rates and how the current system exacerbates those root-cause issues. I am here to discuss how this system impacts the pocketbooks of hardworking taxpayers—including complex (yet avoidable) systemic health care disparities. The fact that private for-profit prisons house nearly 10% of the entire federal/state prison system should give us pause.[90] Montana in particular deserves dishonorable mention, with nearly 50% of its prisons run by for-profit corporations.[91] If we incentivize incarcerations by allowing corporations to monetize off of prisoners, how can we ever seek out true reform?

When compared to the general population, men and women with a history of incarceration are in worse mental and physical health. Data from the Bureau of Justice Statistics found that in 2011, 44% of people who were incarcerated had a mental health disorder.[92] This certainly crosses over to SUDs. In fact, the largest population of mental health patients in one congregate facility is Los Angeles County jail. One study found that within the two weeks following their release, people who were formerly incarcerated were 40 times more likely to die of an opioid overdose than someone in the general population.[93] Moreover, the evidence suggests that when compared to the general population, incarcerated people of both sexes are more likely to have high blood pressure, asthma, cancer, arthritis, and infectious diseases—namely TB, hepatitis C, and HIV.[94,95,96,97,98] We see this trend across the world.

Women with a history of incarceration can face a greater burden of disease than men, especially high blood pressure and infectious diseases (namely viral hepatitis, HIV, STIs, and TB).[99,100] These women are also more likely to have experienced ACEs and physical and sexual abuse than those who are not involved in the criminal justice system, potentially explaining high levels of physical and mental health problems among women who are incarcerated.[101]

The number of older adults (aged 50 years and above) in US prisons is growing.[102,103,104,105] Many correctional facilities, however, are not equipped to address the special health needs of these individuals.[106]

Reintegrating into society also poses special challenges for older adults who were formerly incarcerated. Those who have spent significant time in prison may find it stressful to adjust to the changes that have occurred in society and their specific communities, particularly if family support is lacking.[107] Furthermore, older adults with a history of incarceration are more likely to suffer from abuse and neglect due to a lack of family support when compared to their younger counterparts.[108]

Obviously, the impact on families is tremendous. As discussed in chapter 2, children are especially at risk of negative effects related to parental incarceration. According to 2012 data, more than 5 million children in the United States (approximately 7% of all children in the United States) have experienced the incarceration of a parent whom they resided with at some time.[109] These children are at much higher risk for living in poverty and, particularly, homelessness.[110] These ACEs impact children in so many ways—such as higher rates of learning disabilities, developmental delays, speech/language problems, attention disorders, and aggressive behaviors.[111,112] Additionally, children of incarcerated parents have been found to be up to five times more likely to enter the criminal justice system themselves.[113]

Finally, when it comes to communicable diseases spread through air or droplets, a congregated facility will naturally potentiate the risk of transmission because of overcrowding, poor ventilation, poor sanitation, inadequate medical services, and other institutional factors. In the United States, by August 2020 the 15 largest-known clusters of COVID-19 cases had occurred in prisons and jails, where roughly two-thirds of the population are people of color. Amnesty International reported that the mortality rate recorded by the National Commission on COVID-19 and Criminal Justice in the United States was double that of the general population.

As briefly stated in the section on low-income housing communities, when I was chief medical officer for New York City, we ran a program with the Mayor's Office of Criminal Justice in which we established safe interim sheltering spaces in hotels for people released (through an early release program for low risk "offenders") from city jails like Rikers

Island and local state prisons in an effort to de-densify these facilities and mitigate the risk of disease transmission. The program's objectives were threefold:

1. Reduce the risk of COVID-19 transmission for high-risk communities
2. Connect these communities to integrated primary care-behavioral health programs
3. Connect these communities to permanent supportive housing

While I was quite proud of the principles of this program, the outcomes were very different. We often found many of the rooms defaced or destroyed, and many clients displayed behavior that led or would lead to reincarceration. While I was working for emergency management (made up largely of former law enforcement or fire service personnel), the most common tactic was simply to send a "squad car" down to the hotel to "quiet them down." Those familiar with basic psychosocial theory know that such an approach has the opposite effect, triggering the former trauma of these folks.

We cannot create cages for folks, inundate them with concentrated risk factors, and just assume that once we open those cages they will naturally be rehabilitated. This is a process, and we must rebuild that process starting from the day they are incarcerated (if that is even the "right" solution). We do the same thing when socially complex patients are admitted to our hospital—if the resources are available, we will assign a social worker or case manager to them. If true reform is sought, we must radically transform this process. Until then, our rates of incarceration will continue to surge (along with the associated health care consequences), as will the price tags paid by our average taxpayer (you).

PART II

SYNDEMICS—THE CASCADING IMPACTS OF POVERTY AND PANDEMICS

History of Contemporary Pandemics and Public Health Emergencies of International Concern

Until lions have their historians, tales of the hunt will always glorify the hunters.
—AFRICAN PROVERB

A number of pandemics and public health emergencies of international concern (PHEIC; remember this acronym, as we will use it repeatedly moving forward, especially in the Ebola section) and their socially driven correlates are examined in this chapter, starting with the 3rd Plague pandemic and culminating with the biosocial ingredients that led to the current COVID-19 pandemic. The intention of this chapter is not to perform a deep dive. I am keeping the descriptions of these diseases superficial to ensure they are relatable to readers. What is it? What does it look like? When and where did peaks occur? Which populations were primarily affected? Finally, what were the social determinants? This discussion of the examples is organized as follows:

- Clinical manifestations
- General epidemiology
- Historical timeline
- Sociopolitical determinants

The main objective of this chapter is to illustrate how sociopolitical determinants were common to all examples, which precipitated not only a much wider distribution of disease but also led to far worse outcomes as the underlying system fractured from sociopolitical influences. I'll describe endemic social inequities and connect them to other conditions (e.g., wars and conflicts) that were largely the result of those very inequities and driving forces in corresponding epidemics→ syndemics→pandemics (e.g., Ebola and HIV/AIDS). I'll also provide several case studies starting with the Spanish Influenza and ending with the COVID-19 pandemic.

Definitions are also important. I have applied the following criteria to selecting the pandemics or PHEICs discussed below:

- Occurred in the 20th century (contemporary)
- Took >1 million lives (impact)
- Other exceptional circumstances (relatability)

I will make one exception for Ebola, for circumstances that I'll describe in that section. Most of these examples are encompassed in the timeline of figure 5.1 but not all of them.

But before we move forward, I will consolidate years of public health and epidemiological training into just a few bullet points. People hear the terms *outbreak*, *epidemic*, *pandemic*, *elimination*, and *eradication* thrown about so often in popular culture that many likely seem interchangeable. They're not. This is the simplest way to think about it:

- An *outbreak* is the sudden appearance of a number of cases. The time stamp here is important—emphasis on "sudden."
- *Endemic* describes a disease distribution that is consistently present in one particular geographical area.
- An *epidemic* occurs when the number of cases exceeds the endemic rate (or that which can normally be expected).
- A *PHEIC* occurs when an epidemic has spread in such a way that if not controlled immediately will most likely lead to pandemic distribution. It requires a coordinated international response.

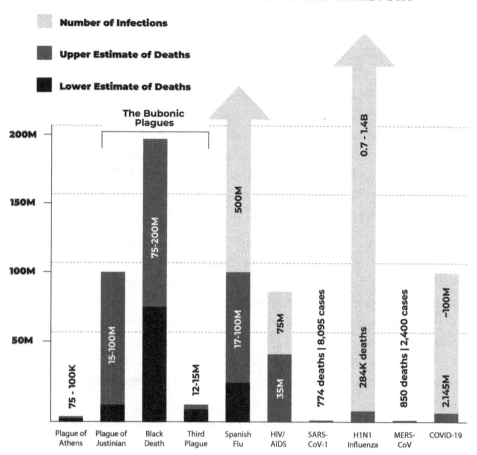

TIMELINE OF THE LARGEST PANDEMICS IN HISTORY

Number of Infections

Upper Estimate of Deaths

Lower Estimate of Deaths

The Bubonic Plagues

200M

150M

100M

50M

75 - 100K | 15-100M | 75-200M | 12-15M | 17-100M | 75M / 35M | 774 deaths | 8,095 cases | 0.7 - 1.4B / 284K deaths | 850 deaths | 2,400 cases | ~100M / 2.145M

Plague of Athens | Plague of Justinian | Black Death | Third Plague | Spanish Flu | HIV/ AIDS | SARS-CoV-1 | H1N1 Influenza | MERS-CoV | COVID-19

500M

FIGURE 5.1. Timeline of pandemics since the fifth century BCE by number of associated deaths claimed. *Source:* Graphic by author.

- A *pandemic* occurs when an epidemic crosses multiple national borders and its replication rate becomes exponential.
- *Syndemic* is a relatively new and timely term that describes a synergistic epidemic of more epidemics colliding and causing an amplified outcome. Syndemics are driven by disparities that are largely socially determined. This section will focus considerable attention on this concept.

- *Epidemiology* is the study of epidemics. More specifically, it studies patterns of disease distribution and the issues that may have contributed to that spread.
- *Disease control* is when we reduce the number of new infections, the number of people currently infected, and the number of people who become sick or die from that disease in a restricted area.
- *Elimination* is stopping the transmission of a disease in a specific geographic area or country but not worldwide.
- *Eradication* is the entire and absolute "elimination" of a disease worldwide. This often requires elimination of the microbe itself. Smallpox is one of the very few examples of this.

Now that we have a working vocabulary of epidemiology, let's get to the point. In order to demonstrate a link between the social conditions described in the previous part and these infectious disease epidemics, we will need a grading mechanism. Let's use the following rubric of five questions, which will allow readers to judge the degree of social determination.

We will return to the topic of a syndemic later, in chapter 7, and readers will notice how the content describing its three levels has been

Rubric for determining the sociopolitical determinants of pandemics and PHEICs

	Sociopolitical determinant-linked questionnaire	Yes	No
1	Is there a sociopolitical link to the original spread of disease?	☐	☐
2	Was there a lack of public and community health infrastructure at the time?	☐	☐
3	If yes, did the lack of infrastructure at the time of spread precipitate more widespread distribution?	☐	☐
4	Was the lack of infrastructure at the time linked to a sociopolitical root cause?	☐	☐
5	Is it treatable? In other words, would building more effective sociopolitical infrastructure mitigate the risk of spread?	☐	☐

incorporated into our rubric. I will ask you to use this grading rubric every time we cover a new infectious disease epidemic. If we achieve 3/5 (60%), there could arguably be a weak correlation; with 4/5 (80%) we can determine that this is a socially determined epidemic (or pandemic); and with 5/5 (100%) there is almost no doubt (though you'll find 100% never really exists in science). Ready to go?

3rd Plague Pandemic, 1855-1960

One of the most well-known terms in infectious disease popular culture is *plague*. It is inextricably connected to pestilence and poverty. Most are unaware that an outbreak existed less than 100 years ago. Three major clinical syndromes are associated with plague: bubonic plague, septicemic plague, and pneumonic plague,[1] with bubonic accounting for the vast majority of cases (i.e., 80–95%). Both bubonic and pneumonic plague were involved with this pandemic.

Clinical Manifestations

Bubonic plague is clinically characterized by the sudden onset of fever, chills, weakness, and headache, followed by intense pain and swelling in a lymph node–bearing area (bubo), which may be preceded by lymph node swelling. Acute buboes are painful and often associated with redness and swelling of the overlying skin. The inguinal (groin) region is the most frequently involved lymph node (in fact, the word "bubo" is a Greek derivative for "groin"), but the armpit and neck may also be involved.

Skin lesions at the site of a flea bite are usually inapparent and thereby ignored or forgotten. Some patients, however, may have necrotic lesions representing gangrene. A minority of patients may develop a fatal clotting disorder. In the absence of treatment, the initial bubonic stage may be followed by a disseminated infection (i.e., sepsis) in approximately 50% of untreated cases, which can lead to complications such as pneumonia (secondary pneumonic plague) and meningitis. Overall, the estimated mortality is 60–100% in untreated plague compared with <15% with treatment.[2]

Epidemiology

Plague is a murine zoonosis; humans are incidental hosts. It is a bacillus (type of bacteria) known as *Yersinia pestis*. Humans acquire plague via bites from rodent (primarily *Rattus flavipectus)* fleas (*Xenopsylla cheopis*), scratches or bites from infected domestic cats, direct handling of infected animal tissues, inhalation of respiratory secretions from infected animals, inhalation of aerosolized droplets from infected humans, consumption of contaminated food, or laboratory exposure.[3,4,5,6,7] Once infected with *Y. Pestis*, *X. cheopis* is unable to digest its food (the rat's blood) and becomes voraciously hungry.[8] After the rat dies of plague, the flea looks desperately around for food and if a human host is available, it will opportunistically move there.

The enzootic (regular nonhuman animal transmission) plague is maintained in nature through flea-borne transmission between partially resistant rodents (enzootic or maintenance hosts). Flea bites are the most common route of transmission of plague to humans, followed by contact with infected animals. More than 200 mammalian species have been reported to be infected with *Y. pestis*, including squirrels, prairie dogs, rabbits, field mice, chipmunks, rats, bobcats, domestic cats, and camels. Intermittently, infection may spread to these more susceptible animals, which function as epizootic (zoonotic outbreak) or amplifying hosts. The incubation period is generally two to eight days.

Casualty patterns indicate that waves of this late 19th-century/early 20th-century pandemic may have come from two different sources. The first was primarily bubonic and was carried around the world through oceangoing trade from transporting infected animals (rodents), humans, or cargoes harboring fleas (the fleas would hibernate for up to 50 days in grain or in soft white items, such as woolen cloth). It's important to note that this is the origin of the term "quarantine," which originates from the Italian "quaranta" (or 40 days, which is the time they would hold certain merchant sailors upon docking). Note that bubonic plague cannot be spread from human to human. The second, more virulent, strain was primarily pneumonic in character with strong person-to-person contagion.

As we discussed above, this pandemic harboring both types of plague spread to all inhabited continents and ultimately led to more than 12 million deaths—primarily in India and China. According to the World Health Organization (WHO), the pandemic was considered active until 1960 when worldwide casualties dropped to 200 per year (nearly all in India).[9] This definition notwithstanding, plague continues to exist globally—albeit at a very low level of transmission and associated mortality.

Historical Timeline

The 3rd Plague pandemic was preceded by two of the most formidable pandemics in history. The first, referred to as the Plague of Justinian (occurring 541–549 ACE), ravaged the Byzantine Empire and claimed between 30 and 50 million lives, persisting in successive waves until the middle of the 8th century. The second plague, notoriously known as the Black Death (1334–1353 ACE), claimed 75–200 million lives, which represented at least one-third of Europe's population. This pandemic recurred regularly until the 19th century (figure 5.2).

So what happened between 1353 and 1855? The bubonic plague remained endemic in populations of infected ground rodents, the primary vector, in central Asia and was a known cause of death in that region for centuries (especially among migrants). Increasing waves of migratory populations of Han Chinese seeking minerals (primarily copper) in the second half of the 19th century continued to come into proximity with plague-infected flea/rat combinations. Other scholars have presented evidence that the increasing spread could have been furthered by a number of other globalizing events, including the growing and lucrative opium trade, which began after about 1840. This deadly

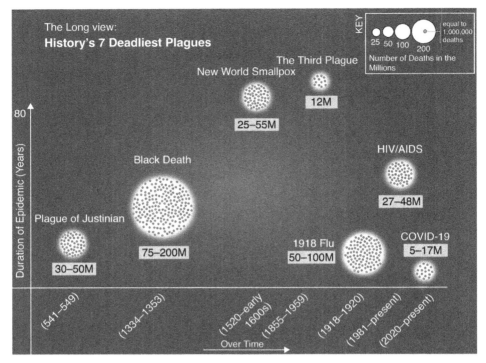

FIGURE 5.2. A chronology of the deadliest pandemics since the sixth century CE.
Source: "History's Seven Deadliest Plagues," GAVI, the Vaccine Alliance, November 15, 2021, https://www.gavi.org/vaccineswork/historys-seven-deadliest-plagues.

combination continued to migrate with these human populations and penetrated more urban territories, causing episodic outbreaks.[10]

The third iteration originated in the Yunnan region of southwest China, where plague caused multiple outbreaks beginning in 1772. In 1894, plague reached Canton (discovered there in May 1894 and identified in a hospital clerk) and then spread to the Pearl River Delta, including Hong Kong, where the disease took over 2,000 lives in a matter of weeks, leading to the exodus of approximately one-third of the population. This exodus caused it to rapidly spread by ships leaving Hong Kong en route to Japan, Singapore, Taiwan, and the Indian subcontinent. The earliest-known European cases occurred in September and October 1896, when two sailors from Bombay died of plague on ships docked on the Thames River in London. Over the next few years, it spread to many cities around the world: Bombay, Singapore, Alexandria, Buenos Aires, Rio de Janeiro, Cape Town, Honolulu, San Francisco, and Sydney, among others.[11] Before 1959, approximately 12 million people across the world (half of them in India) would be casualties of this pandemic.

Sociopolitical Determinants

As we can imagine, the 3rd Plague pandemic either revealed or exacerbated major sociopolitical drivers. First of all, many of the ports infected during the plague were British-held colonies at the time. The British Empire had a known network and practice of enforcing Western hygiene and medical practices and radical quarantine measures in countries and provinces such as India, South Africa, and Hong Kong. Many of these imposed Western sanitary measures were new to these areas and precipitated natives' fear and apprehension of the British government. Such blowback was well documented in ports in British-controlled India, Hong Kong, and South Africa.

Several examples can be drawn from. In India, harsh quarantines were initially implemented by the British government, leading to Indian resentment of those measures and further polarization of existing inequities.[12] In South Africa's Cape Colony, the British government caused a large group of native South Africans to move out of a supposed slum into areas on the outskirts of the city, which many historians argue was a racially motivated move by white South Africans to segregate African-born countrymen in other parts of the city.[13] In Hong Kong the British enforced many locally unfamiliar medical practices, such as floating plague victims in boats onto the water and cooling plague victims with ice, which further precipitated the exodus described above.

An example of sociopolitical determinants in the United States was the governmental response to the plague in Honolulu, where one building in Chinatown was ordered to be burned, which quickly spread, rendering over 7,000 Chinese and Japanese residents homeless. On the mainland, when the plague reached San Francisco, the medical board of the city implemented a strict quarantine of the entire Chinatown district after discovering only one case of the plague; this has led many to question whether this measure was motivated by racial bias among medical professionals, who may have believed Chinatown to be unsanitary and hence already infected by the plague.[14] Many of these drivers either helped to create conditions of de novo infections or further exacerbated the magnitude of the epidemic or the inequities associated with the response.

Shall we grade the sociopolitical determinants of this 3rd Plague pandemic according to our rubric? (Try to keep this handy for future sections.)

To summarize, this is a pandemic spread by pestilence, poverty, migration, trade, war, and drugs—much of which was structurally chartered by the vessels of colonialism. The great medical historian Sheldon Watts writes of the "transitional years" (1880s–1930s) that led to the "full medicalization of the West, and coincided with the great age of European and North American imperialism."[15] This period caused this iteration of the plague pandemic to become further inflamed, as the West enforced new medical measures that the impacted areas were not familiar with and further polarized existing racial preconceptions on both sides. Coming out of the scramble for Africa and

3rd Plague Pandemic: Rubric for determining the sociopolitical determinants of pandemics and PHEICs

	Sociopolitical determinant-linked questionnaire	Yes	No
1	Is there a sociopolitical link to the original spread of disease?	☐	☐
2	Was there a lack of public and community health infrastructure at the time?	☐	☐
3	If yes, did the lack of infrastructure at the time of spread precipitate more widespread distribution?	☐	☐
4	Was the lack of infrastructure at the time linked to a sociopolitical root cause?	☐	☐
5	Is it treatable? In other words, would building more effective sociopolitical infrastructure mitigate the risk of spread?	☐	☐

China was the new discipline of tropical medicine. Watts writes that tropical medicine was an instrument of empire intended to enable the white races to live in, or at the very least exploit, all areas of the globe.

If we are to use our rubric, my interpretation would be that nearly every box would be checked. We might argue that there was some public or community health infrastructure evolving at the time in the areas where spread was taking place (e.g., India, Hong Kong). But according to Watts's theory, this infrastructure was not really meant for the natives and therefore actually had the opposite effect of its supposedly intended implementation.

If we are to review the conditions set forth in chapter 2, it's clear that economic instability played a substantive role in these determinants as employment, food security, housing security, and, of course, poverty were all in significant flux during this time of widespread colonialism. Of course, neighborhoods/built environments played a key role in determining this pandemic, with recurrent and episodic periods of crime, violence, and war throughout the world. Finally, discrimination continues to play a salient role in determining access for communities ruled by empire (one with very different values and ideologies). We saw many examples described in chapter 4.

6th Cholera Pandemic, 1899–1923

Cholera is a quintessential public health problem—one that helped John Snow found the field of epidemiology. It is also strongly associated with poor sanitation and poverty and is well placed here. Its outbreak in India in the late 1880s and into the decades that followed marked the first pandemic of the new 20th century.

Clinical Manifestations

Infection results in a spectrum of disease, ranging from asymptomatic intestinal colonization to severe diarrhea.[16] Abdominal discomfort and vomiting are other common symptoms, particularly in the early phases of disease. Among those with severe disease, most complications are related to the substantial volume and electrolyte loss from diarrhea. This is the main distinguishing factor. Cholera stools may contain fecal matter and bile in the early phases of disease.[17] The characteristic symptom of severe cholera (cholera gravis) is the passage of profuse "rice-water" stool, a watery stool with flecks of mucus, typically with a fishy odor.

The diarrhea is usually painless. Stool output is exceedingly voluminous. The total volume loss over the course of the illness may be up to 100% of body weight.[18] That's a lot. In addition, compared with other causes of childhood diarrheal illness, stool from cholera patients contains a higher concentration of sodium, as well as significant amounts of potassium and bicarbonate (these are other mineral salts). Cholera patients with severe hypovolemia may have sunken eyes, dry mouth, cold clammy skin, decreased skin turgor, or wrinkled hands and feet (also known as "washerwoman's hands"). Patients are frequently apathetic and lethargic. Fever is uncommon. It has a typical incubation period of one to two days.[19,20,21] In the early stages of the cholera epidemic in Haiti, the median time between onset of symptoms and death in individuals who died before presentation to a cholera treatment center was 12 hours.[22]

Epidemiology

Cholera primarily occurs in settings where there is inadequate access to clean water and sanitation. It continues to remain endemic in approximately 50 countries (defined as having reported cholera cases in at least three of the five past years), mostly in Africa and Asia.[23] *Vibrio cholerae* is a bacterium (specifically, two serogroups—O1 and O139) that produces a toxin that leads to the infection we know as cholera in humans. It is primarily acquired by ingesting contaminated food or water. In endemic regions, *V. cholerae* in the water is an important reservoir of the organism. While exposure to environmental *V. cholerae* is significant, direct person-to-person transmission plays an important role. Organisms that were recently shed from infected individuals appear to be transiently more infectious than organisms isolated from the aquatic environment.[24]

Patterns of cholera transmission and infection differ between historically endemic areas and areas experiencing cholera epidemics. In areas with high chronic rates (we call this endemicity), the incidence of *V. cholerae* infection follows a seasonal distribution, with peaks before and after rainy seasons and with breakdowns in safe water, hygiene, and health services contributing further to the epidemic transmission of cholera. Mathematical models suggest these epidemics are also dependent on fluctuations in population-based immunity and climate.[25,26] In areas of high endemicity, the incidence of cholera is highest in children younger than five years of age, likely reflecting the lack of protective immunity.[27] In areas with more limited immunity in the population, massive epidemics may occur, with similar attack rates in children and adults.[28]

Large cholera epidemics often occur in populations impacted by natural disaster or human conflict.[29] These associations reflect the underlying mode of transmission via contaminated food and water. In areas where cholera occurs sporadically, most cases are associated with shellfish consumption. Other risk factors for *V. cholerae* infection and cholera reflect the biological interaction between the host and pathogen, including blood group O (associated with more severe cholera) and partial gastric resections. Breastfeeding, on the other hand, has been shown to be consistently protective against cholera.

The mortality of cholera in untreated patients may reach 50–70%.[30,31] The administration of appropriate rehydration therapy can reduce the mortality of severe cholera to <0.5%.[32] Let me repeat this for dramatic effect: We can literally cut a disease down from killing 50–70% of people it infects to less than 1% with simple intravenous (IV) fluids. In areas where cholera is endemic, the mortality risk is sadly increased in children, where it is 10 times greater than in adults.[33,34]

The 6th Cholera pandemic (preceded by the fifth just ending a few years before and lasting between 1881 and 1896) was attributed to the classical strain of O1.[35] It lasted from 1899 to 1923 and was ultimately responsible for the loss of over 5 million lives. Prior to this, cholera emerged in epidemic form in India in 1817, where it spread beyond the Indian subcontinent, resulting in six worldwide cholera pandemics between 1817 and 1923. Between 1849 and 1854, London physician John Snow proposed that cholera was a communicable disease and that stool contained infectious material. He suggested that this infectious material could contaminate drinking water supplies, resulting in the transmission of cholera. This was a transformative discovery and fundamentally disrupted our understanding of infectious disease epidemiology.

At the start of this iteration in India in 1899, over 800,000 lives were lost that year alone. Cholera has remained endemic since.[36] Initially, there were major outbreaks in Calcutta and Bombay in 1899–1900, followed by a spike in cases in the south (primarily around the port of Madras) until 1904. Since 1900, cholera had begun spreading from India to other countries primarily through British colonial trade routes— especially via mass global commercial trade established by global trading giants, such as the East India Company. This began with a westward expansion into Afghanistan and the Persian Gulf areas and into Burma and Singapore shortly after that in 1901. Simultaneously with this spread to the east, cholera was carried in 1902 by the maritime route, presumably by pilgrims who left Madras en route to the city of Mecca in Saudi Arabia. Mecca has been described as a "relay station" for cholera, with 27 epidemics recorded during this time period and 4,000 and over 20,000 Haj (the famed pilgrimage to Mecca) pilgrims dying in the 1902 and 1907–1908 Haj pilgrimages, respectively.[37]

Cholera was especially lethal in Russia. Historians link this migration mostly through wartime routes. An invasion of Syria taking place via the Sinai Peninsula in 1903 was responsible for the appearance of cholera in the same year not only in Palestine, Asia Minor, and on the

Black Sea coast but also in Mesopotamia and Persia, from where it seemed to be imported in the spring of 1904 by caravans via Samarkand into Baku on the Caspian Sea and ultimately into western Siberia. It soon penetrated urban centers such as Leningrad (now St. Petersburg) and Kiev in 1909–1910. In total, more than 500,000 people died of cholera in Russia from 1900–1925, which was a time of extreme social disruption as the result of revolution and warfare.[38]

The 1902–1904 cholera epidemic claimed 200,000 lives in the Philippines, including their revolutionary hero and first prime minister Apolinario Mabini.[39] More than 34,000 people died in Egypt in a three-month period alone. There was a resurgence of cholera in some countries between 1908 and 1910, which some historians linked to the increase in cases in India during 1905–1908, where an average of over 500,000 died each year. The mortality in India once more exceeded half a million annually in 1918 (556,533 deaths) and in 1919 (565,166 deaths). The decade 1909–1918 was particularly challenging due to the syndemic coexistence of both cholera and plague, causing nearly 800,000 deaths. The WHO shows global total deaths from cholera at 3.8 million in 1910–1919 and then precipitously declining in the 1920s to less than half that amount starting in the 1930s.

The pandemic failed to have much impact in the Americas and caused only small outbreaks in some ports of western Europe because of advances in tropical medicine, sanitation, and public health (as described in the section on plague). This protection notwithstanding, extensive areas of the Ottoman Empire (i.e., Italy, Greece, Turkey, and the Balkans) were severely affected. In 1913 the Romanian Army, while invading Bulgaria during the Second Balkan War, suffered a cholera outbreak that resulted in 1,600 deaths.[40] The last outbreak of cholera in the United States was in 1910–1911, when the steamship *Moltke* brought infected people from Naples to New York City. Vigilant health authorities isolated the infected in quarantine on Swinburne Island. Eleven people died, including a health care worker at the hospital on the island.[41]

Cholera remains a major cause of morbidity and mortality worldwide, with an estimated 2–3 million cases and >100,000 deaths each year, with recent key epidemics taking place in Zimbabwe (2008–2009, with >100,000 infected and >4,000 dead, respectively); Haiti (2010, with over 600,000 cases and 7,000 deaths, respectively), and Yemen (2016–2017, with >500,000 cases and >2,000 deaths, respectively), as well as a number of current outbreaks taking place throughout the sub-Saharan African continent.[42]

Sociopolitical Determinants

Given the temporal overlap of the early 20th century with the 3rd Plague pandemic and the Spanish flu, we will see similarities from a sociopolitical determinant standpoint—particularly commonalities related to colonialism and World War I. The 6th Cholera pandemic was clearly driven globally mostly by British colonialism but then connected to other population-level risk factors (e.g., religious mass gatherings). We also saw a correlation with a shift in the Western biomedicine paradigm and the seminal work of John Snow and other pioneers of infectious disease epidemiology and tropical medicine. That work would have been culturally at odds with many colonized nations and triggered a sense of anxiety regarding the underlying reasons for a changing public health practice among the ruling class.

These similarities notwithstanding, cholera is a very different disease from influenza and plague, with unique transmission properties. Water supplies are key. Mass gatherings (including overcrowding), particularly those involving large congregations of people with insufficient safe water supplies and poor sanitation, enhance the spread of cholera and may be followed by further dissemination when attendees return home. Poor public health infrastructure, including logistical obstacles to appropriate case management, also contributes to a high case fatality rate (CFR) in epidemic settings.

The trifecta of chronic inadequate water and sanitation infrastructure combined with war and natural disasters that disrupt public health facilities (e.g., cyclones and earthquakes) creates the perfect recipe for a cholera pandemic given the introduction of a pandemic cholera strain.

A large part of the cholera burden occurred (and continues to occur) in urban settings, given the high propensity for human-human transmission. Other high-population density situations with insufficient water and sanitation, such as in refugee camps or camps for internally displaced persons and among marginalized communities in congregate settings such as prisons or psychiatric institutions, will create highly pressurized scenarios for cholera outbreaks.[43]

These conditions were common in the areas affected between 1899 and 1923—especially Russia, the Ottoman Empire, and the Philippines (with the ending of the Spanish-American War). South Asia's core drivers seem to be clearly linked to poor infrastructure amplified by seasonal tropical storms (e.g., cyclones, monsoons) and the plight of colonialism. In Eastern Calcutta, the sociodemographic variables that increase the risk for cholera are poverty, use of unsafe water, and proximity to canals. In Bangladesh a lack of education and household density were linked with a higher risk for adults. In children under five, the risk factors were older age, lower socioeconomic status, and lack of breastfeeding.[44] Also in Bangladesh, water temperature and depth, rainfall, and copepod (small crustaceans that increase the risk of the spread of cholera) counts were shown to correlate with the occurrence of cholera toxin–producing bacteria.[45]

The social construction of disease in these areas also further polarized class, religious, and racial differences through xenophobic practices (sometimes state sponsored). As the perception of the disease model changed during the turn of the century, it created a scientific basis for blaming others for the introduction of disease. In Italy some blamed Jews and Romani, while in British India numerous Anglo-Indians ascribed transmission to the migration patterns of Hindu pilgrims. In the United States, many accused Filipino immigrants of introducing the disease. With the recent use of public health law in the United States, such as Title 42, we clearly see that not much has changed.

A current cholera pandemic (the seventh) began in 1961. We have seen many of the conditions described above continue to precipitate a number of outbreaks globally—especially in continents not impacted as heavily (e.g., the Americas, Africa). As described above, the destruction of Yemeni infrastructure, health, water, and sanitation systems and facilities by Saudi-led coalition air strikes led to the spread of cholera in 2017. In addition, ongoing commercial blockades resulted in shortages of fuel and food, leading to famine. In 2019 torrential rains and widespread flooding across Yemen worsened the humanitarian disaster.

In addition to the Arabian Peninsula, we are seeing a number of unprecedented outbreaks on the African continent. The number of African countries reporting indigenous cholera cases to the WHO rose from 16 in 1970 to 45 in 2006 and fell to 14 in 2017, with a recent spike in 2021.[46] With underreporting and inadequate surveillance systems, the number of cholera cases in Africa is probably much higher than what is officially reported. A large number of outbreaks occur in a context of societal vulnerability and often become humanitarian emergencies leading to the collapse of health structures, including surveillance systems.[47]

So, it's time to break out our red pens yet again. How did we do? It should be clear that the cascading impacts of colonialism (primarily British), a shift in the biomedical paradigm, pervasive carnage, vast migration (including forced), and infrastructure disruption and decimation were the core sociopolitical drivers. In addition, we have chronically poor water, sanitation, and hygiene infrastructures (often referred to with the acronym WASH) in many of these nations even today, which amplifies pandemic potential. While we could reduce the CFRs to nearly zero with proper infrastructure and treatment (I did so while working in South Sudan), the cascading impact of the aforementioned factors leads to a level of population stress that prevents systems from applying basic disease control measures, causing the number of cases and associated deaths to far exceed reasonable expectations. Of course, the most historically marginalized will suffer the worst. Making sense? I would give us a score of 100% here, but please grade it for yourself.

6th Cholera Pandemic: Rubric for determining the sociopolitical determinants of pandemics and PHEICs

	Sociopolitical determinant–linked questionnaire	Yes	No
1	Is there a sociopolitical link to the original spread of disease?	☐	☐
2	Was there a lack of public and community health infrastructure at the time?	☐	☐
3	If yes, did the lack of infrastructure at the time of spread precipitate more widespread distribution?	☐	☐
4	Was the lack of infrastructure at the time linked to a sociopolitical root cause?	☐	☐
5	Is it treatable? In other words, would building more effective sociopolitical infrastructure mitigate the risk of spread?	☐	☐

Spanish Influenza, 1918–1920

The Spanish Influenza (a social construction) pandemic is one of the most infamous and lethal pandemics in history. Until 2019 its reference was often arcane. Since COVID-19 it has become the most common referent and deserves a great deal of attention—especially considering it was the first of four flu pandemics in a hundred years.

Clinical Manifestations

I'm sure we're all too familiar with a "flu-like illness," but as the terms "flu" and "common cold" are so frequently used interchangeably, I'll just share some basic disease principles, as the same principles will be used in the next four pandemics.

To begin with, let me be clear: Influenza (or flu) and a "common cold" (upper respiratory infection, or URI) are definitely not the same. A common cold or URI is caused by a number of different types of viruses— namely, rhinovirus (notably, alpha-coronavirus being one of them, but not to be confused with COVID-19 and SARS, which are beta-coronaviruses). While a flu can have "cold-like symptoms" and a cold can have "flu-like symptoms," in general influenza (especially pandemic flu) is a far more severe infection (that was, until SARS and COVID-19).

Infected individuals may be asymptomatic or present with a range of manifestations including mild focal illness (e.g., conjunctivitis or "pink eye"), URI, or fulminant (severe) pneumonia with multiorgan failure.[48] Complications may include acute kidney injury, muscle breakdown, severe clotting disorders, meningoencephalitis (brain infection), and coinfection with bacterial or fungal pathogens (bugs). Signs and symptoms may include fever, cough, shortness of breath, chest pain, and muscle aches; fatigue, headache, diarrhea, and sore throat can occur but are less common. Gastrointestinal, or GI (which has many other references, including belly, gut, tummy, or stomach) manifestations (e.g., abdominal pain, vomiting, and diarrhea), are variable.

While the symptoms of Spanish influenza often started like other influenza outbreaks, its lethality was found in the unique way that it damaged the respiratory tract so as to increase the person's vulnerability to secondary (bacterial) pneumonia infections. Sometimes within hours, patients succumbed to complete respiratory failure. Autopsies would classically demonstrate hard, red lungs drenched in fluid. A microscopic analysis of the lung tissue would reveal that the lungs' typically air-filled cells were so full of fluid that victims literally drowned. The slow suffocation began when patients presented with a unique symptom: mahogany spots over their cheekbones. Within hours these patients turned a bluish-black hue indicative of cyanosis, or lack of oxygen. In fact, when triaging scores of new patients, nurses often looked at the patients' feet first, which would be a triage indicator of who was "worth" saving at the time. Black feet put you in the unfavorable bucket. The incubation period is generally 3–5 days but may be as long as 7–10 days.[49,50]

Epidemiology

The outbreak of Spanish influenza was caused by an H1N1 virus with genes of avian (bird) origin. (Keep this in mind for the 2009 swine flu section.) First, let me briefly break down what these letters and

Human Seasonal Influenza Viruses

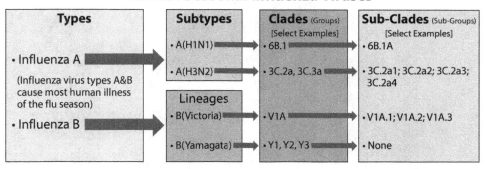

FIGURE 5.3. Types of influenza. *Source:* "Types of Influenza Viruses," Centers for Disease Control and Prevention, September 18, 2024, https://www.cdc.gov/flu/about/viruses-types .html.

numbers actually mean. I'll try not to overcomplicate it, but I think this explanation is important.

Influenza viruses come in four types: A, B, C, and D (figure 5.3). Influenza A and B viruses cause seasonal epidemics of disease in people (e.g., flu season, typically from October–March in the United States). Influenza A viruses are the only ones known to cause flu pandemics. What causes a pandemic? One occurs when new or mutated influenza A viruses crop up that have the ability to spread efficiently among people and against which people have little or no immunity.

Influenza pandemics tend to either spread more efficiently or have higher mortality (cause more death). They rarely do both (evolution would not allow it). This is important to remember. Influenza B can also be responsible for seasonal influenza—but never pandemics. Influenza B viruses generally change more slowly in terms of their genetic and antigenic properties. Influenza C virus infections generally cause mild illness and are not thought to cause seasonal or epidemic outbreaks in humans. Influenza D viruses primarily affect cattle with spillover to other animals but are not known to infect people to cause illness.

Influenza A viruses are divided into subtypes based on two proteins on the surface of the virus: hemagglutinin (H) and neuraminidase (N) (figure 5.4). There are 18 different hemagglutinin subtypes and

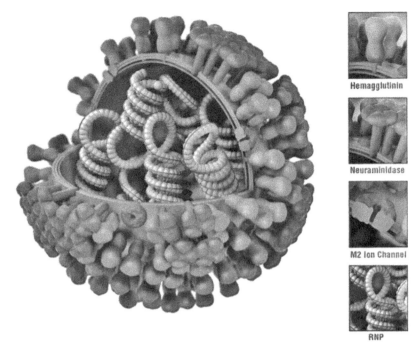

Hemagglutinin

Neuraminidase

M2 Ion Channel

RNP

FIGURE 5.4. A schematic drawing of an influenza A virus that models its biochemistry. *Source:* Centers for Disease Control and Prevention, March 18, 2024, https://www.cdc.gov/flu/about/viruses-types.html.

11 different neuraminidase subtypes (i.e., H1–H18; N1–N11, respectively). While more than 130 influenza A subtype combinations have been identified in nature (primarily from wild birds), potentially many more influenza A subtype combinations have the propensity for virus "reassortment." *Reassortment* is a process by which influenza viruses swap gene segments. Reassortment can occur when two influenza viruses infect a host at the same time and swap genetic information. Current subtypes of influenza A viruses that routinely circulate in people include A (H1N1) (seen in the 1918 and 2009 pandemics) and A (H3N2) (seen in the 1968 pandemic; figure 5.5). Influenza A subtypes can be further broken down into different genetic clades and subclades.

Confirmatory numbers were challenging because of the lack of technological capacity and especially disease control back at that time.

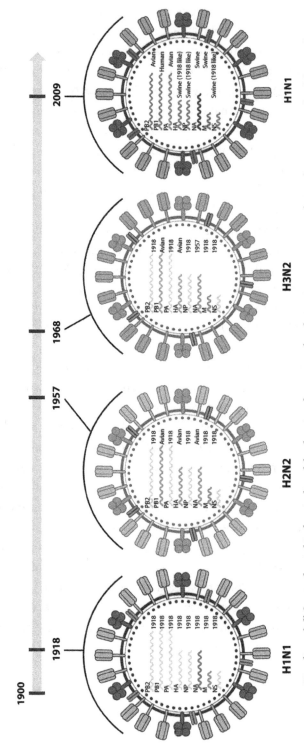

FIGURE 5.5. Timeline of all flu pandemic biochemical models, showing the temporal and genetic reassortment relationships among each of the pandemic influenza subtypes. *Source:* Walter N. Harrington et al., "The Evolution and Future of Influenza Pandemic Preparedness," *Experimental & Molecular Medicine* 53 (2021): 737–749, https://doi.org/10.1038/s12276-021-00603-0.

While the 1918 H1N1 virus has been synthesized and evaluated, the properties that made it so devastating are not well understood. To begin with, we had hardly any control measures, lacking vaccines, known supportive treatment (this is a term for therapeutic measures aimed at mitigating symptom severity but not necessarily addressing the cause), and antibiotics to treat the secondary bacterial infections (usually pneumonia) associated with influenza infections. While measures such as isolation, quarantine, good personal hygiene, use of disinfectants, and social distancing were effective, they were applied unevenly. Understanding this application better may have been a helpful precedent to our management of the COVID-19 pandemic.

While the 1918 Spanish Influenza was by far the most devastating influenza pandemic in recorded history, mortality reports vary widely.[51] It is estimated that about 500 million people (or 33% of the world's population at the time) became infected with this virus. Of that number, scholars estimate that between 17.4 million and nearly 100 million died, with about 675,000 of those deaths occurring in the United States.

The exceptionally high mortality is the combined result of the extremely high infectiousness of the disease and of a case-fatality rate of >2.5%, which is high compared to the <0.1% characterizing other influenza pandemics.[52] I know I just said that these two traits should not coexist—this is one key exception. Mortality was particularly high in people younger than 5 years old, 20–40 years old, and 65 years and older (figure 5.6). While the bimodal (two peaks) distribution of the younger and older populations could be easily explained as a common feature of respiratory diseases, the high mortality in the presumably healthy 20–40-year age group was a unique feature of this pandemic. The pandemic lowered the average life expectancy in the United States by more than 12 years. (For comparison, COVID-19 reduced this by less than 2 years). A comparable death rate has not been observed during any of the known flu seasons or pandemics that occurred either prior to or following the 1918 pandemic (figure 5.7).

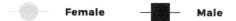
Female   ■— Male

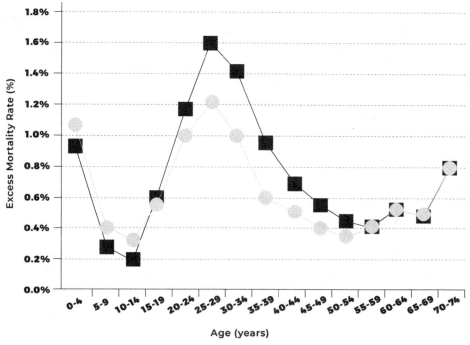

FIGURE 5.6. Age-specific mortality rates for influenza A. *Source:* Graphic by author.

Historical Timeline

Let's start here with the history of this eponymous pandemic. From an etymological (origin of naming, not to be confused with entomology, which is the study of insects) standpoint, the irony is that the 1918 influenza outbreak wasn't restricted to Spain, nor did it even originate there. The earliest recorded outbreak of the Spanish influenza was actually at Fort Riley, Kansas, in March 1918 among US military personnel.[53] Overcrowding and unsanitary conditions created a fertile breeding ground for the virus. Within one week, 522 men had been admitted to the camp hospital suffering from the same severe influenza.

Shown are global mortality estimates from different research publications

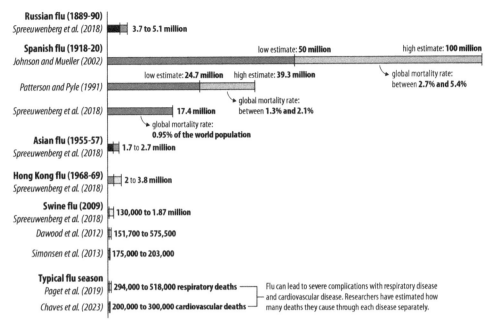

FIGURE 5.7. Global death toll from influenza pandemics, 1918–2009.
Source: Saloni Dattani and Fiona Spooner, "How Many People Die from the Flu?," Our World in Data, March 18, 2024, https://ourworldindata.org/influenza-deaths.

Soon after, the US Army reported similar outbreaks in Virginia, South Carolina, Georgia, Florida, Alabama, and California. Navy ships docked at East Coast ports also reported outbreaks of severe influenza and pneumonia among their crews. The flu seemed to target military personnel and not civilians, so the virus was largely overshadowed by hotter current affairs such as Prohibition, the suffragette movement, and the bloody battles in Europe.

By May 1918, influenza began to subside in the United States. But the ordeal was by no means over. Soldiers at Fort Riley, now ready for battle, incubated the virus during their long, cramped voyage to France. Once they hit French shores, the virus exploded, striking the Allied forces and Central Powers with equal force. A number of varied references applied until one stuck. The Americans fell ill with "three-day fever" or "purple death." The French caught "purulent [puss-filled] bronchitis." The Italians suffered "sandfly fever" (there was no correlation). German hospitals filled with victims of *Blitzkatarrh* (also known as Flanders fever).

From the battlefields of Europe, the epidemic quickly evolved into a pandemic, as the disease spread north to Norway, east to China, southeast to India, and as far south as New Zealand. Even islands weren't safe. Hitching rides on naval ships, merchant vessels, and trains, the virus traveled to the four corners of the earth. By the summer of 1918, it had hit Puerto Rico, the Caribbean, the Philippines, and Hawaii. Within four short months, the virus had rounded the globe and returned once more to US shores.

The influenza epidemic occurred in at least three waves, as visualized in Europe and America, with the second and third slamming the United States in the cold-weather months of 1918. This time civilians were not immune. Globally, the effects were probably exacerbated by the end of World War I, with soldiers returning home and the resumption of commerce. Even in a much less-connected world the virus eventually reached extremely remote places such as the Alaskan wilderness and Samoa in the middle of the Pacific—at times, wiping out nearly its entire adult population.[54] Indigenous communities in the United States, particularly Native Alaskans, suffered disproportionately. Urban dwellers fared poorly too, with New York City and Philadelphia burying 33,000 and 13,000 victims, respectively, in a matter of weeks.

So why was it coined the "Spanish flu"? Spain was neutral in World War I (1914–1918), which meant it was free to report on the severity of the pandemic. At the same time, other countries involved in active conflict were attempting to suppress reports on how the pandemic impacted their populations to maintain morale. Thus, we see how readily misappropriation and labeling can stick, permanently,

Sociopolitical Determinants

The sociopolitical determinants for the cataclysmic impact of the 1918 influenza pandemic are relatively straightforward. The most violent world war in history was coming to an end. The war naturally exacerbated the preexisting social inequities that led to the fighting. That in turn created the perfect recipe for a highly infectious virus to undergo immunologic mutations and precipitate as syndemic,[55] enabling it to travel with soldiers across the world. It was highly infectious among victims globally who had no prior immunity to mitigate the spread.

The spread of the three waves is telling. From its identified origin on a military base in Kansas during World War I (figure 5.8), it spread with American troops throughout the nation and overseas on crowded trains and troop ships. The US public health system was overstretched at the time. The war not only precipitated an unusually high degree of population among troops but also caused the substantive refugee migrations that accompany any major conflict. The mixture of these populations created an immunological opportunity that was sociopolitically determined.

There were important differences in how the disease manifested between races at the time. Eugene Opie, a pathologist and lieutenant

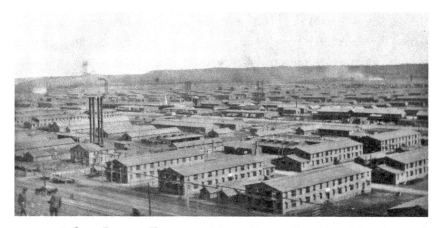

FIGURE 5.8. Camp Funston, Kansas, 1918. *Source:* Margaret Humphreys, "The Influenza of 1918," *Evolution, Medicine, and Public Health* (2018): 219–229, https://doi.org/10.1093/emph /eoy024.

colonel in the US Army medical corps, studied these variations in pneumonia (a typical secondary superinfection of the 1918 influenza pandemic). He noted that "pneumonia of this period has in considerable part affected newly drafted negro troops from southern states, namely Louisiana and Mississippi." Among the 5,982 Black men arriving over four days in late June were 69 cases of pneumonia, whereas among the 12,000 white draftees who arrived in June, only one case of pneumonia occurred. A further cohort of 5,997 Black men arriving in July developed 20 cases of pneumonia, while only 8 cases arose among the 15,000 white recruits in that month.[56] Upon further investigation, part of the reason behind these differences seemed to be related to conditions that were more prevalent in the US South, where race (and access) was likely a contributing factor.

With a saturated US public health system, there was no effective way to contain the distribution of disease, and the second wave moved quickly through the congested military camps of Europe and on to East and South Asia, infecting all sides of the conflict without regard for nationality. This first wave was a minor outbreak but not a major killer. Those who were infected early on were fortunate, as this apparently offered some immunizing protection for the virulent variants of the pathogen to come.[57] That second wave appeared at several locations spontaneously toward the end of August 1918. Thousands of miles apart, military men across multiple continents were quickly febrile, and soon many were overtaken by this mysterious infection. As it made its way back through the United States, it also infected civilians, as described above.

Important socially determined differences were noted among US civilians during that second wave. A brilliant systematic review performed by D'Adamo and team at Johns Hopkins University found only eight articles that assessed outcomes in the 1918 pandemic in relation to socioeconomic status, specifically illiteracy, homeownership, occupation, apartment size, and unemployment. Grantz and colleagues were able to identify a number of social drivers of differences in disease distribution in Chicago. Census tract-level social factors, including rates of illiteracy, homeownership, population density, and unemployment, were assessed as predictors of pandemic mortality (linked to either influenza or pneumonia) in Chicago in 1918–1919. A biostatistical model showed that influenza and pneumonia mortality increased, on average, by 32.2% for every 10% increase in illiteracy rate.[59] In other words, the less literate someone was the higher their likelihood of death from infection from influenza and pneumonia, respectively. That something so seemingly unrelated as literacy should correlate so directly to public health is deeply telling.

Clay and colleagues looked at socioeconomic factors across US cities and found that, compared to cities with the lowest percentage of illiterate residents, cities with the highest percentage of illiterate residents had 21.3 additional deaths per 10,000 during the pandemic.[54] This is a very similar read to Grantz. Mamelund examined individual- and household-level socioeconomic factors in Norway and found that influenza mortality rates were 49% higher in individuals in the "deprived" social class compared to the class considered "advantaged" in terms of income, education, and employment. In addition, Bengtsson et al. examined differences in excess mortality in Norway by individual-level social class and found that among occupational groups (white collar, skilled, low skilled, unskilled, farmers), low-skilled workers had the highest excess mortality rate, and skilled workers had a significantly lower death rate than unskilled and low-skilled workers during the pandemic.[60]

D'Adamo also found five articles exploring racial/ethnic disparities in the 1918 pandemic in the United States. Økland explored military, survey, and insurance data in the United States and found heterogeneous disparities. Interestingly, Black soldiers had a 2.3-times lower influenza incidence but higher excess mortality and CFRs than white soldiers. Using insurance data for the general population, the same article also reported that during the second pandemic wave, while excess mortality was higher for Blacks than whites aged 1–14 years, there was actually no difference in mortality by race for those aged 15–19, and mortality was, interestingly, even higher among whites than Blacks for those aged 20–early 50s. Moreover, Britten examined outcomes among US localities during the 1918 pandemic and found that across almost all cities, white populations experienced higher rates of influenza than Black populations, after adjustment for age and sex.[61] Does that make sense? It's surprising. In other words, the Black population experienced lower influenza incidence and morbidity. Black populations did experience higher CFRs (meaning that of those who did fall ill, a higher percentage died) than whites (e.g., attributed to increased baseline lung disease, malnutrition, inadequate access to care, lower socioeconomic status [SES], and poor housing conditions).[62]

These unlikely outcomes may be explained by policies linked to structural racism. D'Adamo suggests several explanations. First, the lower incidence among Black individuals may be due to poorer scientific access among Black populations at the time. A recent study examining current socioeconomic biases in seasonal influenza surveillance found that measures used for both surveillance and research may be biased against poor communities, as well as those of color. This type of bias may have been even more pronounced in 1918, when surveillance and vital registration systems were far less developed. Second, according to Krishnan, segregation may also have prevented Black individuals from coming into close contact with whites during the 1918 pandemic, reducing their risk of contracting influenza.[62]

Krishnan also hypothesizes that protective immunity from greater exposure to a less virulent early wave, as a result of living in congregated high-exposure risk areas, potentially led to lower susceptibility among Black populations to the deadlier fall/winter wave. Brewer also suggests that the poorer living conditions in tents for Black military members may have (ironically) created conditions for more limited spread because of the likelihood of less overcrowding in tents compared to buildings. In a very recent study, Eirmann et al. tested these hypotheses and among other findings, determined that Black

Spanish Influenza: Rubric for determining the sociopolitical determinants of pandemics and PHEICs

	Sociopolitical determinant-linked questionnaire	Yes	No
1	Is there a sociopolitical link to the original spread of disease?	☐	☐
2	Was there a lack of public and community health infrastructure at the time?	☐	☐
3	If yes, did the lack of infrastructure at the time of spread precipitate more widespread distribution?	☐	☐
4	Was the lack of infrastructure at the time linked to a sociopolitical root cause?	☐	☐
5	Is it treatable? In other words, would building more effective sociopolitical infrastructure mitigate the risk of spread?	☐	☐

populations' exclusion from health care and public health systems may have encouraged greater community-based education and prevention, encouraging behaviors that reduced exposure to infections.[63]

When we are able to break down and analyze some of the conditions described here, it seems difficult to argue against the idea that a number of sociopolitical determinants drove the distribution of spread and death highly unevenly throughout the world. Let's turn to our rubric.

According to my grading, I would score 100% here. From an economic stability perspective, I suspect that most war historians would agree that nearly every driver was impacted by a world war of this magnitude—including employment, food insecurity, housing insecurity, and poverty. Clearly, both the United States and other areas ravaged by H1N1 experienced health care access issues as wartime conditions overstretched the public health systems both before and during the multiple waves, creating stark inequities in terms of access. Neighborhoods or built environments were certainly impacted by war, primarily from a perspective of crime/violence as well as housing, with most men in various countries being conscripted and the labor force falling to levels that made it impossible to create or sustain an adequate housing market. Educational disparities—namely illiteracy—was cited as a correlative feature of infection. All these conditions created the perfect recipe for a pandemic. This one seems like a "no brainer" to me.

Let's move on to our next flu pandemic.

Asian Flu, 1957–1958

What came to be known as "the Asian Flu" first emerged in China in 1957, rapidly spreading across the continent and then the world within a few months. For our purposes, it is notable for marking the first time that the rapid global spread of a modern influenza virus was available for laboratory investigation, given the advances in science and technology.

Clinical Manifestations

Most of the symptoms here are the same as the H1N1 outbreak in 1918 (Spanish flu).[64] As the science advanced, we started to observe some notable complications, including acute kidney injury, muscle breakdown, severe clotting disorders, meningoencephalitis (brain infection), and coinfection with bacterial or fungal pathogens.

Epidemiology

Tests defining the specific antigens of the virus showed it to be unlike any previously found in humans. In animal studies the new H2N2 viruses did not behave that differently from earlier influenza A subtypes. It was first reported in southern China and Singapore in February 1957, in Hong Kong in April 1957, and in coastal cities in the United States in summer 1957.[65]

Although secondary bacterial infections of the lung (pneumonia) were found to be a prominent feature of fatal cases in 1918, they were not as common in Asian flu. Risk factors for adverse consequences included rheumatic heart disease and pregnant women in the third trimester.[66] The global mortality rate of the 1957–1959 influenza pandemic was moderate relative to that of the 1918 pandemic but for context was approximately 10-fold greater than that of the 2009 pandemic. The estimated number of deaths was 1.1 million worldwide, with 116,000 deaths in the United States alone.

Historical Timeline

After the influenza pandemic of 1918, influenza went back to its usual pattern of regional epidemics of lesser virulence in the 1930s through the early 1950s. While surveillance infrastructure was still in its nascent stages in 1957, attentive investigators in Melbourne, London, and Washington, DC, soon had the virus in their laboratories after the initial recognition of a severe epidemic, followed by the publication in *The New York Times* of a 1957 article describing an epidemic in Hong Kong that involved 250,000 people in a short period.[67] Three weeks later, a virus was recovered from the outbreak and sent to the Walter Reed Army Institute for Research in Washington, DC, for study. With the exception of people >70 years of age (those who had experienced the 1918 pandemic), the public was confronted with a virus with which it had no real-world experience, and it became evident that the virus alone, without bacterial coinvaders, was lethal.[68]

The first reported cases are disputed secondary to the People's Republic of China's (PRC) unique reporting practices (note similarities to COVID-19). Some reports are first seen in Guizhou (southern China) in early 1957.[69] Interestingly, the PRC was not a member of the WHO at the time and did not inform other countries about the outbreak.[70]

In late 1957 a second wave of the flu took place in northern China—especially in rural areas.[71] In the same year, as a response to the epidemic, the Chinese government established the Chinese National Influenza Center, which published a manual on influenza in 1958.

By April, approximately 250,000 (or 10% of Honk Kong residents) were receiving treatment. The recent influx of about 700,000 refugees from mainland China had intensified authorities' fears of epidemics and fires due to crowded conditions, and according to a report received by the US Influenza Information Center on May 3, the disease was said to be occurring mainly among these refugees.[72]

By the end of April (or as early as February according to the US Centers for Disease Control and Prevention [CDC]), Singapore also experienced an outbreak, which peaked in mid-May with 680 deaths. By the end of May, the outbreak had spread across Southeast Asia and also involved Indonesia, the Philippines, and Japan.[73] In Taiwan, 100,000 were affected by mid-May.[74] India (sadly, often vulnerable in these pandemics) experienced over a million cases by June.[75] In late June the pandemic reached the United Kingdom and the United States.[76]

The US experience was interesting from a public health perspective. Since the 1918 pandemic, epidemiological infrastructure in the United States had expanded considerably. The Armed Forces Epidemiological Board and its Commission on Influenza were established in 1941, marking the beginning of US military involvement in the control of influenza.[77] Among other activities, the board maintained surveillance of influenza-like illness (ILI) around the world—operating 176 stations by 1957.[78] The Commission on Influenza also conducted studies into vaccination, which was considered highly effective by many subject matter experts at the time.[79]

Moreover, the Communicable Disease Center (today the US CDC) was formed in 1946, initially for the control of malaria within military installations in the southeastern United States. In light of developing Cold War–era concerns over biological warfare, the Epidemic Intelligence Service (EIS) was created in 1951 at the CDC as a combined service and training program in the field of applied epidemiology, with the purpose of investigating certain disease outbreaks, among other activities.[80] It's a very cool program that created the next generation of "disease detectives" or "virus hunters" and one I nearly completed

(I still have my regrets). At the time that I interviewed, my mentors suggested that I not pursue the program given my extensive field experiences and additional graduate education. Admittedly, I was also impatient and wanted to complete my graduate training and get to work. Alas, had I had another opportunity, I would have jumped at the chance.

The 1950s were a tumultuous time in public health in the United States. After the incidence of poliomyelitis peaked in 1952,[81] the first vaccine against it was licensed in 1955. Its rollout that year was marred by an incident in April involving Cutter Laboratories, one of the manufacturers of the inactivated (dead) vaccine, in which some lots actually contained live virus, resulting in tens of thousands of vaccine-derived infections and several cases of paralytic polio. Oveta Culp Hobby, the first secretary of the Department of Health, Education, and Welfare, resigned over this matter that July,[82] and Marion B. Folsom replaced her shortly thereafter. On January 20, 1957, Dwight D. Eisenhower was sworn in for a second term as president. This was the backdrop to the US public health response to Asian flu.

The notion that an influenza pandemic was developing in the Far East first occurred to American microbiologist Maurice Hilleman, who was alarmed by pictures of those affected by the virus in Hong Kong published in *The New York Times* on April 17, 1957.[83] At the time Hilleman was head of the Department of Respiratory Diseases at the Walter Reed Army Institute of Research.[84] He immediately sent for virus samples from patients in the Far East, and on May 12 the first isolate was sent out to the vaccine manufacturers in the United States. Hilleman predicted an epidemic would strike the United States when schools reopened in the fall.[85] He was thereafter instrumental in stimulating the development of the pandemic vaccine. The day after Hilleman's announcement, the Division of Foreign Quarantine began to monitor travelers from the Far East for signs of respiratory illness.[86] All EIS officers and other CDC relevant personnel were alerted of the priority of investigating cases and outbreaks of ILI at that time.[87]

The Public Health Service formally began its participation in the national effort against the flu in late May 1957. The disease was noted for its mild presentation, though high rates of attack in various settings. (Note that it differed significantly from the Spanish influenza, which had had high rates of pathogenicity or disease severity, explained partly by coinfectivity with pneumonia.) It was recommended that the US Department of Defense purchase about 3 million doses of monovalent vaccine targeting the pandemic virus. The Commission on Influenza was asked to propose the composition of the polyvalent vaccine to be used as well.[88]

Some of the first people affected were US Navy personnel aboard destroyers docked at Newport Naval Station and new military recruits elsewhere. The first wave peaked in October and affected mainly children who had recently returned to school after summer break (as Hilleman predicted). The second wave (in January and February 1958) was more pronounced among elderly people and therefore far more fatal.[89]

At the same time that the US public health chops were being activated, the global public health response was starting to coalesce. The Asian flu pandemic was the first influenza pandemic to manifest since the creation of the WHO in 1947. And memories of the 1918 pandemic were still present. In recognition of the worldwide threat of epidemic influenza, the WHO launched its Global Influenza Programme in 1947 with the establishment of the World Influenza Centre at the National Institute for Medical Research in London.[90] This eventually gave rise to the Global Influenza Surveillance Network in 1952 to facilitate global scientific collaboration and fulfill the objectives of the program.[91]

Unfortunately, as China was not a member of the WHO, it was not part of the influenza surveillance network. Consequently, it took several weeks for the news of a Chinese outbreak to reach the WHO, by which time the virus had already spread into Hong Kong and then to Singapore. (Note the similarities experienced in terms of public health transparency with the first reports of COVID-19. This fact would be lamented repeatedly after the pandemic and was taken as reinforcement of the importance of a truly worldwide network of epidemiological surveillance.)

After receiving the report out of Singapore in early May, the WHO reported on the developing outbreak for the first time in its *Weekly Epidemiological Record* published on May 9, 1957. Within three weeks laboratories around the world had concluded that the cause of these epidemics was a new variant of influenza A.[92]

On June 14, the WHO declared that attempts at large-scale quarantine were ineffective, reiterating that all reports it had received emphasized the mildness of the disease in most cases, with the very few deaths having occurred mainly in elderly victims suffering from chronic bronchitis.[93]

(Side note: Isolation and quarantine are quite different. Isolation is intended for those who have been infected and is intended to separate them from others. Quarantine [remember "quaranta"] separates people who have possibly been exposed to the disease.)

On July 11, the term "Asian Flu" finally stuck at an informal meeting of scientists during the Fourth International Poliomyelitis Congress in Geneva. On October 11, the WHO announced that the virus had spread to all populated parts of the world aside from "a few islands or territories having no contact with the outside world."[94] It was, indeed, a pandemic.

Following the main phase of the pandemic, the WHO reflected on its performance as part of its review of the first 10 years of the organization in 1958. It concluded that "the WHO influenza programme fulfilled the major task allotted to it," which allowed "many parts of the world to organize health services to meet the threat and for some countries to attempt to protect priority groups by vaccination." It acknowledged, however, that had its influenza surveillance network been "truly worldwide" (note the PCR exclusion), then preparations could have begun two months earlier and far more disease prevented.[95]

The pandemic of 1957 provided the first opportunity to observe vaccination response in that large part of the population that had not already been primed by novel antigens that were not cross-reactive with earlier influenza A virus antigens. As recurrent infections occurred in 1958–1960, mean initial antibody levels in the population increased, meaning that vaccine-induced antibodies were still present in people's systems and they were partially primed, demonstrating a response to vaccination. This meant that efforts to mount a mass immunization campaign had been partially effective, thereby providing a foundation for future mass immunization campaigns. This would serve as a basis for a mass immunization response over 50 years later with the 2009 pandemic.

Sociopolitical Determinants

The Asian flu paints a very different experience from the past three pandemics previously described. Of course, it was a very different time—post colonialism and after the carnage of the first two world wars. Importantly, it was also a time when the world had developed some important public health infrastructure—namely, with institutions like the US CDC and the WHO. The fact that certain nations (those primarily involved with these pandemics) abstained from participation is telling.

Before we examine this further, it's important to note a relative paucity of disparities or sociological research on both the 1957 and 1968 pandemics, so much of our discussion is speculative and suffers from something described as ecological fallacy. This means that the inferences we are making are based on large populations as opposed to more specific data analysis on individuals. Interestingly, in 2023 D'Adamo et al. conducted a systematic review on disparities research on pandemics and found only 29 articles: 12 and 16 of which focused solely on the 1918 and 2009 pandemics, respectively, and one on the 1918, 1957, and 2009 pandemics. No articles examined the 1968 pandemic.

That said, let's be clear. The virus that caused the 1957 Asian Flu pandemic may have infected more people than the 1918 Spanish influenza, but it was quickly identified, and public and community health programs and antibiotics to manage opportunistic secondary infections were widely available (albeit largely unnecessary) in the West, where vaccines were rolled out by August 1957. The CFRs were relatively low, partly attributed to a lower coinfectivity with pneumonia. The elderly had the highest rates of death, as would be expected. What did take place was a clear disparity in response to the pandemic. The vast majority of mortality took place in China (with disproportionate rates suspected among refugees)—and much of that was likely underreported. This is a unique case better explained by a narrative reminiscent of *A (Public Health) Tale of Two Cities.*

As such, if we bring our grading pens out, we'll find a different experience here. Was there a sociopolitical link to the original spread? We do see a significant infusion of refugees into Hong Kong at the time, which could help explain the origin of the epidemic. Was there a lack of public and community health infrastructure? This is difficult to judge, as we are not clear on what was available in China at the time, although the delays in reporting suggest that access was limited. By contrast, access seems to have been established in the United States and Europe. I would argue that the lack of infrastructure in China (namely, China not engaging with the WHO or the Global Influenza Surveillance Network) was related to a sociopolitical root cause. We do know that this pandemic was mostly preventable and treatable. My calculations give me a 60% here, which is not quite passing. Let's flag this for future discussion and move on to yet another "Asian flu" over 10 years later.

Hong Kong Flu, 1968–1970

As in 1957, a new influenza pandemic arose in Southeast Asia and acquired the sobriquet "Hong Kong" (another social construction) influenza on the basis of the site of its emergence. Once again, the daily press sounded the alarm with a brief report of a large Hong Kong epidemic in the *Times* of London. A decade after the 1957 pandemic, epidemiologic communication with mainland China was even less effective than the decade prior.

Asian Flu: Rubric for determining the sociopolitical determinants of pandemics and PHEICs

	Sociopolitical determinant-linked questionnaire	Yes	No
1	Is there a sociopolitical link to the original spread of disease?	☐	☐
2	Was there a lack of public and community health infrastructure at the time?	☐	☐
3	If yes, did the lack of infrastructure at the time of spread precipitate more widespread distribution?	☐	☐
4	Was the lack of infrastructure at the time linked to a sociopolitical root cause?	☐	☐
5	Is it treatable? In other words, would building more effective sociopolitical infrastructure mitigate the risk of spread?	☐	☐

Clinical Manifestations

Again, general signs and symptoms were very similar to prior flu pandemics such as in 1918 and 1957 (noted above). Predominant findings of H3N2 among uncomplicated cases included fatigue, fever, muscle aches, cough, headache, sinus congestion, and sore throat. During the initial outbreak in Hong Kong, symptoms were mostly mild, without observable excess mortality. In a British Royal Air Force study, half of those with serological evidence of infection had no recorded illness at all. A survey of nearly 7,000 US high school students indicated that the median duration of illness was five days, although cough and prostration in some cases persisted as long as three weeks.[96] Severe disease did occur, however. Some outbreak areas reported complications including pneumonia, myocarditis, and pericarditis. Pulmonary complications in adults included localized primary viral or secondary bacterial pneumonia or diffuse bilateral pneumonia occurring early or late in the clinical course, mostly among persons with underlying comorbid conditions.

Epidemiology

As discussed above, all flu pandemics are caused by influenza A. This time, however, through the genetic reassortment of the Avian virus, we would see the H3N2 version first identified in the United States in September 1968. (Note that it differed slightly from the H2N2 version of just 10 years prior.) The estimated number of deaths was between 1 and 2 million worldwide, with about 100,000 of those in the United States. Most excess deaths were in people >65 years (much like the 1957 pandemic).[97] Since the Hong Kong virus expressed some similar antigenicity to that of 1957, researchers speculated that its more sporadic and variable impact in different regions of the world were mediated by differences in prior antigen immunity. Therefore, the 1968 pandemic has been aptly characterized as "smoldering."[98]

Although the estimated morbidity and mortality of this pandemic was only a small fraction of that associated with the 1918 H1N1 pandemic, the ongoing impact of influenza A (H3N2) virus on public health has been profound. In addition, children were more commonly ill than in the 1957 pandemic—with especially more hospitalizations for coinfections of pneumonia, bronchiolitis, bronchitis, and croup (barking cough). Importantly, it has stuck around, and beyond 1972 this subtype (H3N2) has circulated as a seasonal influenza A virus associated with more sustained and severe annual epidemics than those caused by its counterparts—the influenza A (H1N1) and influenza B viruses.

Historical Timeline

The first recorded instance of the outbreak appeared on July 13, 1968. While it was first officially reported in Hong Kong, it has been speculated that multiple preceding outbreaks occurred on the mainland. Due to a lack of evidence on causal relationships, however, mostly as a result of a strained relationship between Chinese health authorities and other nations at the time (and poor communication and epidemiologic reporting mechanisms as well), it cannot be ascertained whether the Hong Kong virus was truly the origin.[99]

Origin notwithstanding, the outbreak in Hong Kong reached its maximum intensity in two weeks,[100] and it lasted around six weeks in all, affecting about 15% of the population ($n > 500,000$) with a low mortality rate and mild clinical symptoms.[101] The reported data were very limited due to the Cultural Revolution taking place.[102] At the time of the outbreak, the Hong Kong flu was also known as the "Mao flu."[103] The name Hong Kong flu was actually not used within the colony, where the press instead dubbed it the "killer flu" after the first several deaths.[104] There was significant concern about the stigma that would be associated with Hong Kong as a result and how it would impact economic trade.[105] Of course, it was also in Hong Kong that just 10 years prior an influenza pandemic's initial cases were reported. Sixty years later we continue to point fingers and pathologize ethnic communities and associated geographical regions during times of epidemiological outbreaks.

The National Influenza Center at the University of Hong Kong isolated the new virus on July 17 and sent it immediately to the World Influenza Center in London. (The delays seen in 1957 were not reproduced.)[106] Additional specimens were sent to the International Influenza Center for the Americas in Atlanta, Georgia (a component of the National Communicable Disease Center, now the US CDC). Confirmation that the virus strain was a distinct antigenic variant of contemporary influenza viruses prompted a WHO warning on August 16. At this time the virus became available to research and to vaccine production laboratories.

An outbreak of ILI in Singapore during the second week of August 1968 was the first indication of spread outside Hong Kong.[107] Specifically, outbreaks were occurring in other Asian nations— namely, Southeast Asia, including the Philippines, Malaysia, and Vietnam. As the Vietnam War was at its height at the time, this infiltration was soon to have far-reaching global impacts.

Outside of Asia, the first known cases were in the United Kingdom in early August, where it was identified in an infant and her mother in London with no history of travel or known contact. More isolated cases soon followed. In September 1968, cases were reported in India, northern Australia, Thailand, and other parts of Europe. Air travel by an estimated 160 million persons during the pandemic facilitated rapid transmission worldwide.[108] The same month the virus entered the United States. As to be expected, the virus was imported by troops returning from the Vietnam War but, interestingly, did not become widespread in the country until December 1968.

As irony would have it, during the second week of September the 8th International Congresses on Tropical Medicine and Malaria took place in Tehran, with delegates from nearly 100 countries. An outbreak soon erupted, afflicting at least a third of them. The convention was the apparent origin of a broader outbreak within the capital city, which thereafter spread rapidly throughout Iran and other involved nations.[109] I find this particularly curious, as I had a similar experience in early February 2020 while en route to attend the national Conference on Retroviruses and Opportunistic Infections in Boston, essentially the biggest US-based scientific conference on HIV. At the time there was widespread news of a new coronavirus, and after much deliberation, the conference was ultimately canceled. Imagine if it hadn't been!

The development of the pandemic at first resembled that of the 1957 pandemic, which spread unencumbered throughout the spring and summer and had become truly worldwide by October, by which point nearly all countries were experiencing their first or even second wave. The two experiences eventually diverged within a couple of months after their initial outbreaks. In 1968 many countries (e.g., the United Kingdom, Japan) did not immediately see outbreaks despite repeated introductions of the virus throughout August and September. Additionally, after September there was little evidence of continued spread in new areas, despite similar importations of the virus into those areas. Epidemics did eventually develop during the winter months, but these were often mild (especially when compared to the US experience). In some countries (again, such as the United Kingdom and Japan) it was not until the following winter of 1969–1970 that truly severe epidemics developed.[110]

Worldwide deaths from the virus peaked in December 1968 and January 1969, when public health warnings and virus descriptions were widely issued in the scientific and medical journals.[111] During these winter months, extreme measures were necessary. In Berlin the excessive number of deaths led to corpses being stored in subway tunnels, and in West Germany, garbage collectors had to bury the dead because of a lack of undertakers. This reminded me of arriving in Sierra Leone during the Ebola outbreak in 2015 to find the bodies just piled up due to a lack of sanitarians and undertakers. In total, Germany registered approximately 60,000 estimated deaths. In some areas of France, half the workforce was bedridden, and manufacturing suffered large disruptions because of absenteeism.[112]

As this epidemic progressed, initially throughout Asia, important differences in the pattern of illness and death were noted. In Japan epidemics were small, scattered, and desultory until the end of 1968. Most striking were the high illness and death rates in the United States following introduction of the virus on the West Coast. This experience stood in contrast with the experience in Western Europe, in which increased illness occurred in the absence of increased death rates.

On September 2, a respiratory specimen from a marine who had just returned to San Diego, California, from Vietnam produced the first US isolate. Before leaving Vietnam, the marine had shared a bunker with a friend recently returned from Hong Kong. As expected, a cluster of ILI manifested shortly thereafter. Concurrently, military physicians reported outbreaks in Hawaii and Alaska among personnel recently returned from Southeast Asia. Before the end of the week, influenza surveillance was heightened all across the country, and summaries of the data were thereafter reported regularly by the CDC each week. On September 6, the National Communicable

Disease Center officials requested cooperation from all state health officers, epidemiologists, and laboratory directors for "monitoring the importation of the virus and in conducting surveillance for influenza."[113]

Public health investigations reported in the *Morbidity and Mortality Weekly Report* identified influenza A (H3N2) virus in travelers to the United States from Asia. Increased surveillance in the United States continued over the next year, expanding upon systems implemented during the 1957 pandemic and including reports on school and workplace absenteeism, school closings, hospital admissions, and outpatient visits, as well as reported cases and outbreaks.

Initially, cases occurred primarily among persons returning from Asia, but US influenza activity increased dramatically in October. The first reported civilian outbreak in the continental United States was identified in Needles, California, with more than one-third of its population reporting ILI. ILI reports in Colorado increased 10-fold in one week in early November. In addition, the first outbreaks in eastern states occurred around the same time. The epidemic became widespread in December, involving all 50 states before the end of the year. Outbreaks occurred in colleges and hospitals, with the disease sometimes attacking upward of 40% of their respective populations. Reports of absenteeism among students and nurses grew. School and college closures occurred in 23 states, and 31 saw elevated worker absenteeism. For example, schools in Los Angeles reported rates ranging from 10% to 25%, whereas the Greater New York Hospital Association reported absenteeism of 15–20% among staff and urged its members to impose visitor restrictions to safeguard patients.[114]

Peak influenza activity for most states likely occurred in the latter half of December and then declined throughout January. Excess pneumonia-influenza mortality passed the epidemic threshold during the first week of December and increased rapidly over the next month, peaking in the first half of January. A second, albeit less severe, pandemic wave of illness in the United States occurred late in the following season (1969–1970). Over these two seasons, 70% of excess pneumonia and pandemic influenza deaths in the United States actually occurred during the 1968–1969 season, which was opposite to most other countries, where the initial 1968 wave tended to be less severe but was followed by an increasingly severe wave in 1969–1970.[115] Following the epidemic of influenza A, outbreaks of influenza B began in late January and continued until late March. Most elementary school children were affected. This influenza B activity fits within the pattern of epidemics every three to six years, but the 1968–1969 flu season became the first documented instance of two major influenza A epidemics occurring in successive seasons.[116]

It became apparent once the extent of antigenic variation in the virus was recognized that a new vaccine would be needed to protect against it. But hopes of efficient production were limited as the manufacture of the previously recommended vaccines in the United States had concluded by July 1968, and the supply of fertilized chicken eggs (which is how we grow many flu vaccines) was also challenged. Nevertheless, collaboration and planning efforts triumphed, and the first cultures of the virus were provided to manufacturers in August by the National Institutes of Health (NIH), as well as a strain isolated in Japan shortly thereafter. Fortunately, the private sector (i.e., Merck and companies) had also projected the likelihood of pandemic potential similar to the 1957 precedent and began early production of vaccines in 1968. Merck would go on to produce over 9 million of the nearly 21 million doses of vaccine produced. The other half was produced by a private collaborative (e.g., Eli Lilly, Lederle Laboratories, Parke-Davis [a subsidiary of Pfizer], and Wyeth). Notably, all but Wyeth had been involved in the production of the 1957 vaccine.[117]

On November 15, just 66 days after the production strain became available, the first batch of 110,000 doses of vaccine was released, most of which went to the US Armed Forces. Notably, this represented a quicker turnaround than the release of the first doses of the 1957 vaccine, which took 3 months after its production strain became available. By the end of the year, over 10 million doses had been released.[118] At this point, influenza was widespread in the country, but its severe manifestations were largely attenuated, a victory that can be attributed to the efficient rollout of the vaccine effort. This was certainly a win for public health.

Sociopolitical Determinants

The year 1968 is remembered for a number of sociopolitical associations and general upheaval—namely, the military conflict in Vietnam, civil rights activism, the assassinations of prominent leaders, and widespread public demonstrations, as well as significant scientific achievements such as heart transplant surgeries and manned space flights. Certainly remembered less frequently is this pandemic.

At the height of the outbreak in December, 1968, *The New York Times* described the pandemic as "one of the worst in the nation's history," yet schools and businesses, for the most part, continued to operate as normal. The pandemic raged over three years yet is largely forgotten today, commented *The Wall Street Journal*. Unfortunately, there has been a paucity of research on sociopolitical contributing factors to the 1968 pandemic (as was also the case with the 1957 pandemic). Some researchers suspect that there was less media coverage of these pandemics because health care professionals at the time worried about causing public panic and fear.[119] We can only speculate.

With that said, let us think through these factors and judge for ourselves. What made this pandemic even more concerning than prior ones was that it was the first to exhibit an accelerated spread due to extensive air travel. Despite the prevalent spread of the virus and its associated disruptions, the public health response at both the federal and global level was relatively minimalistic, with many of the affected countries operating as usual (which was certainly the case with the United

States). This was ironic, given its spread into the White House, where even President Lyndon B. Johnson and members of his cabinet were thought to have been infected. Fortunately, low disease severity and mortality rates caused many public health professionals to believe that more costly population-scale public health interventions (e.g., lockdowns, school closures, or community-level quarantines) were largely unnecessary.[120] Although 23 states underwent school and university closures, the United States did not implement any broad social distancing or containment measures.

Vaccines were eventually developed but not in time to blunt the initial spread of the virus. Instead, infection control measures were relatively biomedical in nature and did not necessarily incorporate the sociopolitical dimensions to disease response. These largely included a combination of vaccinations, hospitalizations for severe cases, and antibiotics to treat secondary (bacterial) pneumonia. In most countries, vaccines were not available until after the pandemic had peaked. Meanwhile, surges in hospitalizations caused problems in some areas, with an excess hospitalization rate of 150% reported in certain cities. Hospitalization was significantly more likely among the elderly and occurred at a rate that would be impossible to accommodate today (due to population growth).[121] The characteristics of this pandemic indicated a lack of progress in public health intervention strategies and medical science between the 1957 and 1968 pandemics. Only 10 years prior, we also lost over a million lives but seemed to reproduce many of the same mistakes.

Consequently, while vaccine production was accelerated and scientific collaborations were far better than prior epidemiological "attacks," we could have done a lot better. So why didn't we? To begin with, the world was largely divided over the Vietnam War at the time, and the salient racial / ethnic disparities in the United States (and across the world) precipitated fierce and formidable protests across the globe. Great political divides and associated distrust of systems were ongoing at the time. The world was a tinderbox and so subsumed by moral indignation that both the communities and the government may have wanted to brush this "little bug" under the proverbial rug. Fortunately, the relatively low morbidity and mortality (especially after the first wave in the United States) and the virus's predilection for the very young and old made it easier for us to do that.

Moreover, some prior immunity may have been generated by the 1957 pandemic, despite the formidable antigenic drift (table 5.1). This happens every year with certain viruses, when particles that compose the virus change enough to escape the immune system of the hosts it infects, which is why an effective vaccine for flu is an ongoing challenge. All this was chance and helped to prevent outcomes similar to the 1918 precedent but was far in excess of what it could have been. Moreover, as racial/ethnic riots were pervasive at the time and the United States was generally affected by "population stress," the ability of certain communities to protect themselves from disproportionate impacts was certainly affected. Unfortunately, that level of detail regarding the disparity of epidemiological outcomes along sociopolitical lines is unclear, as the research was simply not available at the time, as D'Adamo and team pointed out.[58]

Table 5.1. Comparison of antigenic shift and drift among influenza viruses

Drift	Shift
Minor change within subtype	Major change, new subtype
Point mutations	Exchange of gene segments
Occurs in A and B subtypes	Occurs in A subtypes only
May cause epidemics	May cause pandemic
Example: A/Fujian (H3N2) replaced A/Panama (H3N2) in 2003–2004	Example: H3N2 replaced H2N2 in 1968

Source: S. Al Hajjar and K. McIntosh. "The First Influenza Pandemic of the 21st Century." Annals of Saudi Medicine 30, no. 1 (2010): 1–10. https://doi.org/10.4103 /0256-4947.59365.

Given the analysis above, let's review our rubric (below), shall we? Is there a sociopolitical link to the original spread? Between the initial spread of the disease in China, given the impact of the Cultural Revolution on both spread and mitigation, as well as the Vietnam War fomenting the spread back from Asia to the United States (and beyond), this piece is irrefutable. But was there also a lack of public and community health infrastructure? This question is more challenging to address, as the answer is mixed.

We can acknowledge some accelerated surveillance and vaccination efforts globally but at the same time flag this development as not uniform or universal (namely, not in China) and muted as a result of the Vietnam war and Cultural Revolution, respectively. Then the response was not substantively improved by a nearly identical global distribution of disease just 10 years prior, suggesting that the infrastructure was lacking. We'll let the reader determine this for themself. If we assume that the former was true, I believe it is implied that this did spread, or, at the very least, dilute mitigation or control. Was the lack of infrastructure sociopolitically linked? Absolutely. Could we have done better? It is difficult to dispute that better information to communities (including better bidirectional dialogue with governmental

Hong Kong Flu: Rubric for determining the sociopolitical determinants of pandemics and PHEICs

	Sociopolitical determinant-linked questionnaire	Yes	No
1	Is there a sociopolitical link to the original spread of disease?	☐	☐
2	Was there a lack of public and community health infrastructure at the time?	☐	☐
3	If yes, did the lack of infrastructure at the time of spread precipitate more widespread distribution?	☐	☐
4	Was the lack of infrastructure at the time linked to a sociopolitical root cause?	☐	☐
5	Is it treatable? In other words, would building more effective sociopolitical infrastructure mitigate the risk of spread?	☐	☐

and scientific institutions and agencies), more effective and equitable distribution of resources, and more transparency would have led to far fewer infections and related deaths. In summary, depending on the reader's interpretation of number 2, I would score this between 60% and 100%. What do you think? Let's move now to the current century with yet another flu pandemic and assess how the development and response changed, shall we?

Swine Flu, 2009–2010

In April 2009 a new, fast-spreading influenza virus jumped from pigs to humans, becoming a global pandemic in just a few months. Its porcine source inevitably led to the memorable moniker "the swine flu." This time the reservoir was different from the birds of the past (figure 5.9).

Clinical Manifestations

Much like the clinical manifestations seen in prior influenza pandemics, those of the novel 2009 influenza A (H1N1) virus varied from asymptomatic infection to serious fatal illness that included worsening of other underlying conditions or severe viral pneumonia with multiorgan failure. The CDC defined cases as ILI as a fever of >37.8°C (>100°F) plus cough and/or sore throat in the absence of a known cause other than influenza. In the 2009 outbreak of the "swine flu" pandemic in New York City, 95% of virologically proven cases satisfied the ILI definition. Vomiting and/or diarrhea occurred in up to 38% of outpatients in the United States. Symptoms usually lasted 4–6 days. Young children sometimes had atypical influenza illness with the absence of fever and cough. One case study described 89 children with confirmed H1N1 who required hospitalization in Birmingham, United Kingdom. The most common symptoms were fever (81%), cough (73%), and diarrhea (62%).[122] Infants often presented with fever and lethargy.

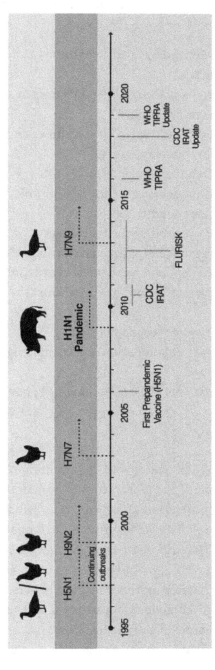

FIGURE 5.9. Flu pandemics and their animal reservoirs. Combined timeline indicates the temporal relationships between emerging potential pandemic strains (with accompanying animal reservoirs) and steps taken to improve pandemic preparedness. *Source:* Walter N. Harrington, "The Evolution and Future of Influenza Pandemic Preparedness," *Experimental & Molecular Medicine* 53 (2021): 737–749, https://doi.org/10.1038/s12276-021-00603-0.

Three categories of clinical presentations were seen during the 2009 pandemic:[122]

1. Mild illness characterized by fever, cough, sore throat, diarrhea, myalgias, and headache
2. Progressive illness characterized by mild illness in addition to the following signs or symptoms:
   a. Chest pain, rapid breathing, or labored breathing in children
   b. Hypotension (low blood pressure)
   c. Confusion or altered mental status
   d. Severe dehydration or exacerbation of a chronic conditions (e.g., asthma, heart conditions)
3. Severe illness characterized by the following:
   a. Profound hypoxemia (low oxygen levels in the blood), abnormal chest X-ray, and mechanical ventilation
   b. Encephalitis (brain infection) or encephalopathy (brain disease)
   c. Shock and multisystem organ failure
   d. Myocarditis (heart inflammation) and rhabdomyolysis (muscle explosion)
   e. Invasive secondary bacterial infection (e.g., pneumonia)

Epidemiology

Evidence of the person-to-person spread of swine-origin influenza viruses (SIVs) is very limited, and most swine-to-human transmissions have been epidemiologically dead-end events (i.e., onward transmissions are incredibly rare). The H1N1 virus was a known exception. (Remember where the H and N come from in the 1918 pandemic description; see figures 5.2 and 5.3.) In the spring of 2009, it was first detected in the United States and spread quickly across the world. This new virus contained a unique combination of influenza genes not previously identified in animals or humans. This virus had two genes from influenza viruses that normally circulate in pigs in Europe and

Asia and three genes that normally circulate in North American pigs, as well as genes from influenza viruses from birds and humans. Few young people had any existing immunity against this virus (as detected by antibody response), but nearly one-third of people >60 years old did, likely from prior exposure to an H1N1 virus earlier in their lives.[123] Vaccination with seasonal influenza vaccines offered little cross-protection against infection with this virus, even though they contained H1N1 strains.

Although this virus is likely of swine origin, it has not (to date) been detected in pigs prior to its appearance in humans. Human infections with swine influenza have been sporadically detected (or at least published in the literature) since the late 1950s. These findings usually occurred in people with direct and indirect exposure to pigs (i.e., people working in pig farms, etc.) The first significant outbreak of an avian A (H1N1) influenza virus lineage occurred in 1979 and led to the establishment of an avian-like A (H1N1) virus lineage in European pigs. So contrary to popular opinion, despite being informally called swine flu the H1N1 flu virus cannot be spread by eating pork products. Who comes up with this stuff? Similar to other influenza viruses, it is typically contracted through respiratory droplet transmission.[124] The incubation period range is one to four days (mean of two days).

As described in the 1918 flu pandemic section, the emergence of the 2009 pandemic A(H1N1) virus was a result of a reassortment event between a North American *triple-reassortment* swine influenza virus and a European avian-like A(H1N1) (H1avN1) influenza virus. Since its introduction into the European swine population, it has reassorted broadly with the circulating swine A(H1N1), A(H3N2), and A(H1N2) subtypes. The pH1N1 HA had evolved from the avian-origin 1918 pandemic influenza H1N1 virus, which is thought to have entered human and swine populations at about the same time but to have evolved into distinct lineages in pigs and in humans. Early serologic (blood-based) studies suggested that many older adults had some cross-reactive immunity to the pH1N1 HA due to prior infection with related strains

Table 5.2. Timeline of genetic reassortment of H1N1 from 1918 to 2009

Time	Event
1918–1919	H1N1 pandemic also affected swine
1930	First isolation of H1N1 in pigs
1968	H3N2 infect swine in Asia after human pandemic
1976	Outbreak of new H1N1 swine strain of A/New Jersey/1976 occurred in military personnel at Fort Dix, New Jersey
1998	Triple reassortant viruses were isolated from pigs
1958–2005	37 human swine-origin influenza viruses were reported
2005–2009	11 sporadic triple reassortant swine influenza viruses were reported in humans
2009	New quadruple reassorted swine influenza H1N1 strain (A/California/07/2009) emerged in human populations and caused a global influenza pandemic

Source: S. Al Hajjar and K. McIntosh. "The First Influenza Pandemic of the 21st Century." *Annals of Saudi Medicine* 30, no. 1 (2010): 1–10. https://doi.org /10.4103/0256-4947.59365.

(dating back to 1918). Children and most young adults, however, were immunologically naive (no prior antibodies). Sorry, I know it's a lot of numbers and letters, but this is relevant for this pandemic, you'll see. Stay with me. The timeline in table 5.2 will help.

The A(H1N1) influenza virus from 2009 contained genes from pig, bird, and human influenza viruses in a combination that had not been reported before in any part of the world. Following the emergence of the 2009 pandemic, this virus was also isolated from pigs in multiple areas of the world (including Europe), and it is currently circulating in pigs in several European countries. The infections in swine were initially due to transmission from infected humans and then subsequently spread through pig-to-pig transmission.

As with prior flu pandemics of the 20th century, the 2009 swine flu pandemic demonstrated wave behavior, with timing varying geographically. In Mexico, for example, a three-wave pandemic profile was identified, with spring, summer, and fall waves. Pandemic peaks in the rest of North America were more consistent with a two-wave profile, with spring–summer (March 29–August 2, 2009) and fall (August 2–December 31, 2009) waves.[125] Within one week in April 2009 in the United States, 10 cases had been confirmed in three states, and investigations of probable cases were underway in six additional states. This first wave peaked during June 2009, and by August influenza activity levels had decreased substantially in most states, although activity was sustained throughout the summer months at levels substantially above what is normally seen during the summer for seasonal influenza. The second pandemic wave began in the southeastern United States as children returned to school in mid-August and early September. Over the following two months, the disease became geographically widespread throughout the United States. Illness occurring during this fall wave ultimately accounted for the majority of US cases seen during the pandemic. The fall wave peaked in late October, and since that time, although the circulation of pH1N1 virus has continued, influenza activity has decreased and remained below what is expected in the winter months.[126]

Several research groups have made estimates of the global death toll from the swine flu, which range from 130,000 to 1.87 million people worldwide.[127] An estimated 284,400 people died from infection during the first year alone.[128] Between April 2009 and April 2010, the CDC estimated there were more than 60 million cases, 274,000 hospitalizations, and 12,000 deaths in the United States. Globally, 80% of deaths were estimated to have occurred in people <65 years of age, which differs substantially from typical seasonal influenza epidemics (approximately 70–90% are ≥65 years).[129]

Historical Timeline

While the 2009 outbreak represented the appearance of a new virus, the swine flu had been around in some form since 1919. Memorably, an outbreak in 1976 had caused then-president Gerald Ford to order a mass immunization program in the United States.

Although the most straightforward explanation was that the new virus originated in swine in Mexico (it was first identified in a 5-year-old boy in a rural town in Veracruz), several studies suggested that this was unlikely because key genetic components of the virus had never been detected in the Americas. Much like the first few cases in Mexico, on April 15, 2009, the first case of the H1NI virus in the United States was identified in a child (a 10-year-old boy in Southern California); two days later, a second case was confirmed in a 9-year-old girl in an adjacent county in California. Why? As most parents know, children are intractably drawn to poop. During the subsequent two weeks, additional cases of infection with this new virus were detected in Mexico, California, Texas, and other states.[130]

In response to the swine flu virus, in late April 2009 the WHO declared its first-ever PHEIC and on June 11 declared it a pandemic. The extent of global trade and travel allowed swine flu to spread as widely in 6 weeks as past pandemics had in 6 months (recall it had been 40 years since the last flu pandemic). By July, infection was reported in 122 countries, with 134,000 laboratory-confirmed cases and 800 deaths.[122] Ultimately, it would be reported in 212 countries and overseas territories.

Fortunately, the response to the 2009 H1N1 pandemic, particularly in North America and Europe, demonstrated a significantly improved level of preparedness relative to past pandemics. This was the result of a number of factors, including heightened public health emergency preparedness efforts catalyzed by the earlier SARS outbreak of 2002–2003 and persisting fears surrounding H5N1 avian flu. Containment efforts employed a combination of pharmaceutical and nonpharmaceutical (supportive) interventions. The swine flu pandemic notably marked the first pandemic response combining both vaccination and antiviral use (as antiviral technology was largely lacking 40 years prior). In the United Kingdom, for example, an aggressive containment campaign combined school closures and voluntary isolation with antiviral treatment for suspected cases and mass prophylaxis of potential contacts; these interventions helped control the outbreak until more information could be gathered.

In Canada the largest mass immunization program in the nation's history was carried out, with the federal government investing $400 million to purchase 50 million doses. Recommendations were subsequently made by the CDC Advisory Committee on Immunization Practice (ACIP). Based on their guidance, high-priority groups were the first to receive vaccination, before it was expanded to all just a few weeks later (as more supply became available; recall this same practice with COVID-19). While Canada celebrated the impressive public health feat of covering approximately 33–50% of its population over the remainder of the pandemic, vaccination coverage was lower in the United States (with state averages from 12.9% to 38.8%) and much of Europe, with the exception of Norway (45%) and Sweden (59%). Again, we see more examples of the toxic effects of vaccine hesitancy. Unfortunately, there was little use of antivirals before September 2009, though awareness campaigns targeting primary care physicians increased their use to treat patients later in the pandemic.[131]

Nonpharmaceutical measures applied in response to past pandemics were again widely implemented to help contain the pandemic. The most common among these were recommendations for hand hygiene and voluntary isolation of symptomatic individuals. The United States, United Kingdom, and Australia did recommend and implement school closures, for example. While understanding of the influenza virus's properties and transmission was by this point fairly advanced, weaknesses in maintaining consistent diagnostic protocols presented challenges for surveillance efforts. Officials tracking data on hospitalization, intensive care admission, and mortality struggled to generate relevant surveillance data to inform decisions in real time. This was the case in a number of countries.[131]

The mass vaccine efforts this time were impressive—especially in the United States. The US Food and Drug Administration (FDA) had approved multiple formulations of the vaccine in mid-September 2009;

a national vaccination program was initiated in October. In July 2009, estimating that initial vaccine supplies could be insufficient to meet demand, the ACIP recommended priority groups for the vaccination program. This same practice would famously play out again in 2020 with COVID-19.

As the science had improved by leaps and bounds since the 1968 pandemic, studies were actually able to determine how many lives were saved as a result of the vaccine effort. In one study conducted by Borse et al., they estimated that from October 3, 2009 to April 18, 2010, the mass immunization program was 62% effective in directly preventing 712,908–1,458,930 clinical cases, 3,923–10,393 hospitalizations, and 201–520 deaths in the United States. A million lives were spared of infection in the United States alone.[132] That's not bad, but could it have been better? Borse et al. also calculated the effects of earlier vaccine administration on the number of clinical cases prevented and found that if the vaccine program had begun one, two, or eight weeks earlier, the number of clinical cases prevented would have increased by 27%, 59%, and 306% compared with the base estimate, respectively.

The pandemic began to taper off in November 2009, and by May 2010 the number of cases was in steep decline. On August 10, 2010, the director general of the WHO, Margaret Chan, announced the end of the H1N1 pandemic.

Sociopolitical Determinants

As presented during the section on the 1918 pandemic, D'Adamo et al. conducted a systematic review on the disparities between flu pandemics of the 20th / 21st centuries and demonstrated some consistent and compelling findings. Eight studies had examined socioeconomic factors in the 2009 pandemic, with data far more advanced and specific, based on the recency of this pandemic. Balter et al. reported hospitalization rates two times higher in high-poverty neighborhoods than in low-poverty neighborhoods in New York City.[133] Similarly, Rutter et al. found that influenza mortality rates were three times higher in the least affluent compared to the most affluent areas of England. One study examining neighborhood-level factors in Ontario, Canada, found that during the first and second 2009 pandemic waves, hospitalized individuals were more likely to have a lower education level and live in deprived neighborhoods than those who were not hospitalized and lived in such neighborhoods.[134] Similarly, in a study examining the association between education level and hospitalizations in New York City, adults with no education beyond high school had a 4.5-times greater chance of hospitalization than adults with some college education, and those without a high school education had 32 times higher chance than those with some college education. Get it? The poorer and less educated you are, the higher the likelihood of getting flu, becoming hospitalized, or dying.

That research also found 13 studies exploring racial / ethnic disparities in the 2009 pandemic, compared to 0 for the 1968 pandemic. Across included studies on the 2009 pandemic in the United States, minority communities generally had higher incidence, mortality, or hospitalization rates than whites. Hispanic populations also experienced an elevated risk of exposure to pandemic influenza in 2009 compared to all other groups. Individuals of low SES, or living in areas of low SES, also experienced worse outcomes, including higher mortality in 1918.

During the 2009 pandemic, both SES and race / ethnicity predicted influenza incidence, hospitalization, and intensive care unit (ICU) stay. For example, factors that low-income minority populations tend to disproportionately experience, such as household overcrowding, inability to engage in social distancing because of work, a lack of sick leave and paid time off, and job insecurity, predict influenza-like-illness incidence. These same factors (as well as more limited access to health care and greater susceptibility to severe disease because of underlying structural inequities) likely contributed to the persistent socioeconomic and racial disparities identified in the included articles. For example, neighborhood disinvestment has led to a range of structural housing conditions and employment with inadequate protections and crowded working conditions, which potentially increase the risk of exposure to the viruses that cause pandemic influenza. Additionally, non-white populations that experience overcrowding, lower household income, and lower educational attainment than their white counterparts tend to lack information on preventive measures and are at an increased risk of hospitalization.

Black and Hispanic populations in the United States had generally worse outcomes in the 2009 pandemic as compared to the white population. One study based in Illinois reported that hospitalization rates were two to three times greater for Black and Latinx populations than white populations. Moreover, in Wisconsin the hospitalization rates were highest among Black, Hispanic, and Asian residents, especially in Milwaukee. Two nationwide studies in the United States also found that the Hispanic population most often lacked access to health care and were at higher risk of exposure. Pediatric deaths were also highest among Hispanic residents and lowest among white residents in the United States. Castrodale et al. examined mortality rates among 10 US states and found that American Indian / Alaska Native individuals experienced a mortality rate four times higher than those in all other racial / ethnic groups combined during the pandemic. A study by Quinn et al. of the US population found that Black individuals had the highest susceptibility to complications based on a prevalence of chronic conditions compared to white and Hispanic individuals. The study by Navaranjan et al., based in Canada, found that those who tested positive for influenza were more likely to be of East / Southeast Asian, South Asian, and Black ethnicity compared to test-negative controls.

D'Adamo et al. only found one study comparing multiple pandemics (including 1918, 1957, and 2009 flu pandemics) in New Zealand, which analyzed mortality rates for Indigenous peoples (Māori), as compared to people of European ancestry. The Māori had mortality rates 7.3, 6.2, and 2.6 times higher than persons of European ancestry during the 1918, 1957, and 2009 pandemics, respectively.

Time for the grading pens again, but I hope this one will be simpler. Was there a sociopolitical link to the original spread? Not this time.

Cases first emerged in Mexico (arguably) and shortly thereafter in the United States. There were no relevant world wars or mass sociopolitical events taking place at the time. Was there a lack of public and community health infrastructure? Absolutely. As the multiple studies have consistently demonstrated, poverty, education, race / ethnicity, and all other social determinants listed in part I (and included again here as a refresher) seem to have had a formidable influence on this pandemic, including the following:

- Economic stability
- Education access and quality
- Health care access and quality (health equity)
- Neighborhood and built environment
- Social and community context

As the research suggests, these factors clearly had an effect here with these significantly higher rates of infection, hospitalization, and death among certain groups. Hopefully, the rest of the rubric is easier to judge this time with all of this contemporaneous research to help guide our thinking. The social epidemiological research of the 21st century has been a game changer in terms of highlighting the need for more

Swine Flu: Rubric for determining the sociopolitical determinants of pandemics and PHEICs

	Sociopolitical determinant–linked questionnaire	Yes	No
1	Is there a sociopolitical link to the original spread of disease?	☐	☐
2	Was there a lack of public and community health infrastructure at the time?	☐	☐
3	If yes, did the lack of infrastructure at the time of spread precipitate more widespread distribution?	☐	☐
4	Was the lack of infrastructure at the time linked to a sociopolitical root cause?	☐	☐
5	Is it treatable? In other words, would building more effective sociopolitical infrastructure mitigate the risk of spread?	☐	☐

interventions. Hopefully, the next three pandemics will help to concretize this thinking. By the way, I grade this as an 80% likelihood of sociopolitical determination, but it's up to you to agree with me or not.

HIV/AIDS, 1981–

It's time to transition from flu to a completely different type of virus. Around 1980, and much to their own astonishment, physicians detected the existence of a disease that seemed "new" because they thought they had never seen it before. HIV/AIDS would go on to become a defining feature of the next three decades, with massive social, cultural, and political implications in addition to its obvious public health impact.

AIDS is a disease emanating from infection with HIV. According to the definition imposed by the CDC at the beginning of 1983 and later adopted by the WHO, AIDS was characterized by the onset of a syndrome of either malignancy or infectious manifestations from opportunistic organisms, or by the two together, in adults under 60 years of age with no previous underlying pathology or immunosuppressive therapy. The virus was isolated in 1978–1979, but its role as a causal agent for AIDS was only truly realized beginning in 1984.

Clinical Manifestations

Okay. This one is complicated. There are so many stereotypical images of this disease—most of which are erroneous. Let's try to simplify it. First of all, HIV infection can be divided into the following stages:

- Acute HIV infection (also called primary HIV infection or acute seroconversion syndrome, among other terms)
- Chronic HIV infection, which can be further subdivided into the following stages:
  - Chronic infection, without AIDS
  - AIDS, characterized by a CD4 cell count <200 cells/μm (microliter) or the presence of any AIDS-defining condition

Acute HIV Infection

An estimated 10–60% of individuals with early HIV infection will not experience symptoms at all. In patients who have acute symptomatic infection, the usual time from HIV exposure to the development of symptoms is 2 to 4 weeks, although incubation periods as long as 10 months have been observed.[135]

A variety of symptoms and signs may be seen in association with acute symptomatic HIV infection. This constellation of symptoms is also known as acute retroviral syndrome. When symptoms do appear, the most common findings are fever, swollen lymph nodes, sore throat, rash, muscle and joint aches, diarrhea, weight loss, and headaches.[136,137,138,139,140,141]

A generalized rash is also a common finding in symptomatic acute HIV infection. The eruption typically occurs 48–72 hours after the onset of fever and persists for 5–8 days. Since the GI tract is a primary target during acute infection, patients with acute HIV infection often complain of nausea, diarrhea, anorexia, and weight loss averaging five kilograms. More serious GI manifestations are rare and include pancreatitis and hepatitis.[142,143] Finally, headache, often described as eye pain exacerbated by eye movement, frequently accompanies acute HIV infection.

Chronic HIV Infection

Following primary infection, seroconversion (generating antibodies to the virus), and the establishment of the viral set point is a period of chronic HIV infection characterized by relative stability of the viral level and a progressive decline in the CD4 cell count (or white blood cells, otherwise known as your *T cells*). I like to describe this as the immunological "defense army" or "brick wall" intended to protect from outside microbial invaders (i.e., lurking microbes that typically would not get into your house). In the absence of highly active antiretroviral therapy (HAART; the mainstay of treatment for HIV), the average time from HIV acquisition to a CD4 cell count <200 cells/ μm is approximately 8–10 years.

Most folks with HIV have few to no symptoms prior to developing severe immunosuppression (when the CD4 count declines to <200 cells/µm). Some patients experience generalized / nonspecific symptoms and signs such as fatigue, sweats, persistently swollen lymph nodes, or weight loss. The quintessential image of AIDS made famous in the 1980s and early 1990s in movies such as *Philadelphia* is (generally speaking) no longer relevant in the Global North. For the most part, 80% of our patients are well controlled. It is the 20% who are not that we must worry about—most of which is socially driven. The Global South has come leaps and bounds since the 1980s but still has room for improvement until it matches the success of its northern counterpart.

AIDS is the outcome of chronic HIV infection and consequent depletion of CD4 cells (T cells). It is defined as a CD4 cell count <200 cells/µm or the presence of any AIDS-defining condition (generally opportunistic infections, or those bugs generally lurking around that would never get into the house, or other unique conditions, such as cancer) regardless of the CD4 cell count. The term "advanced HIV infection" is often used to refer to infection when the CD4 cell count is <50 cells/µm. The good news is that the dystopian term "AIDS" is reversible. When a patient's CD4 cell count increases to >200 cells/µm with ART and they have no AIDS-defining conditions, they are no longer considered to have AIDS.

Prior to the introduction and widespread use of combination HAART, AIDS-associated illnesses were the principal cause of morbidity and mortality associated with HIV infection. Some classic ones are *Pneumocystis jirovecii* pneumonia, which helped define the disease in an edition of the CDC's *Morbidity and Mortality Weekly Report* on June 5, 1981, in a cluster of rare pneumonias among patients at the University of California, Los Angeles, hospital, most of whom identified as gay males.[144] This was the proverbial "shot heard around the world." Some others are TB, *Mycobacterium avium* complex infections, and oral and esophageal candidiasis (or thrush), respectively (table 5.3).

While mortality from opportunistic illnesses has become much less common with the widespread use of effective HAART, death from AIDS

Table 5.3. A list of acquired immune deficiency syndrome (AIDS)-defining conditions

Bacterial infections, multiple or current

Candidiasis of bronchi, trachea, or lungs

Candidiasis of esophagus

Cervical cancer, invasive

Coccidioidomycosis, disseminated or extrapulmonary

Cryptococcosis, extrapulmonary

Cryptosporidiosis, chronic intestinal (>1 month's duration)

Cytomegalovirus disease (other than liver, spleen, or nodes), onset at age >1 month

Cytomegalovirus retinitis (with loss of vision)

Encephalopathy, HIV-related

Herpes simplex causing chronic ulcers (>1 month's duration) or bronchitis, pneumonitis, or esophagitis (onset at age >1 month)

Histoplasmosis, disseminated or extrapulmonary

Isosporiasis, chronic intestinal (>1 month's duration)

Kaposi's sarcoma

Lymphoma, Burkitt (or equivalent term)

Lymphoma, immunoblastic (or equivalent term)

Lymphoma, primary, of brain

Mycobacterium avium complex or *Mycobacterium kansasii*, disseminated or extrapulmonary

Mycobacterium tuberculosis of any site, pulmonary, disseminated, or extrapulmonary

Pneumocystis jirovecii pneumonia

Pneumonia, recurrent

Progressive multifocal leukoencephalopathy

Salmonella septicemia, recurrent

Toxoplasmosis of brain, onset age at >1 month

Wasting syndrome attributed to HIV

Source: B. R. Wood. *The Natural History and Clinical Features of HIV Infection in Adults and Adolescents*. Adapted from UpToDate. https://www.uptodate.com/contents/3724.

still occurs in individuals with late diagnosis and those who have difficulty engaging in care or adhering to HAART. In the absence of effective HAART, the median survival time for patients with advanced HIV infection (CD4 cell count <50 cells/μm) is 12–18 months.[145,146] With effective treatment, however, the prognosis for an individual with AIDS or advanced HIV improves dramatically. In fact, most recent studies demonstrate nearly no difference in survival (between an HIV+ person when compared to the general population) if early treatment takes place.

Epidemiology

The molecular description of HIV can be complex, so I will try to simplify as much as possible. Worldwide, there are two types of HIV: HIV-1, which originated from simian immunodeficiency virus (SIV) strains in apes, and HIV-2, which originated from an SIV strain in sooty mangabey monkeys. Yes, it did originate from apes and monkeys. HIV-1, by far, is the most prominent type and is further divided into different groups and subtypes. The main clinical implications of these different types of HIV are that infection with HIV-2 appears to have a slower natural history than HIV-1 and is intrinsically resistant to certain antiretroviral agents. HIV-2 is endemic to West Africa and is rarely seen in the United States. It is estimated to cause approximately 5% of global HIV infections.

By the end of 2021, the reported statistics on the global burden of HIV were as follows:[147,148]

- 38.4 million adults and 1.7 million children (<15 years old) were living with HIV/AIDS.
- 1.5 million adults and 160,000 children were newly infected with HIV that year.
- 552,000 adults and 98,000 children died of AIDS that year.

The overall prevalence of HIV globally appears to have stabilized (at 0.7%) but continues to rise in some countries (ironically, this is a good thing), likely due to increased survival of infected people because of HAART. Nearly 60% of the world's population that has HIV is in sub-Saharan Africa (this is down from nearly 80% in the late 1990s). Countries in sub-Saharan Africa and the Caribbean have the highest national rates of adult HIV prevalence, exceeding 25% in some sub-Saharan countries.[147,148] The highest HIV prevalence rate in the world is in Swaziland (27.2%). In terms of sheer numbers of the population with HIV within sub-Saharan Africa, 25% are in South Africa and 13% in Nigeria.[149]

Children bear a substantial proportion of the burden of HIV, both directly and indirectly.[147,148] When we look at new infections, 70% were born in sub-Saharan Africa, 25% in Southeast Asia, and the remainder in Latin America and the Caribbean.[147,150] Additionally, it is estimated that 25 million children have been orphaned by AIDS.

One of the motivating factors for me to enter the world of medicine in the late 1990s / early 2000s (especially infectious diseases) was interning in sub-Saharan Africa (SSA; namely Uganda and South Africa) and seeing hundreds of children . . . babies . . . infected with this "viral grim reaper." It's heart-wrenching. Fortunately, with major advancements in obstetric care in addition to the improvement and equitable access of HAART, these numbers have dramatically declined. Those achievements notwithstanding, even one is tragic, and the current numbers are far higher than that. In fact, over 2 million infants are born to women with HIV annually (this includes breast milk).

Globally, HIV/AIDS was one of the top-10 causes of death from the 1990s to 2010s, mainly driven by the mortality associated with HIV in SSA, where it was the primary cause of death.[151] Due to a marked increase in access to HAART, however, AIDS-related mortality has declined by 45% since 2010. Wow. Pause on this for a minute. Approximately 10% of the world's population lives in SSA, but the region is home to almost two-thirds of the global HIV burden.[152]

After SSA, the Caribbean has the second-highest HIV prevalence rates in the world.[147,148] In 2021, the 16 countries in the Caribbean region accounted for 330,000 people living with HIV; overall HIV prevalence was 1.1%. An estimated 6 million individuals with HIV (15% of the global total) live in Asia and the Pacific islands.

Nevertheless, low prevalence in massive Asian populations can result in substantial HIV burdens. As an example, don't be fooled by India's low national adult HIV prevalence rate of 0.2%, as it translates into an estimated 2.4 million people. In fact, this is one of the highest figures in the world (and was the highest when I worked there in 2004 with United Nations International Children's Emergency Fund [UNICEF] or the UN Children's Fund). The HIV epidemic in the Middle East and North Africa (MENA) is growing (one of the only areas in the world where it is actually worsening). It has increased in prevalence by 33% since 2010.[147,148] Moving across the globe, there are 1.8 million HIV infections in the Eastern European and central Asia region (including the Russian Federation), where there is an urgent need to scale-up HIV prevention services.[147,153] HIV prevalence averages 0.9%, but Eastern Europe / Central Asia is one of only three regions (along with the MENA) where the HIV epidemic is growing (an increase in prevalence of 48% since 2010 and AIDS-related deaths by 24%). In the United States, we have an estimated 1.2 million persons living with HIV.

How is HIV transmitted? Unfortunately, this has been so poorly understood historically by lay communities worldwide. Through decades of dedication from battalions of educators, we have certainly made great strides in terms of the world's understanding of the disease—and especially mitigating the associated stigma. Let's reflect on the origins of our framing of this disease. The earliest names of "morbus Gallicus," "gay pneumonia," "gay-related immune deficiency (GRID)," or "gay compromise syndrome" were radically inappropriate and inaccurate. For historians these names are interesting, precisely to the extent that they reveal medical bias and either national or moral prejudice. Once the universality of this disease was recognized, a more accurate system of nomenclature substituted the former—AIDS (which still was not even entirely sufficient as a stand-alone disease).

Today, the major modes of acquiring HIV infection are as follows:[154,155]

- Sexual activity
- Needles (predominantly among people who inject drugs)
- Mother-to-child

The relative importance of these different modes of transmission in driving the HIV pandemic varies geographically and has evolved over time. The risk of getting HIV varies widely depending on the type of exposure or behavior (such as sharing needles or having sex without a condom). Some exposures to HIV carry a much higher risk of transmission than others. For some exposures (e.g., oral sex), while transmission is biologically possible, the risk is so low that it is not possible to put a precise number on it. Risks add up over time, however, so that even behavior with relatively small risk can accrue and lead to a high lifetime risk of HIV infection (table 5.4).

More than 80% of infections worldwide occur through heterosexual (male-female) transmission, and over 50% of all people with HIV in the world are female.[156] These statistics reflect the situation in SSA (where most HIV exists) and where heterosexual transmission is the main contributor to the HIV pandemic.[157,158]

Conversely, males are far more likely to be infected in the Global North. This, in part, reflects the epidemic among men who have sex with men (MSM), who are 19 times more likely than the general population to have HIV.[159] In some resource-rich settings, despite high rates of testing and access to HAART the incidence of HIV infection among MSM has increased, while the incidence from other modes of transmission has trended downward. Currently, MSM transmission accounts for approximately 70% of newly diagnosed HIV infections in the United States. The HIV epidemic is particularly pronounced among MSM throughout Latin America and in certain Caribbean countries (e.g., approximately 30% of MSM in Jamaica are living with HIV).[147,148]

Table 5.4. Estimated risk for acquisition of HIV by exposure route

Type of exposure	Risk per 10,000 exposures
Parenteral	
Blood transfusion	9,250
Needle-sharing during injection drug use	63
Percutaneous (needle stick)	23
Sexual	
Receptive anal intercourse	138
Insertive anal intercourse	11
Receptive penile-vaginal intercourse	8
Insertive penile-vaginal intercourse	4
Receptive oral intercourse	Low
Insertive oral intercourse	Low
Other*	
Biting	Negligible
Spitting	Negligible
Throwing body fluids (including semen or saliva)	Negligible
Sharing sex toys	Negligible

Source: Centers for Disease Control and Prevention. *HIV Risk Behaviors*. November 13, 2019. https://www.cdc.gov/hiv/risk/estimates/riskbehaviors.html.

Note: Factors that may increase the risk of HIV transmission include sexually transmitted diseases, acute and late-stage HIV infection, and high viral load. Factors that may decrease the risk include condom use, male circumcision, antiretroviral treatment, preexposure prophylaxis. None of these factors are accounted for in the estimates presented.

* HIV transmission through these exposure routes is technically possible but unlikely and not well documented.

While the rates of sexual transmission have historically been the most formidable, there are increasingly more outbreaks among injecting drug users (IDUs)—especially in the southern United States. This is a big focus of mine currently. Actually, outside of SSA, IDUs account for approximately 30% of new HIV infections—driven especially by increasing epidemics in Central and Eastern Europe and in some countries of Asia.[160] It is also a major concern in industrialized nations and MENA, which is what is largely driving those spikes as described above. We can effectively prevent these outbreaks if we focus on what works.

Historical Timeline

While AIDS was only recognized in 1981 (June 5 in that famed CDC *Morbidity and Mortality Weekly Report*), molecular studies indicate that HIV was present in Central and West Africa beginning in the early 1900s, likely in localized populations.[161] The current pandemic may have emerged from these populations in the mid-1900s with improved access to transport and other societal changes.[162] This probably took place in Zaire (currently the Democratic Republic of the Congo, or DRC). Additional molecular studies suggest that HIV evolved from SIV, which has been found in some subspecies of monkeys on Bioko (an island off the African coast) and some subspecies of chimpanzees in Cameroon.[163,164] Researchers believe that all the SIV strains infecting primates across Africa diverged from a common ancestor between 32,000 and 78,000 years ago.[164]

Let's be clear. AIDS is a disease emanating from infection with HIV. According to the definition imposed by the CDC at the beginning of 1983 and later adopted by the WHO, AIDS was characterized by the onset of a syndrome of either malignancy or infectious manifestations from opportunistic organisms, or by the two together, in adults under 60 years of age with no previous underlying pathology or immunosuppressive therapy. The virus was isolated in 1978–1979, but its role as a causal agent of AIDS was only truly realized beginning in 1984.

Earlier, we discussed some of the differences between HIV-1 and HIV-2. The first epidemic (caused by HIV-1) was identified in 1981. The second epidemic (caused by HIV-2) would most likely have gone unnoticed if the weight of the first had not sharpened the attention of physicians and guided the research of virologists.[165]

It is tempting to propose a single place of origin for the HIV-1 epidemic and to situate it in Africa. It still remains to be seen how the virus exactly escaped, however. It is as easy to imagine plausible scenarios as it is difficult to demonstrate their actual occurrence, but three pathways continue to dominate scientific speculation: Haiti, Cuba, and the Peace Corps.

Despite the long-standing existence of HIV-1 in Africa, its manifestations were relatively discrete, limited to sporadic cases, and most likely limited to one or more low-level endemic zones. AIDS in epidemic form is a recent phenomenon. We can track some outbreaks of aggressive Kaposi's sarcoma (KS; the skin cancer classically associated with AIDS) cases in equatorial Africa beginning in the 1950s. It became especially salient in the early 1960s among migrant workers who came down to South Africa from the central regions with highly malignant KS complicated by fatal meningitis (brain infection) and pneumonia.

The second epidemic (HIV-2) flared up in West Africa (independent of the first one), namely Senegal, The Gambia, the Cape Verde Islands, and especially the Republic of Guinea-Bissau, from which it spread to the Ivory Coast, Mali, and the Central African Republic. The disease was recognized in 1981 among these countries' refugees seeking medical care in Portugal and France, but its precise nature and the extent of its primary focus were not clear until somewhat later.

The viral isolations were key to control, as it allowed us to create serological screening exams in 1985 for HIV-1 (when ELISA, which became the gold-standard assay, was approved by the FDA). Testing was a game changer, and you'll see the importance of this when we discuss the future of syndemic management in chapter 7. The advent of Western blotting later improved the sensitivity of diagnostic tests, as it was available only two years later. Only after HIV-2 was isolated at the end of 1985 were specific serological tests available to perform systematic epidemiological studies.

Sociopolitical Determinants

In terms of models of how sociopolitical conditions determine the shape and fate of pandemics, HIV/AIDS is one of the most helpful in terms of crystallizing the connections. As SSA has been so heavily hit, it makes sense for us to examine some core ingredients that led to the sustained generation of this pandemic. This will take a bit more time than the other pandemics, so buckle up.

In the SSA of the 1980s, epidemiologists and public health specialists in development agencies greatly underestimated the potential magnitude of HIV/AIDS.[166] The risk-group paradigm fostered belief that
HIV/AIDS would largely be an urban disease in both biomedical and
popular circles. High risk was believed to be limited to bounded networks of "core transmitters." These included sex workers and their clients, the military, and long-distance truckers, all of whom were recognized as having multiple sex partners. Consequently, rural areas with
"traditional" sexual morality and practices would be spared. Since many
of SSA's populations were mainly rural, it was believed that the impact
of HIV/AIDS would be restricted. Certain critical social scientists, however, argued against this perspective, pointing to the multifactorial
constellation of forces that would likely cause HIV/AIDS to explode
across the subcontinent, including over a century of extensive colonialism, Christian ideologies, migrant labor exploitation, urbanization,
tribal customs, gender inequality and violence, and the practice of
Western biomedicine and epidemiology in African contexts (without
the appropriate time dedicated to cultural integration).

To add to the complexity of this spread, HIV is obviously sexually
transmitted (I like to say life is too), and these infections continue to
remain at the quintessence of the social determinant paradigm. A modern "plague" has a greater chance of spreading if it can be transmitted
during the most intimate and compulsive of human activities.[167] On few
occasions in history have laws successfully stopped people from having
sexual relations with each other. Precisely because the virus is transmitted sexually, it makes government and ensuing public health interventions particularly fraught. Perhaps no other single human behavior
is as heavily surrounded by cultural sensitivities and opinion differences
as the sexual transmission of HIV/AIDS—until 2019 anyhow.

Let's define a new concept. The social construction of disease is the
social, economic, political, cultural, and historical processes that contextualize or frame interpretations of social reality in various, distinctive ways. To be clear, the production (determinant) and construction
are different but connected. Our perception of disease is inextricably

linked to the determinants, particularly those that relate to sexuality, as society has often been divided by its outlook upon this extremely sensitive and misunderstood topic. This is especially the case with HIV in Africa given the Global North's hegemony, which has pigeonholed the truth about African sexual practices and ideologies throughout the 20th century. Sex is sex.

The social construction of HIV/AIDS attitudes that continue to persist today emanates from its initial discovery in the early 1980s. Due to HIV/AIDS classic modes of transmission in the Global North (i.e., intravenous use and sexual transmission, namely homosexual), it was originally constructed that "individuals such as you or me" were impermeable to the potential danger that it represented. Conversely, only people stigmatized in advance either by their behavior, ethnic origin, or some other sociopolitical determinants were the "ones truly in danger." In fact, during the time of its initial discovery some American epidemiologists coined the most susceptible groups as the "4-H Club": homosexuals, heroin addicts, Haitians, and hemophiliacs despite the fact that in 1983–1984, only 6% of Americans with HIV/AIDS were Haitians, and fewer than 1% were hemophiliacs (recall this is where the eponymous Ryan White programming would be transformative). Some replaced the last group with hookers, or simply added an additional number, bringing the fateful "club" to a membership of five. I would argue that the sixth H would be human beings.

We merely have to turn to the present and to perceptions of the "African AIDS pandemic," however, to recognize that these social constructions continue to retain extreme popularity and that a century of colonial rule and of a medicalized discourse on the "African" has had long-lasting effects. Rosenberg asserts that just as a playwright chooses a theme and manages plot development, so a particular society constructs its characteristic response to an epidemic.[168] The history of sexually transmitted infections (STIs) in Africa is deeply rooted in racism that is intrinsic to European conceptions, attitudes, and fantasies of Black sexuality. The fact that STIs were perceived to be so rampant in the SSA population (or Africans in general) led to the gross misunderstanding that Africans were by nature promiscuous and hence constitutionally predisposed to immorality. Let's be honest. This was the colonial mindset. In fact, early in the identification of HIV/AIDS, the scientific and medical community (i.e., the WHO) constructed a definition for "African AIDS" distinct from that of the West.

So let's reflect back to part I and consider some of the current sociopolitical drivers of HIV across the continents. In SSA, for example, a substantial proportion (roughly one-fourth; I'm simplifying, of course) of new infections are among special (we call them "key" populations and their sexual partners. Specifically, transgender women and sex workers represent high-risk groups.[169] In a study in eight sub-Saharan African countries, 33%, 28%, and 27% of transgender women said they had been physically attacked at some point, had been raped, or were too afraid to use health care services, respectively.[170] Studies on sex workers on the continent have reported similar findings. I'm currently working on a project on sexual and gender-based violence (SGBV) in the eastern DRC, an area some have tragically dubbed the "rape capital of the world."[171]

Respect for human life is commonly eviscerated within these caustic environments of perennial war (often precipitated by centuries of colonialism, which we will discuss below), thereby legitimizing murder and desensitizing rape. Militarized groups often use rape as an instrument of terror. Yet little of the world is aware of this epidemic. In a contemporary era now acutely aware of gender-based discrimination (#MeToo), how are such women forgotten? Such pervasive acts infect communities and provoke a constant state of fear and an internalized sense of weakness and hopelessness. This culture of violence bleeds into a feeling of collective inadequacy and humiliation among men (exacerbated by a lack of economic security), leading to a drive to procure a sense of power and domination.

India's social drivers are not materially different. In India, barriers to pandemic control include the lack of social acceptance of condoms and the legal ramifications of being gay that limit access and adherence to best-prevention practices.[172] I worked on an HIV project with UNICEF in the early 2000s in southern India on the perception of HIV among adolescents (specifically in Tamil Nadu). It was a beautiful project that allowed me to connect with thousands of youths, their educators, and their families. We quickly determined, however, that it was nearly impossible to conduct our research with clarity given the taboo on sexual education and discourse. How could we ask about the risk of HIV when we could not speak openly about the number one risk factor? A high HIV prevalence has also been found among the LGBTQIA+ (lesbian, gay, bisexual, transgender, queer / questioning, intersex, and asexual / aromantic / agender) population in other Asian countries, including Cambodia (9% among MSM and transgender females), Thailand (15%), and India (18%).[173] Of course, these numbers are classically underreported. High prevalence among sex workers is also a major contributor to the spread in this region, where it exceeds 20% in certain urban centers throughout Asia (e.g., Mumbai, Hanoi).[147,148]

In Europe the HIV epidemic is strongly driven by IDUs and is dominated by two countries, Russia and Ukraine (81% and 9% of new infections, respectively). The fact that these two nations are currently at war (as I write this) will surely only exacerbate any gaps in prevention services. In the MENA, cases are highly concentrated among special populations and their sexual partners. IDUs accounted for 43% of new HIV infections in 2021 and gay men and other MSM for another 23%.[147] Women are particularly vulnerable to SGBV, stigma, and discrimination, resulting in limited access to HIV services. Coverage of services for the prevention of mother-to-child HIV transmission is among the lowest in the world.

HIV continues to have a disproportionate impact on certain populations in the United States, HIV prevention and treatment programs are not adequately reaching those who could most benefit from them, and certain groups such as MSM, people of transgender experience, and Black, Indigenous, and people of color (BIPOC) communities continue to be disproportionately affected. The highest mortality rates among people with HIV are reported among Black Americans (accounting for 45% of all HIV-associated deaths, compared to 32% and 16%, respectively for white and Latinx populations, respectively).[174] From 2014 through 2018, the number of HIV diagnoses actually increased for transgender adults and adolescents. Among transgender male-to-female adults and adolescents with new HIV diagnoses in 2018, those aged 25 to 29 years composed the largest percentage (27%), followed by those aged 20 to 24 years (25%).[175]

As we discussed in part I, as well, geography matters. HIV diagnoses in the United States are far from evenly distributed across states and regions. The highest rates of new diagnoses occur in the southern United States. Special populations and their sexual partners are disproportionately impacted, accounting for 99% of new HIV infections. High levels of stigma and discrimination faced by the LGBTQIA+ population continue to impede the provision of effective prevention services. In addition, high levels of physical, sexual, and emotional violence toward women and girls are also significant barriers.

But we must dig deeper. It's not enough to say people of color, sex workers, transgender women, and IDUs are the ones that are disproportionately impacted. While these (key) populations do remain at much higher risk of infection and control than other groups, the majority of the disease still lives in Africa, and over half of those infected are heterosexual women. Let's explore some core historical developments that created a foundation for these current sociopolitical events in SSA. We will explore three core determinants and explain how they led to the production of the largest concentration of HIV/AIDS in the world—colonialism, migrant labor, and apartheid. Importantly, when we look at an epidemiological map of Africa (figure 5.10), we can see that the vast majority of HIV/AIDS prevalence is concentrated (in epidemiology, red is usually bad) in southern Africa. Let's explore why . . .

First, colonialism played a substantive role in the pandemic spread of HIV/AIDS. The parceling out of territories to colonial governments and the ensuing damage to traditional economies was followed by additional injury with decades of internecine war. Colonialism in southern Africa was formalized in 1652 when the Dutch East India Company established a fort at Table Bay as part of its expanding network of trade

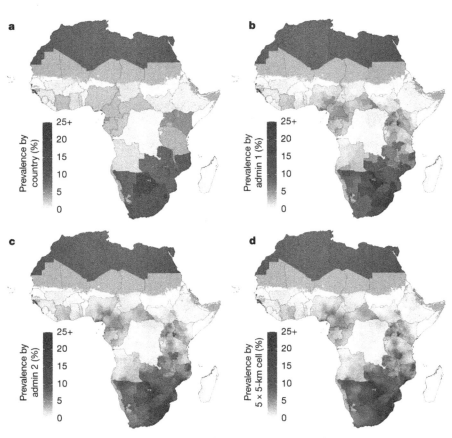

FIGURE 5.10. HIV epidemiological map showing HIV seroprevalence concentration gradients across sub-Saharan Africa. *Source:* Laura Dwyer-Lindgren et al., "Mapping HIV Prevalence in Sub-Saharan Africa Between 2000 and 2017," *Nature* 570 (7760): 189–193, https://doi.org/10.1038/s41586-019-1200-9.

in the Indian Ocean and changed shifts in 1795, when the Cape became a British colony.[176] As late as the 1870s, the subcontinent was divided into a large number of polities, chiefdoms, colonies, and settlements of widely diverging size, power, and racial compositions yet lacked political unity or cohesion. Yet within fifty years, a unified and distinctively capitalist empire had been formed, as an integral part of the British Empire. Subsequently, this land was ruled by white hands and ideologies and had firmly entrenched colonial and settler interests.

Second, the crucial significance of the discovery of diamonds on the Vaal-Hartz River junction in 1867, the ensuing rush to the Kimberly diamond fields, and the subsequent massive growth of mining crystallized the catalysis of this colonial movement in southern Africa. The discovery of valuable mineral deposits and the need to procure labor supplies to mine them caused the southern African interior to become a highly coveted region for the British to control directly. Direct control over this area would enable a variety of settler and colonial interests to secure and regulate African labor. By the end of the 1880s, the British had effectively exerted control, either directly or through their colonies in the Cape and Natal, over a large number of African societies. The Anglo-Boer War of 1899–1902 marked the completion of the process of conquest begun in the 1870s.

Southern Africa's HIV prevalence (the highest in the world at one point) is rooted in the social changes that began with this "mineral revolution." These mineral discoveries marked southern Africa's transition from a precapitalist, rural backwater to an industrial, capitalist economy shaped by the mining industry and its irreducible dependence on inexpensive migrant labor. The special hazards of the mining operations, as well as prolific impoverishment in the countryside, together had abrupt and devastating implications for the physical well-being of workers, both Black and white.[177] For these workers, the health costs of this process were high.

Southern Africa's dependence on mineral extraction and its position in the world economy meant that the effects of uneven development were also felt in the towns that developed in the wake of the mineral discoveries. The most significant growth was in the port towns as well as on the Rand, where industries were heavily dependent on the demands of the mines. Moreover, the accelerating spread of disease to more distal regions of the colony resulted from a combination of the health hazards of the mining industry, the migrant labor system, and the low-wage urban economy, along with the simultaneous and connected impoverishment of the countryside.

In a similar vein, Sidney Kark's statements regarding migrant labor may be added to this argument in illustrating the relative absenteeism of fathers and sons from the rural economy, leaving mothers and daughters to fend for themselves and, at times, leaving them with no other option than sex work.[178,179] Furthermore, the loss of protection of the male role created a stratospheric increase in SGBV, especially gang rape. The association between STIs, prostitution, and migrancy reflected the consequences of the broader processes of landlessness, poverty, proletarianization, and urbanization on familial relationships and sexual mores for men and women.

As reserve conditions worsened, a dependence on migrancy began to dominate rural economies. The long absences of men from their homes, wives' dependence on inadequate remittances, and fear of abandonment imposed greater strains on marital relationships. In summary, the institutionalization of the migrant labor system along with rapid urbanization reflected the gradual collapse of rural economies, as well as the accompanying anomie of the rural society in general.

Southern Africa's industrialization was made possible by the constant movement of large numbers of sexually active men from town to countryside and back, bearing their diseases with them, resulting in the impoverishment of the countryside and the marginalization of women and children. It is a pattern in which the rewards have been largely reaped by whites who are citizens, and the costs have been largely borne by the vast majority (i.e., Blacks). For them, it has spelled poverty and powerlessness, as well as relative and absolute misery.

Finally, it's important to explore a national policy that sealed the deal in terms of the sociopolitical determination of this pandemic. Apartheid, one word, emanating from the linguistic fusion of Dutch and French (Afrikaans), translating to a state of separation, is at times difficult to separate from the connotation of terror, evil, mayhem, irrationality, and insanity. The seeds of apartheid were sown as early as 1910 as a means of solidifying the cross-class Afrikaner alliance, which had been consciously forged in the preceding decades. The cornerstone of apartheid was the division of all South Africans by race. Race laws touched every aspect of social life, beginning with the prohibition of "mixed marriages" (1949) and the Immorality Act (1950), which extended the existing ban on sex between whites and Africans outside marriage. Complete racial division in the future was the ultimate goal.

In the course of the late 1970s and 1980s, the rigid nationalist model developed during the apex of apartheid began to break down at the same time that civil volatility peaked. Because of preexisting structurally racist policies beginning in 1867, however, the erratic population movements induced the requirements for the mutation and migration of HIV. Furthermore, the civil volatility that emanated from the overt oppression during the era of apartheid caused a rapid acceleration of the spread—albeit in a latent form. Throughout this same period of South Africa's relative global isolation, globalization was nearly ubiquitously underway, drastically transforming the context of global production and distribution and, ultimately, the way of life. Yet apartheid was impermeable to this process and simply propagated a relatively stagnant form of oppression and marginalization.

As the apartheid regime melted to give way to the inextricable processes of democratization, capitalism, and neoliberal market-driven policies, however, the jack-in-the-box was vehemently sprung free, and the HIV/AIDS epidemic began to identifiably metastasize throughout the continent. Though it is irrefutable that conditions remarkably improved for the oppressed populations in 1994, globalization accompanied by neoliberal policies and markets effectively polarized these preexisting circumstances. Moreover, relative poverty was accentuated as over a decade of international money poured into the "other" side of the rainbow.

This situation subsequently spurred further frustration, hostility, and ensuing violence. The aggression of this conditioned violent society changed from one that was largely politically stemmed to one that turned inward to communities and families with residual prolific SGBV. This was simply the result of desperate attempts by African men to reassert patriarchal domination in a rapidly changing society (as we saw with the DRC). This has proven all the more intractable because long before the last phase of the struggle, South Africa had been a profoundly violent society.

Curiously, the apartheid state, due to its international status as a sociopolitical pariah, actually acted as a buffer against Western encroachment. Therefore, the manifestation of the silent epidemic that at the time was bursting at the seams due to the centuries of civil instability that preceded it was also suppressed. It was only until this buffer was neutralized that the threshold for volatility was manifestly reached with the HIV/AIDS pandemic. It was in 1994 that population stress caused all infrastructure to buckle, releasing the biological missile without any countermeasures in place to protect the populace.

Southern Africa was an ideal stop along the trajectory of the globalized networks of trade expanding between the 17th and 19th centuries. South Africa, specifically, has long retained a continental leadership role within a globalized economy, mainly emanating from the attraction of the mining industry—leading to an intractable network of migration. The "mineral revolution" created a devout need for low-paid, unskilled migrant labor and subsequently caused a rupture of the social cohesion that largely rural communities experienced prior to the advent of colonialism. Together these created an impeccable mutative route for the retrovirus to travel. It is through these very microniches that HIV/AIDS has exploded so vehemently, placing southern Africa at the forefront of the pandemic.

South Africa is but one example, but the developments across postcolonial Africa in general in the 20th century spurred years of confusion, frustration, hostility, violence, volatility, and ensuing insurgencies among structures based upon race, class, and gender—namely, race. These sociopolitical determinants conjunctively created the perfect recipe for pandemic distribution. Again, the evolution of this virus was nearly in lockstep with the concurrent sociopolitical factors taking place in southern Africa (and other nations) at the time. The virological seeds of the pandemic were sown over the course of centuries—beginning systematically with colonialism.

Hopefully this helps to illustrate that while HIV was first discovered in 1981, the viral evolution had been baking and brewing for decades, and the sociopolitical determinants that exhausted any social cohesion and inflamed population stress to its apex had been developing throughout centuries of Western encroachment and exploitation. These external forces began with the conquest of colonization and were further exacerbated by forcibly imposing a physical and ideological "system" of culture, religion, economics, and politics, leaving behind a drastically marginalized and unequal society. There should be little question as to why something spread through such culturally sensitive means (sexuality) was so vulnerable to influence by a culmination of cultural changes layered in by Christian missionaries, foreign militaries, and Western biomedical interventions. The precolonial African ideologies, particularly those surrounding sexuality, would be shattered forever.

What is particularly intriguing is how the combination of sociopolitical determinants that emerged in the 1980s and 1990s demonstrates nearly a flawless correlation with the increase of HIV/AIDS incidence rates. Yet at the same time, the 1960s and 1970s should have theoretically demonstrated a similar association so that when HIV was initially identified in 1981, the epidemic in Southern Africa would have been conspicuously prolific. South Africa should have been among the first, not the last, of the countries to suffer from its ravages. Paradoxically, this was not the case. South Africa was not heavily afflicted with the globalizing epidemic in the early to mid-1980s, as were other sister African countries. In fact, the pandemic did not appear to proliferate until 1994. Subsequently, I argue that this anachronistic finding is due to two occurrences—the internal machinery of the apartheid state and the external process of globalization. And then there is always bad data.

Still today, South Africans of absolute poverty are unable to access HAART, primary schooling, and quality primary health care. In fact, South Africa is the most unequal nation in the world according to the Gini coefficient, which measures income inequality.[155] Sadly, this has not changed since 1994, toward the end of apartheid, when this duality was made visible by the different Human Development Index scores (otherwise known as the "happy index") for Black and white South Africans, where "white South Africa" ranked 24th and "Black South Africa" ranked 123rd.[166] The levels of crime, poverty, disease, and social decay amidst the marginalized areas of the world may cause many whites to feel threatened and many Blacks, in turn, to feel resentment that nothing is being done. There is a fundamental Manichean distinction at the heart of public ideals about race in the world (as we discussed in chapter 4 on our section on minority race)— particularly in SSA and the Caribbean, curiously the same regions with the largest prevalence of HIV/AIDS.

The question fundamentally addressed here is why did it take the international community so long to overcome the epistemic barriers and realize the potential of this pandemic? As we will discuss further in part III, when it comes to biomedicine, the facts must be promulgated by those who are socially authorized to do so. As Greg Behrman argues in his book *The Invisible People*, in the domain of epidemic disease that authority is conventionally given to epidemiologists, biomedical researchers, and physicians in public health.[180] The authority to contextualize and describe infectious disease has traditionally precluded social scientists and ethnographers, who use qualitative methods to examine social relations, meanings, and their surrounding contexts. It is because of this failure to properly recognize and describe the influence of the core sociopolitical seeds that helped shape the HIV/AIDS pandemic (especially in SSA) that it took us so long to get it right. It was only until the new millennium that the conventional "scientists" started to listen, which is ultimately why we have made such important advancements in the control of this pandemic. I think we're close, and hopefully this book helps spread the right narrative. Alas, we are not out of the proverbial woods yet.

It's time to grade this pandemic once again. This is an easy 100% for me, but I'm interested to hear from folks who disagree.

HIV/AIDS: Rubric for determining the sociopolitical determinants of pandemics and PHEICs

	Sociopolitical determinant-linked questionnaire	Yes	No
1	Is there a sociopolitical link to the original spread of disease?	☐	☐
2	Was there a lack of public and community health infrastructure at the time?	☐	☐
3	If yes, did the lack of infrastructure at the time of spread precipitate more widespread distribution?	☐	☐
4	Was the lack of infrastructure at the time linked to a sociopolitical root cause?	☐	☐
5	Is it treatable? In other words, would building more effective sociopolitical infrastructure mitigate the risk of spread?	☐	☐

Ebola (West Africa, 2014–2016; Democratic Republic of the Congo, 2019–2020)

Ebola is a word that provokes profound reactions from both the lay and academic communities. This parabolic relationship reflects fear balanced with intrigue. The enigma and catastrophic potential surrounding it have been most commonly cited as the most emotive factors. Yet never before did we have a sustainable caseload to follow and study its etiologic factors. In fact, starting in 1976 the cumulative mortality for all previous outbreaks until the West African one on record was less than 2,000. That was all to change in 2014, as it captured the attention of the Western world in a way that few epidemics had before. Although it technically does not meet the definition of a pandemic (i.e., it did not cause >1 million deaths nor reach global distribution), I have included it because of its lethality and the contemporary and popular understanding surrounding it.

Clinical Manifestations

Patients with Ebola virus disease (EVD) typically have an abrupt onset of symptoms 6–12 days after exposure (range, 2–21 days).[181,182,183] There is no evidence that infected persons who have not yet developed signs of illness are infectious to others. The number of 21 days is very important because during the West Africa epidemic, this number was doubled to determine when an area was considered to be "ebola-free." In terms of symptoms, fever is the hallmark of the disease. Other common signs and symptoms include fatigue, headache, vomiting, diarrhea, abdominal pain, and loss of appetite.[184,185,186,187] The GI symptoms may be the most impactful and if not controlled can lead to severe hypotensive shock and ultimately death. Reports have also described weakness, muscle aches, and rash.

Despite the traditional name of Ebola hemorrhagic fever, major bleeding is not found in most patients (despite what popular fiction suggests), and severe hemorrhage tends to be observed only in the late stages of disease. Some patients develop progressive hypotension and shock with multiorgan failure, which typically results in death during the second week of illness. Neurological findings occasionally manifest, with examples such as meningoencephalitis (brain infection) occurring. Serious cardiac and respiratory manifestations can arise and (if not managed with basic supportive conditions) lead to death. Finally, a number of reports have mentioned eye involvement (even following resolution of the infection), causing blurred vision, photophobia (pain associated with light), and even blindness.

Epidemiology

Ebola is unique from all other pandemics listed; in West Africa and the DRC, it was officially a PHEIC (recall this reference from our discussion of the swine flu in 2009). But it has been carved out from the qualifying criteria we have set forth for all other pandemics described for the following reasons:

1. It is contemporaneous with ongoing outbreaks.
2. It has such a profound visceral effect.
3. It has an incredibly high CFR.
4. I was there (twice).

The Ebola virus is a part of the family Filoviridae, which includes its "cousin" Marburg virus.[188,189,190] The Ebola virus consists of six types: Zaire, Sudan, Bundibugyo, Tai Forest, Reston, and Bombali.[191] Of these, only the first four have caused recognized disease in humans; all but the Reston virus are indigenous to Africa. The Zaire species was the first to be discovered.[192] From 1976 through 2013, Ebola caused multiple outbreaks in the DRC and neighboring countries in Central Africa, with CFRs (as a refresher, number of people killed / number of people infected) often approaching 90%. The silver lining of the high CFR of EVD, however, is that it burns out quickly and nearly always takes place in rural areas, where population density is low. In fact, these outbreaks with the Zaire species usually involved $n < 100$ cases and were contained within a period of weeks to a few months.

In 2014 the Zaire virus appeared in West Africa, producing an epidemic in Liberia, Guinea, and Sierra Leone that took more than two years to control.[193] There were nearly 29,000 total cases (suspected, probable, or confirmed), of which more than 15,000 were laboratory confirmed, and the overall CFR was approximately 40%. Since then the Zaire species has been responsible for additional epidemics, including several outbreaks in the DRC.[194,195] A subsequent outbreak in Guinea in early 2021 appears to have resulted from persistent human infection since the 2014 West African epidemic, though the manner of persistence could not be determined.[196,197]

The Sudan species of Ebola virus was also discovered in 1976.[198] In five outbreaks in Uganda and Sudan, including one that ended in January 2023, CFRs have averaged approximately 50%. Compare this to most flu pandemics (excluding the 1918 one), where CFRs < 1%. The Bundibugyo species has been responsible for small outbreaks in Uganda and the adjacent DRC,[199] while the Ivory Coast virus has caused one nonfatal case.[200]

Outbreaks typically begin when a human comes into contact with an infected animal or its body fluids.[201,202] The persistence of the virus in persons who have recovered from EVD may also potentially be a source of infection for new outbreaks.[203,204,205] Person-to-person transmission is based upon direct physical contact with the body fluids of individuals who are ill with EVD or have died from the infection, in the absence of personal protective equipment (PPE).[206,207,208] Studies in laboratory primates, however, have found that animals can be infected with EVD through droplet inoculation of the virus into the mouth or eyes. Persistence of the virus (beyond 6 months post resolution) in semen can also transmit infection. In other words, it can actually be an STI. Those who provide hands-on medical care or prepare a cadaver for burial are at greatest risk (because the viral load is highest at death).

Single infections or small clusters of cases may occur frequently within an enzootic (animal to animal, in this case, bats) region, but since human-to-human transmission requires direct physical contact with the virus-containing body fluids of a sick person, these introductions may "burn out" without being diagnosed. The most infectious body fluids are blood, feces, and vomitus. Infectious virus has also been detected in urine, semen, saliva, aqueous humor, vaginal fluid, and breast milk.[209,210,211,212,213] Epidemics are typically recognized only after several generations of transmission have occurred, weeks after the initial infection, when a severely ill patient is treated in a medical facility.

Prior to the epidemic in West Africa, outbreaks of EVD were, again, typically controlled quickly. This outcome was generally attributed to the fact that most outbreaks occurred in remote regions with low population density, where residents rarely traveled far from home. The West African epidemic, however, showed that EVD can spread rapidly and widely as a result of the extensive movement of infected individuals (including undetected travel across national borders), the spread of the disease to densely populated urban areas, the avoidance and / or lack of adequate PPE, and the absence of dedicated medical isolation centers.

The 2014–2016 West African epidemic demonstrated that the mortality associated with EVD may be reduced through adequate supportive care. I was in Sierra Leone in 2015 and what was absolutely critical was the focus on Ebola treatment units (ETUs) and the importance of incorporating basic public health practices of infection prevention and control (IPC)—namely, isolation, quarantine, and good basic hand hygiene. This outbreak also accelerated the investigation of therapies and vaccines for treatment and prevention of the Zaire species of Ebola virus. These were manufactured by a number of pharmaceutical companies in addition to the US government and used in the DRC outbreak. I actually received this series through an NIH clinical trial, and this ultimately became a game changer (mentioning I was "Ebola proof" also often went well at social events).

Historical Timeline

While our focus is on West Africa and the DRC, we'll zoom out a bit and explore three discrete regions where historical outbreaks have taken place since 1976 to give some more context. First, in Central Africa, EVD was first recognized when two outbreaks occurred almost simultaneously in Zaire (hence the name of the subtype) and in Sudan in 1976.[214,215] An epidemic caused by this same Zaire species subsequently caused several hundred cases in 1995 in Kikwit, DRC (formerly Zaire).[216] Additional outbreaks have subsequently occurred in the DRC—primarily since 2018.

An outbreak in the Équateur Province was detected in early May 2018, leading to an intensive response by the DRC Ministry of Health, the WHO, Medecins Sans Frontieres (Doctors without Borders), and other nongovernmental organizations to rapidly establish treatment facilities, case finding, and contact tracing to prevent further transmission. The end of the outbreak was announced on July 24, 2018.[217] There were 33 deaths (a CFR of 61%). Notably, ring vaccination campaigns (this means identifying cases and vaccinating concentric circles around those point cases) were begun less than two weeks after the outbreak was confirmed; nearly 4,000 health care workers, contacts of patients, and their contacts received the vaccine.

A subsequent outbreak was reported on August 1, 2018, in the North Kivu Province (the northeastern region of the country bordering Rwanda and Uganda, where long-term armed conflicts have produced large numbers of refugees).[218,219] One year later on June 11, 2019, the

WHO reported that the outbreak had spread to Uganda (which borders the DRC). All the cases were imported from the DRC, however, and there were no transmission or secondary cases in Uganda. During this outbreak, mobile field laboratories and ETUs were rapidly established, and the vaccination of health care workers and close contacts of patients was initiated.

I worked on this outbreak in the South Kivu area and was shocked to see the degree of violence and even murders against health care workers who were simply trying to help. People could not see that these people simply wanted to help. All they saw were people with the classic Tyvek (hazmat) suits (appearing extraterrestrial) taking people into ETUs with approximately half making it out. There was no trust. There was no system in place. When the epidemic was declared over on June 25, 2020, there had been 3,470 confirmed cases with 2,287 deaths, with a CFR of 66%. Of those cases, approximately 57% were female, 29% were younger than 18, and 5% percent were health care workers. During the North Kivu epidemic, medical workers investigated some 250,000 case contacts, tested 220,000 blood samples, and vaccinated more than 300,000 people. This was the second-largest outbreak in history.

As the North Kivu outbreak was coming to an end, another outbreak was identified in Mbandaka, Équateur Province, on June 1, 2020. In contrast to the earlier outbreak, cases were widely distributed within the province, occurring in 13 of the 18 health zones. By the time it was declared over on November 18, 2020, there had been 119 confirmed and 11 probable cases, with 55 deaths. More than 40,000 people at high risk of infection were given the vaccine. Clearly, the scale was considerably different from that prior, and some of the foundational pieces (including very recent experience with mass vaccinations) helped with mitigation.

On February 7, 2021, another EVD outbreak was identified in the North Kivu region. After the occurrence of 11 confirmed cases and 6 deaths and the administration of 2,000 doses of vaccine to persons at risk, the outbreak was declared over on May 3, 2021. Virus sequencing suggests that it had actually resulted from the transmission of virus from a survivor of the 2014–2016 West Africa epidemic (we will discuss below) and not through introduction from an animal reservoir.[220] In October 2021, a cluster of Ebola cases in the same area was recognized and quickly contained; these cases originated from persistent virus in a survivor of an earlier epidemic in North Kivu.[221] The next year (April 23, 2022), yet another outbreak was declared in the northwestern Equateur Province, which was found to be attributed to a spillover event from an animal source and not from viral persistence in a survivor. This outbreak was declared over in July 2022.

In Northeast Africa, the Sudan species caused an epidemic in the Sudan in 1976 (same time as the above) and has been responsible for several outbreaks in East Africa since that time, including an epidemic of some 400 cases in Gulu, Uganda, in 2000.[222,223] More recently, on September 20, 2022, an EVD outbreak was declared in Uganda.[224]

The deadliest and most well-known to date occurred from 2014 to 2016 in West Africa, which was caused by the Zaire species. It was here (in Sierra Leone) that I spent over a month and endured some of the most frightening experiences of my life. The outbreak technically started in Guinea in late 2013 and was confirmed by the WHO in March 2014. This outbreak was unique in that all prior Ebola outbreaks caused by the Zaire virus had occurred in Central Africa (the DRC mostly, as we just discussed). The initial case is believed to have been a two-year-old child who developed fever, vomiting, and black stools, without other evidence of hemorrhage.[225] The epidemic subsequently spread to Liberia, Sierra Leone, Nigeria, Senegal, and Mali. Sequence analysis of viruses isolated from patients indicated that the epidemic resulted entirely from sustained person-to-person transmission, without additional introductions from animal reservoirs.[226,227]

Nearly 29,000 probable, suspected, and laboratory-confirmed cases of EVD were identified, with more than 11,000 deaths. These cases included 881 infected health care workers, of whom approximately 60% died. The magnitude of the epidemic, especially in Liberia and Sierra Leone, was probably underestimated, due in part to individuals with EVD being cared for outside the hospital setting early in the epidemic—partly because of a lack of access and partly because of a lack of trust in the system.

Guinea, Liberia, and Sierra Leone experienced widespread Ebola virus transmission, and the rate of new infections did not slow significantly until the spring of 2015. Extended periods of disease-free (defined as 42 days without any known cases in the province; just take the relatively arbitrary 21-day incubation period and double it) transmission were subsequently reported. In certain nearby countries (Senegal, Nigeria, Mali), introductions of EVD resulted in short chains of person-to-person transmission, which were quickly terminated.

The end of the epidemic was officially recognized in early 2016. Sporadic cases continued to be detected, which were attributed to sexual transmission from survivors with persistent virus.[228] As was widely televised, cases of EVD occurred in residents and health care workers who were exposed to the virus in West Africa and were then treated in hospitals in the United States and Europe.[229,230,231] On September 30, 2014, the first travel-associated case of Ebola was reported in the United States. A returning physician who was asymptomatic while traveling from Liberia to Dallas, Texas, developed clinical findings consistent with EVD approximately five days after arriving in the United States and subsequently died. Two nurses involved in his care were ultimately infected but ultimately recovered.

In February 2021, a new outbreak of EVD was detected in a region of Guinea affected by the 2014–2016 epidemic. There were 16 confirmed and 7 probable cases, of whom 12 died. The index case was a female nurse, whose family remained healthy. Virus isolates were closely related in sequence to those that had circulated in the area in 2014–2016, suggesting that the outbreak resulted from persistent human infection.

Sociopolitical Determinants

Given the relatively contained outbreaks starting in the 1970s, the question is as follows: What happened in 2014 in West Africa when nearly

29,000 became infected without a prior known reservoir in this region (recall that this was the first outbreak in West Africa)?

Curiously, four studies dating between 1978 and 1982 (later published in 1986) analyzed antibody prevalence to the Ebola virus in frozen blood samples in Liberians and demonstrated anywhere between 6% and 14% prevalence (indicating prior exposure).[232] As such, Ebola was, in fact, not novel to the region at all but instead remained in certain "sanctuary sites" only to emerge (theatrically) three or four decades later. But why did we have this uncharacteristic explosion that took so many lives and that varied considerably from previous ones? Sierra Leone was the hardest hit—with nearly 14,000 total cases and nearly 4,000 dead.[233] Moreover, how did we have the second-largest outbreak on record just two years later in a different region (the DRC)?

It is difficult to display more troubling statistics (resulting from a highly precarious sociopolitical system and an anemic infrastructure) than Sierra Leone. With the lowest recorded life expectancy in the world (at 45.3 years), the fifth-highest maternal mortality rate, the second-highest IMR, and the highest under-5 mortality rate, health care in Sierra Leone is precarious, at best.[234]

Moreover, as quality of health is inextricably connected with access to resources and highly correlated with general quality of life, it is no surprise that they are ranked the sixth-lowest on the Multidimensional Poverty Index,[235] have the third-highest illiteracy rate, and rank 183 out of 187 nations analyzed on the "happiness index." Much like the case with the sociopolitical developments in South Africa, we can draw an interesting association with Western encroachment in that Sierra Leone played a pivotal role in the West African slave trade. Sadly, the country subsequently became an example of the lasting chaos that the slave trade made of many African cultures—a volatile reality that still persists today. Ebola was an opportunistic infection.

Sierra Leone's health care infrastructure was tenuous when Ebola hit. In fact, there were fewer than 60 physicians in the entire nation with absolutely no safety net, meaning nearly all health care resources were out-of-`pocket. So if we want to better understand the formula that calculated an output of so many lives lost due to a previously recorded latent infectious disease, the calculus requires the tenuous (or necrotic) public health infrastructure to be factored in, in addition to the interacting factors of the stark inequalities that led to such an unprecedented explosion of cases.

Such inequality could not be better visualized than in a setting where the horrifying national data reported above are further exacerbated by specific domestic inequalities in the 14 administrative districts that compose the political borders. Some of the worst statistics in the country were in Kono District (where I was based and the 2006 movie *Blood Diamond* was set; figures 5.11a–d). Ironically, this area also contains some of the highest concentrations of diamond mines in the world. The harvesting of these "precious" stones famously fueled one of the bloodiest battles in contemporary African history (where more than 50,000 were killed, well over 1 million displaced, and an estimated 10,000 child soldiers abducted and eviscerated of innocence between 1991 and 2002).[236] As we can see, the confluence of slavery, colonialism, and migrant labor around diamond mines manifests once again in conditions that are ripe for an emerging infectious disease to lead to pandemic proportions.

As a result of a precarious imbalance of power, the control of such minerals has never truly profited the nation in any meaningfully distributive manner but has mostly been absorbed by a small minority of Sierra Leoneans acting as puppets for foreign investment and control. Koidu Holdings is the quintessential example of such an operation, in which a foreign group of investors (mostly South Africans and Israelis) control the most advanced diamond-harvesting operation in the area (i.e., kimberlite mining) and have been further funded by a number of other foreign sources (including Tiffany & Co., which in 2011 entered into a $50 million amortizing term loan in exchange for preferential access to such diamonds at "fair market value").[237] Other smaller transactions and exportation are facilitated mostly by the Lebanese minority residing in Sierra Leone (and may even be associated with such diamonds

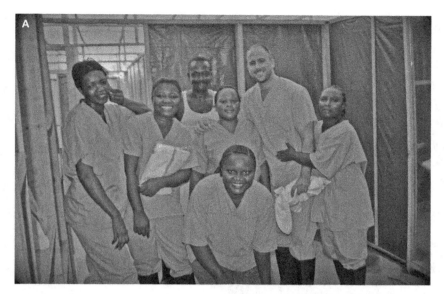

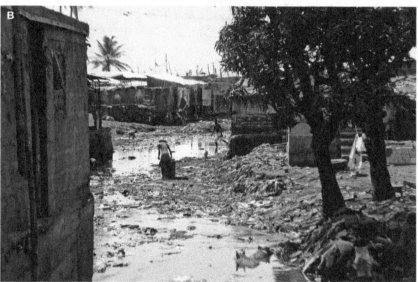

FIGURES 5.11. A–D Assortment of personal photographs from Sierra Leone Ebola response, 2015. A: group photo at Ebola training center (coordinated by WHO and the International Organization for Migration), Freetown; B: water source, Freetown; C: changing shifts at the Ebola treatment unit in Koidu, Kono; D: South African diamond mine run by Koidu Holdings located less than two miles from Kono hospital. *Source:* Photos by author.

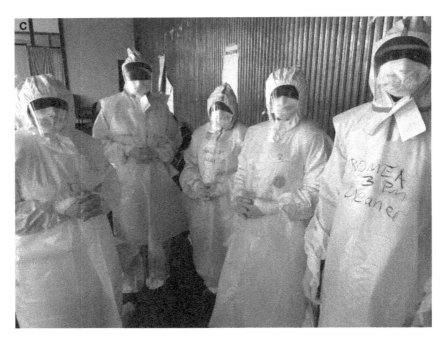

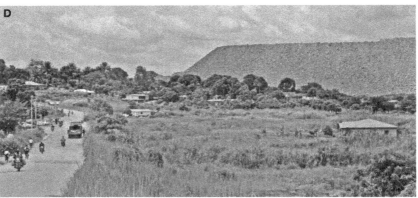

FIGURES 5.11. (Continued)

being traced to Hezbollah, per US State Department reports).[238] All of
this while local Sierra Leoneans working in the mines are making less
than five dollars a day.[239]

The following are some thoughts that I documented while taking
shifts inside the Ebola treatment units (ETUs) in 2015:

The same conditions continue to present themselves. This is the very formula that fuels a dysfunctional public health system. When diseases impact these communities, only a select few will be able to decide their fate. While I was working on Ebola at the regional government hospital in Kono, I also helped with non-Ebola patients—namely pediatric malaria. Patients were admitted with inaccurate diagnoses and management with very little follow up after such admissions (e.g., patients languish for weeks without being seen by a health care professional once admitted), blood transfusions were ordered as a perceived panacea (with frighteningly poor quality in screening and frequent fatal consequences), and those requiring emergent care (including a number of patients in shock) were denied treatment unless they could actually buy the medications and supplies themselves (all treatment must be purchased before administration for all populations other than children under 5 years and pregnant women).

All of these egregious circumstances are not a fault of any one individual or hospital, but rather a system that is deeply fractured by corruption naturally feeding off of poverty that is contorted further by actors who regulate access to essential resources.

Within this milieu, Kono was impacted heavily by Ebola—and the government hospital was largely abandoned. In December 2014, the WHO reported that over 11 days, "two teams buried 87 bodies, including a nurse, an ambulance driver, and a janitor drafted to remove such bodies. . . . One response team also discovered over 25 accumulated dead bodies in a cordoned area of the (government) hospital."[240] It was this hospital that I was working to help strengthen their system. This district was effectively abandoned, yet ironically has the most salient multinational presence (outside of the capital, given the diamond mining industry). There were more than a few dozen languages actively being spoken (and these were not the health care workers). The more supportive systems available, the lower the CFRs. Those that "matter" have access to these systems. Those that "do not matter" will suffer. Root causes need to be addressed, and systems need to be fundamentally redesigned. Global awareness is a critical step to achieve these ends.

In the end, the world continues to profit off of these pretentious minerals, yet the local system is left bankrupt—and, as a result, people die for not being able to afford the necessary $2–$5 for essential fluids and antibiotics. Remarkably, it was still here where I found infants unnecessarily fighting for their last breaths in front of me.... It was where men hemorrhaged from preventable diseases ... and women with basic asthmatic exacerbations simply "pass off" (a term to describe the relative passive state of death) without adequate care in a bankrupt system that has left the people desperate, vulnerable and apathetic. We must do better....

It's time for grading, once again, and I hope that the message is becoming increasingly clearer. Was there a sociopolitical link to the original spread? As the reservoir had been relatively latent, with a disease that never previously caused more than 100 deaths, we see that unique conditions were needed in order to drive epidemic formation. The case that I presented, given some of the most profound disparities in the world, is certainly compelling. Clearly, with fewer than 60 physicians in a country with a population of approximately 2 million, the second and third questions can be easily answered. Why did the lack of infrastructure exist? The reasons are numerous, but the most salient are centuries of affliction from the slave trade, inequities precipitated by the diamond trade, and, finally, a recent war that killed off a sizable number of young workers.

Ebola: Rubric for determining the sociopolitical determinants of pandemics and PHEICs

	Sociopolitical determinant–linked questionnaire	Yes	No
1	Is there a sociopolitical link to the original spread of disease?	☐	☐
2	Was there a lack of public and community health infrastructure at the time?	☐	☐
3	If yes, did the lack of infrastructure at the time of spread precipitate more widespread distribution?	☐	☐
4	Was the lack of infrastructure at the time linked to a sociopolitical root cause?	☐	☐
5	Is it treatable? In other words, would building more effective sociopolitical infrastructure mitigate the risk of spread?	☐	☐

Finally, is it treatable? While EVD has one of the highest CFRs on record, many cases can be managed by supportive measures (e.g., IV fluids). And, of course, the essential component for optimal control of any infectious disease—a vaccine—now exists (but did not at the time of the West African epidemic). I give this one another easy 100%.

COVID-19, 2019–

Let's move on to the present day . . .

For obvious reasons, the COVID-19 pandemic holds some of the most urgent and powerful lessons for understanding the sociopolitical determinants of pandemics. Having served as the chief medical officer for New York City during the COVID-19 pandemic, it is also an area I am well-equipped to discuss from a first-person viewpoint.

Clinical Manifestations

Based on the frequent boluses of media-facilitated information (including misinformation), it is likely that the numbers of COVID-19 lay "clinicians" and "epidemiologists" are higher today than for any previous infectious disease in history. So let me share some objective information.

Among patients with symptomatic COVID-19, cough, myalgias, and headache are the most commonly reported symptoms. Other features, including diarrhea, sore throat, and smell or taste abnormalities are also well described. Mild URI symptoms (e.g., nasal congestion, sneezing) also appear. The incubation period is generally 14 days following exposure, with most cases occurring approximately 4–5 days (median = 4 days) after exposure.[241,242,243]

Much like influenza, pneumonia is the most frequent serious manifestation of infection, characterized primarily by fever, cough, and shortness of breath. Although some clinical features (in particular smell or taste disorders) are more common with COVID-19 than with other viral respiratory infections,[244] no specific symptoms or signs can reliably distinguish COVID-19.[245] Acute respiratory distress syndrome (sometimes requiring mechanical ventilation) is the major complication in patients with severe disease and can manifest shortly after the onset of shortness of breath. Outside of the respiratory system, blood clots are reported more frequently than in other URIs. Blood clots in the legs and lungs are particularly common in severely ill patients in the ICU. Brain infections are a common complication, particularly among critically ill patients.

The time to recovery is highly variable and depends on age, vaccination status, and preexisting comorbidities (other chronic health issues) in addition to illness severity. Folks with mild infections (the majority) are expected to recover relatively quickly (e.g., within 2 weeks), whereas many with severe disease have a longer convalescence (e.g., 2–3 months). This has been categorized as *long COVID-19*. By definition, these broad range of symptoms must continue for ≥2 months (i.e., 3 months from the onset of illness), have an impact on the patient's life, and not be explainable by an alternative diagnosis. The most common persistent symptoms include fatigue, memory problems, shortness of breath, chest pain, cough, and cognitive deficits.[246] Data also suggest the potential for ongoing respiratory impairment and cardiac sequelae.[247,248,249,250,251,252]

Epidemiology

As discussed above in the 1918 flu epidemiology section, coronaviruses have existed for centuries within human populations as a relatively common cause of URIs (again, common colds). Most of these have been in the form of alpha-coronaviruses and represent approximately 5–15% of all URIs. COVID-19 is a novel beta-coronavirus. Another name for the virus is severe acute respiratory syndrome coronavirus 2 (SARS-CoV-2).[253] It was not the first novel beta-coronavirus. Others have cropped up in recent years—including the famed SARS outbreak in 2002–2004. The Middle East respiratory syndrome (MERS) virus, another novel beta-coronavirus, appears more distantly related.[254,255]

Like other viruses, SARS-CoV-2 evolves over time. Most mutations in the SARS-CoV-2 genome have no impact on viral function. Certain variants have garnered widespread attention because of their rapid emergence within populations and evidence for transmission or clinical implications; these are considered variants of concern and are known by many Greek letters, including the famed Delta and Omicron variants.

A joint study conducted in early 2021 by China and the WHO indicated that the virus descended from a coronavirus that infects wild bats and likely spread to humans through an intermediary wildlife host.[256] Most scientists believe the virus spilled into human populations through natural animal-human transmission, similar to the 2002–2004 SARS (i.e., civets) and 2012 and ongoing MERS (i.e., camels) outbreaks, consistent with other pandemics in human history.[257] The likelihood of this type of transmission will continue to increase with ongoing disruption to the climate and natural ecosystems. One study made with the support of the European Union found that climate change increased the likelihood of the pandemic by influencing distributions of bat species.[258]

A minority of scientists and certain members of the US intelligence community believe the virus may have been inadvertently leaked from a laboratory such as the Wuhan Institute of Virology.[259] Subject matter experts in this space have mixed views on the issue,[260] but the overall consensus seems to be that the virus was not developed as a biological weapon and is unlikely to have been genetically engineered.[261] There is no evidence that SARS-CoV-2 existed in any laboratory prior to the pandemic.[262]

Globally, over 600 million confirmed cases have been reported and over 7 million have died to date. The reported case counts underestimate the overall burden of COVID-19, however, as only a fraction of acute infections are diagnosed and reported. One university-based study reported that the global CFR was 1.02% as of March 10, 2023. (If you can recall the definition from our section on Ebola, in other words, a little over 1% of those infected with COVID-19 died; this can be compared to nearly 40% for Ebola).[263] A December 2022 WHO study estimated excess deaths from the pandemic during 2020 and 2021, concluding that 14.8 million excess early deaths occurred. We haven't seen this scale of mortality so quickly since the 1918 Spanish flu.

Person-to-person spread is the main mode of SARS-CoV-2 transmission. It is thought to occur mainly through close-range contact (i.e., within approximately six feet, but the reality is that the distance is almost always less than three feet; we just doubled it to be safe) via respiratory particles (e.g., spit). Virus released in the respiratory secretions when an infected person coughs, sneezes, or talks can infect another person if it is inhaled or makes direct contact with the mucous membranes. SARS-CoV-2 is almost never actually airborne (despite popular opinion), although this still remains controversial.

SARS-CoV-2 has been detected in nonrespiratory specimens, including stool, blood, ocular secretions, and semen, but the role of these sites in transmission is uncertain.[264,265,266,267,268,269,270] The detection of SARS-CoV-2 RNA in blood has also been reported in some but not all studies that have tested for it.[271,272,273,274,275] The likelihood of bloodborne transmission (e.g., through blood products or needlesticks) appears low; respiratory viruses are generally not transmitted through the bloodborne route.

The risk of transmission after contact with an individual with COVID-19 increases with the closeness and duration of contact and appears highest with prolonged contact in indoor settings (i.e., household contacts).[276] Of course, the highest risk is for those who live in multigenerational homes as well as congregate care facilities. When I was the chief medical officer (CMO) for New York City, this was my greatest challenge—trying to mitigate this risk as much as possible through a number of means (e.g., hotels, congregate facility dedensification, etc.).

A question I often received was how infectious is COVID-19? We evaluate this with the basic reproduction number (R_0). The best way to explain this is as follows. If you take one person infected with

COVID-19 and put them in a room, how many other people do they infect? In January 2020, this was between 1.4 and 2.5,[277] but a subsequent analysis claimed that it may have been closer to 5.7 (with a range of 3.8–8.9).[278] Frequently reported clusters of cases after social or work gatherings also highlight the risk of transmission through close non-household social contact.[279,280,281,282]

Even today, superspreading events, in which large clusters of infections can be traced back to a single index case, are thought to be major drivers of the pandemic.[283,284,285] They have been mainly described following prolonged group exposure in an enclosed, usually crowded, indoor space. The risk of transmission with more indirect contact (e.g., passing someone with the infection on the street, handling items that were previously handled by someone with the infection) is not well established and is likely very low. Many individuals with COVID-19, however, do not report having had a specific close contact with COVID-19 in the weeks prior to diagnosis.[286]

Historical Timeline

In December 2019, adults in Wuhan, the capital city of Hubei Province and a major transportation hub of China, started presenting to local hospitals with severe pneumonia of unknown cause.[287] Many of the initial cases had a common exposure to the Huanan wholesale seafood market, which also traded live animals. The surveillance system (put into place after the SARS outbreak, ironically) was activated, and respiratory samples of patients were sent to reference labs for causal investigations. On December 24, Wuhan Central Hospital sent a lung fluid sample from an unresolved clinical case to a molecular sequencing company, Vision Medicals. Three days later, Vision Medicals informed the Wuhan Central Hospital and the Chinese CDC (yes, it's the same name, and the Europeans also share the same convention) of the results of the test, reporting a novel coronavirus.[288] Around the same time, a cluster of suspected pneumonia cases was observed and treated by a pulmonologist in Hubei Provincial Hospital, who informed the Wuhan Jianghan CDC.[289] This was another microbial shot heard around the world.

On December 31, 2019, China notified the WHO of the outbreak (a wholly different occurrence from prior pandemics), and on January 1, the Huanan seafood market was closed. On January 7 the virus was identified as a coronavirus that had >95% homology with the bat coronavirus and >70% similarity with SARS-CoV (SARS outbreak of 2002–2004). Environmental samples from the Huanan seafood market also tested positive, signifying that the virus originated there.[290] The number of cases started increasing exponentially, some of which were not exposed to the live animal market, suggestive of the fact that human-to-human transmission was occurring.[290] The first fatal case was reported on January 11, 2020.

The massive migration of Chinese during the Chinese New Year fueled the epidemic. Cases in other provinces of China, in addition to neighboring nations (e.g.. Thailand, Japan, and South Korea in quick succession), were reported in people returning from Wuhan. Transmission to health care workers caring for patients was reported on January 20. Three days later, the 11 million population of Wuhan was placed under lockdown. Soon this concept would be scaled across the world. Cases of COVID-19 in countries outside China were reported in those with no history of travel to China, suggesting that local human-to-human transmission was taking place there.[290] Airports in different countries, including India, put in screening mechanisms to detect symptomatic people returning from China, placed them in isolation, and tested them for COVID-19. Soon it was apparent that the infection could be transmitted from asymptomatic people and also before the onset of symptoms. On January 30, the WHO declared COVID-19 a PHEIC.[291] By March 11, 2020, the virus had spread to 110 countries, and the WHO officially declared it a pandemic.[292]

Outside China, Italy had its first confirmed cases on January 31, 2020 (linked to two tourists from China)[293] and overtook China as the country with the most deaths on March 19, 2020.[294] By March 26 the United States had overtaken both nations with the highest number of confirmed cases in the world.[295] New York and California originally saw the most cases. Research on coronavirus genomes indicates that the majority of COVID-19 cases in New York City came from European travelers, rather than directly from China or any other Asian country.[296] Certainly, no other nation has been as disproportionately impacted as the United States, where the pandemic ranks first on the list of disasters by death toll[297] and was the third-leading cause of death (across all categories) in 2020, behind heart disease and cancer.[298] In fact, this is the reason I wrote this book, as I now have your attention. Let's unpack this further

So what went wrong? The first US case was reported on January 20, and President Donald Trump declared the US outbreak a public health emergency on January 31. Restrictions were placed on flights arriving from China,[300] but the initial US response to the pandemic was otherwise slow in terms of preparing the health care system, stopping other travel, and testing.[301] The first known American deaths occurred in February. On March 6, 2020, Trump allocated $8.3 billion to fight the outbreak and declared a national emergency on March 13.[302] By mid-April, disaster declarations were made by all states and territories as they all had increasing cases. A second wave of infections began in June, following relaxed restrictions in several states, leading to daily cases surpassing 60,000. By mid-October, a third surge of cases began. There were over 200,000 new daily cases during parts of December 2020 and January 2021.[303]

The Trump administration evacuated US nationals from Wuhan in January.[304] On February 2 the United States enacted travel restrictions to and from China.[305,306] On February 6, the earliest confirmed American death with COVID-19 (that of a 57-year-old woman) occurred in Santa Clara County, California. (This hit home for me, as it was less than 20 miles from my home in the Santa Cruz mountains.) The CDC did not report its confirmation until April 21, by which point nine other COVID-19 deaths had occurred in Santa Clara County.[307] The virus had been circulating undetected at least since early January and possibly as early as November. On February 25 the CDC warned the American public for the first time to prepare for a local outbreak.[308] The next day, New York City saw the sickening of its "patient zero," Manhattan attorney Lawrence Garbuz (then thought to be the first community-acquired case).[309]

A fourth rise in infections began in March 2021 amidst the rise of the *Alpha* variant, one that was far more easily transmissible and first detected in the United Kingdom.[310] That was followed by a rise of the *Delta* variant, an even more infectious mutation first detected in India. Next came the *Omicron* variant (January 2022), first discovered in South Africa, which led to record highs in cases and hospitalizations—with as many as 1.5 million new infections reported in a single day.[311] By the end of 2022, an estimated 77.5% of Americans had been infected with some variant of COVID-19 at least once, according to the CDC.[312]

By the middle of March, all 50 states were able to perform tests with a physician's approval, either from the CDC or from commercial labs. The number of available test kits remained limited, however.[313] At the time I was the CMO for New York City and was helping with the operational stand-up of what we called *T3* (Test, Treat, and "Take Care"). Testing was thought to be instrumental to the control of the disease. We weren't wrong. Sort of.

As cases began spreading throughout the nation, federal and state agencies began taking urgent steps to prepare for a surge of hospital patients, including establishing additional places for patients in case hospitals became overwhelmed. These were referred to as alternative care sites. We also started converting hotels to manage some of the most minimal care requirements.

In March 2020 I was a part of one of the earliest efforts to leverage hotels to manage patients. This was for the last cruise ship on Earth,[314] the *Grand Princess*, which was forced to dock in Oakland and decanted to a Fairfield hotel in San Carlos, California.[315] It was one of the most impressive (albeit somewhat draconian) displays of public health efforts that we had seen in decades, with over 100 "clients" (not quite patients, as many were simply quarantined) "forced" to comply with our efforts, given the presence of US marshals patrolling the premises at all times. I was the only infectious disease physician present amidst a large team of emergency management and medicine professionals. The contrast was curious.

Throughout March and early April, several state, city, and county governments imposed "stay-at-home" quarantines on their populations.[316] By March 26 the number of cases in the United States exceeded any other nation. On April 11 the US death toll became the highest in the world at 20,000, surpassing that of Italy.[317] We had not seen this type of impact from an infectious disease since 1918. On April 28 the total number of confirmed cases across the country surpassed 1 million.[318] I was in the belly of the beast.

By May 27, less than four months after the pandemic had reached the United States, 100,000 Americans had died.[319] State economic re-openings and a lack of widespread mask orders resulted in a sharp rise in cases across most of the continental United States outside the Northeast.[320] A study conducted in May 2020 indicated that the true number of COVID-19 cases in the United States was much higher than the number of confirmed cases, with some locations having 6–24 times as many cases as reported.[321]

In a time when we needed to rely on global solidarity more than ever, on July 6 the United States announced our withdrawal from the WHO.[322] On July 10 the CDC adopted the infection fatality ratio, which is "the number of individuals who die of the disease among all infected individuals (symptomatic and asymptomatic)," as a new metric for disease severity (this replaced CFR, as a case typically included symptoms, by definition).[323] The degree of political tension continued to escalate, with partisan camps inadvertently created based on their position on public health practices (e.g., face masks, stay-at-home orders, vaccines). Once we threw schools and elections into the mix, we had one of the most hotly contested and divisive applications of US public health in history.

On September 22 the United States passed 200,000 deaths.[324] In early October an unprecedented series of high-profile US political figures and staffers announced they had tested positive.[325] On October 2,

Trump announced on Twitter that both he and the First Lady had tested positive and would immediately isolate.[326] Trump was given an experimental Regeneron product with two monoclonal antibodies and taken to Walter Reed National Military Medical Center.[327]

From early 2020, more than 70 companies worldwide (with 5 or 6 operating primarily in the United States) began vaccine research.[328,329] The global competition, naturally, had national security implications for various countries. In preparation for large-scale production, Congress set aside more than $3.5 billion for this purpose as part of the CARES Act.[330] Among the labs working on a vaccine was the Walter Reed Army Institute of Research, which had previously studied other infectious diseases, such as HIV/AIDS, Ebola, and MERS. On August 5, 2020, the United States agreed to pay Johnson & Johnson more than $1 billion to create 100 million doses of another COVID-19 vaccine.[331] The deal gave the United States an option to order an additional 200 million.

On August 31, 2020, the CDC released its outline for how to administer and distribute the COVID-19 vaccine across the entire country. It was interesting explaining this to thousands of anxious people—the term "health care rationing" was used repeatedly. This is always a provocative concept in democratic nations. In October 2020, 44 vaccines were in clinical trials on humans, and 91 preclinical vaccines were being tested on animals.[332] Most of these trials were underway as well.[333] On November 20, 2020, the Pfizer–BioNTech (US–Germany alliance) partnership submitted a request to the FDA for emergency use authorization (EUA), a distinction in which the products are not officially approved but can be used for emergency purposes.[334] The FDA, in turn, announced that its Vaccines and Related Biological Products Advisory Committee—the FDA's vaccine intelligentsia version of the CDC ACIP—would review the request.[335]

On November 9, President-Elect Biden's transition team announced his COVID-19 Advisory Board.[336] This time it was a collection of impressive and highly erudite public health professionals to guide the future of the US public health waters. On the same day, the total number of cases had surpassed 10 million, averaging 102,300 new cases per day.[337] In November, the Trump administration reached an agreement with a number of retail outlets, including pharmacies and supermarkets, to make the COVID-19 vaccine free, once available.[338] This was a game changer—especially for the uninsured.

On December 11, the FDA granted the EUA for the Pfizer–BioNTech vaccine.[339] An initial shipment of 2.9 million doses was scheduled to be distributed rapidly, and Pfizer promised to supply the rest of the 100 million doses through March 2021.[340] Pfizer had adequate stocks available and began this distribution on December 17, 2020, but the federal government reduced the amount Pfizer was allowed to distribute.[341]

One week later the FDA granted the Moderna vaccine EUA,[342] which Moderna had requested on November 30, 2020.[343] The United States planned to rapidly distribute 5.9 million doses. with more to come later.[344] Much fanfare was associated with the release, including an almost "Rockettes" synchronization of Pfizer trucks leaving their mass manufacturing facilities in Kalamazoo, Michigan. The entire public health world seemed to be synchronously holding its proverbial breath as we all awaited the output of the public-private partnership we know all too well in the United States (theatrically and somewhat accurately named Operation Warp Speed). At the time I was the COVID-19 vaccine incident commander (known as the vaccine czar in certain circles) for Marin County and one of the operational leads for the entire Bay Area. I distinctly recall coming into the emergency operations center on the morning of December 27 and finding a number of boxes having been unceremoniously delivered to the door. The timing with the Christmas holidays was curious.

The original vaccines used a relatively new technique referred to as mRNA (messenger RNA; the reality is that we have had this technology for quite some time but had yet to bring it to scale). Some of these also required ultralow temperature storage due to the fragility of the mRNA, which was new for most public health responders. Studies have shown them to be highly protective against severe illness, hospitalization, and death. As a simple comparison with fully vaccinated people, the CDC found that those who were unvaccinated at the time were 5 to nearly 30 times more likely to become either infected or hospitalized. Unfortunately, vaccine hesitancy was soon to emerge as one of the most formidable opponents to centralized public health successes.[345] As we have discussed, much of this phenomenon was sociopolitically determined.

In spite of recommendations by the government, more than 2 million people flew on airlines during the Thanksgiving holidays.[346] On December 8 the United States passed 15 million cases, with about 1 out of every 22 Americans having tested positive since the pandemic began.[347] On December 14 the United States passed 300,000 deaths, representing an average of more than 961 deaths per day since the first known death on February 6. As this served as one of the peaks in mortality, more than 50,000 were reported in the previous month, with an average of 2,403 daily deaths occurring in the previous week.[348]

On February 27, 2021, the Janssen (Johnson & Johnson) COVID-19 vaccine was also granted an EUA. Unfortunately, despite its promise as a one-shot alternative to the mRNA vaccines, this vaccine received considerably poor optics for a number of reasons, including the use of fetal-harvested stem cells in its production in addition to significantly poorer effectiveness (albeit still considerably higher than most other vaccines). We'll discuss this further in chapter 8 regarding the role of interfaith and spiritual leaders. The final straw was the data released on April 13 about the vaccine and the risk of blood clots (which turned out to be relatively uncompelling, as the birth control pill causes exponentially more clots), which, in turn, led the FDA and CDC joint advisory to pause any additional use. Once it was released from this safety hold, it was simply too late. The vaccine climate had fundamentally shifted in the country.

The COVID-19 saga continues at the time of this writing (albeit with much less dramatic vicissitudes). For the purposes of this book, we'll end the historical timeline here.

Sociopolitical Determinants

The pandemic has had far-reaching consequences beyond the disease itself and the efforts to contain it, including political, cultural, and social implications. From the earliest days of the pandemic, incidents of xenophobia and racism against Asian Americans were reported.[348] We all heard a number of attempts to pathologize East Asians (especially the Chinese) once the virus emerged on the scene. Reflecting back to prior pandemics (especially the 1918 Spanish Influenza pandemic, whose origin was, again, not Spanish at all), this is a common theme in pandemic response.

During most of 2020, much of my lens was filtered through New York City, which of course was the epicenter at the time. This also turned out to be the culmination of much of my life's work, as it was irreducibly salient that despite the issues and the capacity of New York City to form an effective response—it simply could not. This is where I came in.

For context, the New York City mayor at the time, Bill DeBlasio, was experiencing political friction with Oxiris Barbot, the New York City health commissioner, and decided to hand over most of the public health emergency contracts to NYC Health and Hospitals (NYC H&H), which is a publicly funded hospital and health center corporation, not a public health agency. In other words, the hospital staff did not have the chops to effectively respond to this emergency. They needed time, despite the fact that the New York City Department of Health and Mental Hygiene had over 6,000 employees. This was where emergency management came in (as it did in many parts of the country). Unfortunately, the New York City Office of Emergency Management (NYCEM) had <5 permanent staff in its health and medical section. The reason for this was simple—most emergency management in the United States (especially in New York City) was weather related. Prior to this pandemic, tropical storms were the focus du jour. COVID-19 changed all that. When the mayor ordered NYCEM to hold down the fort until NYC H&H could effectively take over with its T3 program (it needed approximately two to three months of lead time), it was clear that NYCEM was going to need a bigger boat. It also needed a captain who could take the helm effectively. Someone knew a guy . . .

At the time, I was working to stand up the city's main COVID-19 field hospital at the Billie Jean King US Tennis Association Center. When I received the call, I was taking a run in Central Park. The caller asked if I was interested in applying for this emergency position—the first CMO in New York City. I asked when and they curtly responded "in five minutes." I took the interview and, after three panels later that day, was offered the job the following day. My life was about to change.

During my time in that role, New York City had over 214,000 cases and 21,000 deaths (or approximately 5% of the entire global mortality burden).[349] We saw this disproportionate impact in the city for many reasons—most of which make New York City spectacular and unique. What was to come surprised even the most cynical, however: a rise of protests and associated violence not seen in the city for decades.

I wrote down the following thoughts when I was up late one night shortly after the protests of the shooting of George Floyd in New York City in May 2020:[350]

Infections have always had a predilection for areas of poverty and inadequate access. Rudolf Virchow, a well-known German microbiologist, famously wrote: "As disease is so often associated with poverty, physicians are the natural attorneys of the poor," a mantra that drives many of us social justice-driven infectious disease specialists. Paul Farmer, the author of *Infections and Inequalities*, wrote that "human rights violations are not accidents; they are not random in distribution or effect. Rights violations are, rather, symptoms of deeper pathologies of power and are linked intimately to the social conditions that so often determine who will suffer abuse and who will be shielded from harm."[351,352]

The inequalities we have seen with COVID-19 have been striking and uncompromising. In the United States, we've found both the incidence of infection and mortality to be disproportionately higher among people of color. In certain contexts, unforgivingly so.[353]

As discussed repeatedly, historically marginalized populations across the world, including NYC, are at the highest risk of adverse health consequences based on the woefully inadequate resources provided for people living in poverty. These conditions are endemic and are simply flared with infectious disease outbreaks.

COVID-19 seems to be the gold standard of this amplification of these health inequities. But nearly every infectious disease outbreak of global significance follows a similar narrative. The lack of access to basic sanitation, hygiene, vaccinations and nutrition as well as to the principles of isolation, the distrust of the very governments empowered to facilitate these isolations and the decades of preceding sociopolitical violence led to perfect storms of infectious disease outbreaks and associative violence.

There are countless previous examples demonstrating the association between population stress and infectious disease—e.g., leishmaniasis, cholera, typhus, trench fever, anthrax, tuberculosis, and certainly HIV/AIDS and Ebola. It is likely that fractured health systems worsened by episodic social disruption place inordinate stress on societies and disproportionately impact the most vulnerable in those respective societies. Given such woefully inadequate health care systems unequipped to manage the needs of its citizens coupled with latent microbes existent for decades awaiting perfectly opportunistic moments, we can speculate that stark inequalities may be one of the strongest precipitants of infectious disease outbreaks.

As the circle of poverty and disease continues, population stress can not only be a precedent to outbreaks, but can also be the consequence of such. Months of government-facilitated isolation, quarantine, and separation for COVID-19, disproportionate adverse health consequences, as well as further economic distress on populations predisposed to adversity likely precipitated a pressure cooker scenario that activated frustration from decades of systematic oppression and violence. Social norms and civic boundaries had dissolved, and it is plausible that populations felt more emboldened to express their sense of lived injustice. NYC (like cities across the world) were aggravated by the gross inequities seen in this world. It caused them to take to the streets and demand justice. It further caused thousands to break down the months of progress that social distancing had on the incidence of COVID-19 in NYC. This, in conjunction, with the anger and emotional exhaustion associated with the unjust killing of George Floyd, likely led to a widespread compromise on the immune systems of thousands, placing them at higher risk of infection and poor disease progression.[354] Just in time for subsequent waves of infection, as the cycle of social and political determinants continues.

Weeks into taking this job, the majority of my time was spent setting up isolation and quarantine hotels across four boroughs (Staten Island, unfortunately, was not included), with the "prize" hotels located in the middle of Times Square. I was commanding and writing policies for thousands of nurses and emergency medical services personnel. Fear was contagious. There was no trust—in government or science. New York City had so many agencies that it was difficult to cut through the fat. Outside of the time spent with the teams in the hotels, I spent much of my time describing the differences between isolation and quarantine to city officials. The housing insecure did not want to leave the hotels once they were cleared. It was so difficult to speak to anyone and get anything done. As a result, some of the leaders among the New York City health agencies created an interagency system integration task force with four working groups: IPC; behavioral health, intellectual, and developmental disorders; coordination, planning, and operations; and, of course, the SDoH. I coordinated all four. This was one of my proudest achievements—being able to cut through the proverbial fat and facilitate dozens of agencies to come together in a unified way to help create order for the thousands of communities in a city I loved. Alas, this should have been created ahead of time.

Zooming out beyond New York City, it was inarguable that we saw disproportionate numbers of cases in Black and Brown populations. From 2019 to 2020 in the United States, the life expectancy of Latinx communities decreased by 3 years; for Black communities, 2.9 years; and for non-Hispanic white communities, less than half that at 1.2 years.[355] As of September 15, 2020, Black Americans had COVID-19 mortality rates more than two times higher than the rate for whites and Asians, who had the lowest rates.[356] Black communities also had a greater propensity for infection than white Americans.[357] For instance, a study from April 2020 showed that Black Americans in Chicago accounted for over 50% of COVID-19 cases while composing only 30% of the city's population.[358] In Michigan, Black Americans, who compose 14% of the population, suffered 33% of the state's COVID-19 cases.[359] In April 2020 the Johns Hopkins University and American Community Survey noted from responses by 131 predominantly Black communities in the United States that the infection rate of Black Americans was 137.5 per 100,000 individuals, more than three times that of White Americans.[360]

In a similar vein, the Navajo Nation actually had the highest rate of infections in the United States in May 2020. After two years of the pandemic, American Indians/Alaskan Natives experienced a precipitous drop in life expectancy to 65 years of age, which was a loss of more than 6.5 years since 2019. On par with the average American life expectancy in 1944 and lower than every country in the Americas except Haiti, this decrease was the worst among all racial groups in the United States. High rates of diabetes and obesity, combined with crowded multigenerational housing, added significantly to the risk of higher mortality among US Indigenous populations.[356] In June 2021 the CDC confirmed these numbers, reporting that American Indian or Alaska Native non-Hispanic persons had the highest rates of both hospitalizations and deaths, while Latinx communities suffered the highest infection rates of COVID-19 compared to white persons. Additionally, a study published by the *New England Journal of Medicine* in July 2020 revealed that the effects of stress and weathering on minority groups decreases their stamina against COVID-19.[361]

To be clear, these disproportionate cases were not necessarily the direct result of the infection. As this book argues, the vast disparities seen among Black and Brown communities is the combined result of the flaring up of salient inequities among chronic conditions in addition to poor access to appropriate primary care and prevention programs. These access barriers are multifactorial and are generally the result of either poorly funded public and community health programs in certain areas or the systematic distrust and misunderstanding of these institutions, especially among the poorest communities in the world—especially in the United States. Case in point: Obesity, diabetes, and tobacco use were some of the strongest risk factors when it came to COVID-19 deaths.

Was there something specific about COVID-19 that seemed to really trigger these disparities relative to other pandemics or PHEICs? This is not a "COVID-19 thing." This is a "pandemic thing," and there is a common trend to all of them. Whether 1918 or 2019, the core conditions remain the same. What has changed is that in this current era of information sharing, we have so many more data points connecting these dots that we are exponentially more aware.

As COVID-19 vaccines began to be distributed to the public in December 2020, there was clear inequalities in the rates and patterns of distribution by race and geography. In some states, Black and Brown communities received smaller shares of the vaccinations even if their rates of infection were higher. For example, Colorado had 10% of vaccinations going to Latinx communities even though Latinx accounted for 41% of total cases.[362]

Vaccine hesitancy was at an all-time high during COVID-19 for a number of reasons. Most of the studies around this topic that involved communities of color (including one that I conducted while at Marin County)[363] generally cited distrust as one of the primary reasons they were hesitant to or refusing to be vaccinated. Studying these findings in aggregate allows us to easily see that there are general trust issues with systems of government and science. Of course, some of this can be traced back to the Tuskegee Syphilis Study, in which Black communities were intentionally (and unknowingly) infected with syphilis in order to track its national progression without treatment.[364] In the United States, we saw a very striking similarity with some of the Nazi eugenics experiments.

Curiously, however, it's not just communities of color that share this sense of distrust. In fact, Black communities and registered Republicans (regardless of race) had the highest rates of COVID-19 vaccine hesitancy. The issue of systematic distrust is not specific to the United States. Recently, we have seen similar trends in Hungary, Italy, Russia, Brazil, Turkey, and the Philippines. Many of these nations have been described as illiberal democracies, where the political leadership and populace are often clashing, but the faint scent of democracy at least allows some opinions to be registered.[365]

The rates of misinformation and conspiracy theories during the COVID-19 pandemic were some of the highest ever seen among pandemics or PHEICs. Importantly, these salient discrepancies in truth help to further potentiate the sociopolitical drivers of health care access, highlighting the inherent weaknesses in the US public health system.[366] *We must depoliticize public health. Full stop.*

Let's move to a different topic—how the COVID-19 pandemic polarized the existing inequities in health care access. Indeed, there was a mass reduction of health care services (especially among ambulatory "nonurgent" centers), which disproportionately impacted historically marginalized communities. Fear and systematic distrust further exacerbated this engagement with health care. Health care facilities, staff capacity, equipment, and resources were overstretched—especially in the Global South.[367,368] Researchers have modeled the indirect effects of the pandemic on mortality, including increased child mortality associated with reduced health service use.[369] Conventional ways of providing care (which already suffered from historical inequities) were further impacted and polarized inequities. Innovative methods were sorely needed in order to reach these and other populations (e.g., drug users). This is a lot of what Wellness Equity Alliance does. We specifically look into innovative clinical service delivery models that connect community and public health systems in order to mitigate risk for those most vulnerable.

In addition to the pandemic's direct and indirect disproportionate health effects on certain communities, it also exacerbated general differences in respective public and community health infrastructures through relative economic disruptions. As a case in point: Black and brown communities more often work in the manual labor fields, where they were usually considered "essential" during the initial stages of the pandemic (reflect back on our discussion of this in chapters 2 and 4). In addition, they were often living in multigenerational homes and lacked the general privilege to escape risk by jetting out to their vacation homes or areas of lower population density.

The economic consequences have been profound and attributable to multiple reasons—namely, the outcomes of the disease itself (e.g., families with multiple deaths losing breadwinners, increased poverty due to health expenditures) and the result of behavior changes due to fear of contracting the virus or of stigmatization. Public health and social measures also required businesses and schools to close and restricted cultural and social gatherings and travel. Unequal changes in these circumstances have implications for health inequity. The digital gap, for example, has further negative impacts on equity, whereby some groups can telework, continue schooling, or seek medical advice, including SGBV (domestic), while others cannot. According to the International Telecommunication Union, about half of all people globally are offline, and more women than men have restricted or no access to online information.[370]

The global economy contracted by more than 3% during this pandemic, reducing the income of billions of people and driving close to 95 million people into extreme poverty.[371] Sizable decreases in income affect low-income families first. In Indonesia it was estimated that an additional 1.3 million people were pushed into poverty, returning the level of poverty in the country to that in 2004.[372] A study in 29 European countries indicated an average doubling of the poverty index, to over 9%, a rate of mean loss of earnings for poor workers of 10–16% and an average increase in the Gini coefficient of 3–7%.[373]

Social protection programs were mobilized across the world. The United States activated the American Rescue Plan Act, which was, no doubt, helpful. Social protection is important for health (including a number of other covariates) by ensuring income stability and security in crises and reducing social inequality. Case in point, a cohort study of low- and middle-income households in the United States that lost work during the COVID-19 pandemic showed that receiving unemployment insurance resulted in a 4% decrease in food insecurity.[374] Unfortunately, given the law of unintended consequences, concern has grown that social protection measures have failed to prevent people from falling into poverty and, despite best intentions, have actually widened the gap, given that the most impoverished are often working in the informal economy. A study in China of the positive use of social protection to support households during the pandemic called attention to the common problem of groups that do not qualify for protection, such as undocumented or unregistered migrants and homeless populations.[375] This was also seen in SSA.

Moreover, the greater mobility of the low-paid workers in precarious employment (a job that may be easily lost, is short-term, or is poorly paid and with no or few "benefits" such as paid sick leave or paid annual leave) has increased their risk of exposure to COVID-19. We see this quite a bit in the city of Vernon, California, where I am the public health officer and where over 50,000 mostly low-skilled workers go in every day to punch a clock. Greater food insecurity reduces the feasibility of adhering to public health and social measures and increases mobility, which increases exposure to infection.[376]

Poor protection at work and precarious work arrangements for many essential workers also contribute to the risk of infection. Essential workers are required to be present at their workplaces regardless of their medical vulnerability or lack of protection. One meta-analysis (a study of studies) identified a systematic lack of access to protective equipment in the agricultural and health care sectors, highlighting that BIPOC, migrant, and female workers are disproportionately affected. Similar results were found in studies conducted in Stockholm, Sweden, and Mumbai, India.[376]

Overall, at a system level the high death rates of health care workers are a tragedy on their own but have also increased the strain on health systems and exacerbated the projected global shortage of 15 million health care workers by 2030.[377] When I was running the COVID-19 hotel program in New York City early in the pandemic, most of our

COVID-19: Rubric for determining the sociopolitical determinants of pandemics and PHEICs

	Sociopolitical determinant–linked questionnaire	Yes	No
1	Is there a sociopolitical link to the original spread of disease?	☐	☐
2	Was there a lack of public and community health infrastructure at the time?	☐	☐
3	If yes, did the lack of infrastructure at the time of spread precipitate more widespread distribution?	☐	☐
4	Was the lack of infrastructure at the time linked to a sociopolitical root cause?	☐	☐
5	Is it treatable? In other words, would building more effective sociopolitical infrastructure mitigate the risk of spread?	☐	☐

hotels were set up for health care workers in order to mitigate risk to their families. Unfortunately, it was not enough, and many were still infected and needed to drop out. Early reports from global WHO programs warn of setbacks in controlling diseases such as HIV/AIDS, TB, malaria, dengue, measles, and polio in the future, which will increase demands on public health systems, lead to further population stress, and ultimately cost more lives. Our next and final chapter in this part examines these contemporary issues.

And now it is time for grading again—one last time. As COVID-19 has produced the most data around the sociopolitical drivers of disease to date by far, I will allow the students to become the teachers: Use your knowledge to grade the most contemporary of all pandemics.

CHAPTER 6

The Most Prevalent Infectious Disease Killers Today

The only thing we learn from history is that we learn nothing from history.
—FRIEDRICH HEGEL

We've now discussed every major pandemic or public health emergency of international concern (PHEIC) since 1899 to demonstrate the common sociopolitical drivers of pandemics and the variable effect they play on population stress levels and how that helps determine a number of outcomes—from poor to poorest. This chapter brings these lessons into today's world to better explain why this all matters. While two of these infectious diseases from the microbial hall of fame are still very much present and relevant in today's ecosystem, we will discuss five others in detail and then summarize the sociopolitical determinant rubric and how it can likely be successfully applied to all.

In 2019 the World Health Organization (WHO) estimated that approximately 15% of annual deaths worldwide were attributable to infectious diseases.[1] The good news is that this number had decreased by nearly 10% (23.7%) since 2000—generally because of the impressive reductions in AIDS-related deaths (deaths have fallen by 51% since 2000, moving from the world's 8th leading cause of death in 2000 to the 19th in 2019), as well as deaths attributable to diarrheal diseases, childhood cluster diseases (e.g., whooping cough, measles), and malaria. The bad news is that COVID-19 has significantly increased this proportionate mortality since 2019 (the scale of which we are still calculating).

If we zoom out further for comparative purposes, the world's biggest killer is ischemic heart disease (e.g., heart attacks), responsible for 16% of the world's total deaths. Stroke and COPD are the second and third leading causes of death, responsible for approximately 11% and 6% of total deaths, respectively. Lower respiratory infections (e.g., pneumonia) remained the world's most deadly communicable diseases, ranked as the fourth leading cause of death.[1]

People living in low-income countries are far more likely to die of a communicable disease. Despite the global decline, 6 of the top 10 causes of death in low-income countries are infectious by nature. The "big 3," as they're often grouped together, are malaria, tuberculosis (TB), and HIV/AIDS. Fortunately, all 3 are falling significantly. Diarrheal diseases are more significant as a cause of death in low-income countries (especially in children under 5) and rank in the top 5 causes of death for this income category (figure 6.1).

With that said, COVID-19 and HIV/AIDS are the most formidable infectious diseases we have seen since the 1918 Spanish flu. While pneumonia, pediatric diarrheal diseases, and TB may have directly taken more lives, COVID-19 and HIV/AIDS remain particularly unique, for a few reasons. First, their impact is not necessarily directly seen at times, but they have a particular predilection for vulnerabilities. While one can argue that this is generally the case for infectious diseases, as they prey on either individual or population-level compromised immunities (i.e., population stress), HIV/AIDS specifically attacks the immune system to allow outside invaders to infiltrate, and COVID-19 specifically preys more on the infirm than many other infectious diseases—the poorer, the older, the chronically sicker—at

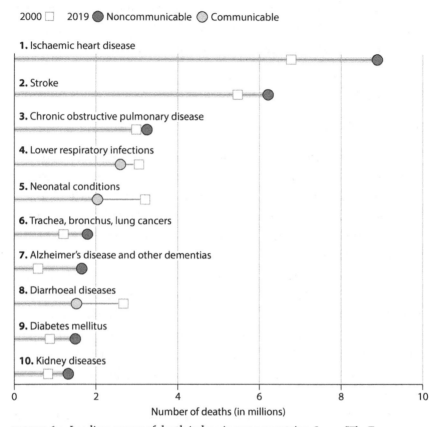

Leading causes of death globally

2000 ☐   2019 ● Noncommunicable   ◔ Communicable

1. Ischaemic heart disease

2. Stroke

3. Chronic obstructive pulmonary disease

4. Lower respiratory infections

5. Neonatal conditions

6. Trachea, bronchus, lung cancers

7. Alzheimer's disease and other dementias

8. Diarrhoeal diseases

9. Diabetes mellitus

10. Kidney diseases

0   2   4   6   8   10

Number of deaths (in millions)

FIGURE 6.1. Leading causes of death in low-income countries. *Source:* "The Top 10 Causes of Death," World Health Organization, December 9, 2020, https://www.who.int/news-room/fact-sheets/detail/the-top-10-causes-of-death.

a greater scale. It is partly for these reasons that I have chosen to focus my career and nearly all my attention on these two diseases, and I am writing this book today largely because of my experience with these diseases and the gross inequities I have seen with both. As we substantially addressed these two diseases in chapter 5, we will skip any granular dive into these and skip over to TB but include them in our general roundup at the end of this chapter. We will also exclude lower respiratory infections, as their clinical manifestations and epidemiological distribution are similar to influenza and COVID-19 and are so multifactorial (multiple microbes or "bugs" can cause them) that they are difficult to discuss as a monolithic sociopolitical issue across the world. Got it? Let's move forward. . . .

Tuberculosis

Clinical Manifestations

TB is a complex disease process that can be either pulmonary (in the lungs) or extrapulmonary (outside the lungs). The disease course can be broken up into three forms—primary, latent, and reactivation.

Reports show that approximately 15–20% of TB is extrapulmonary, but much of that is underreported.[2] In fact, some experts believe this number could be closer to 50%. Primary TB describes new TB infections or active disease in a previously naive host. Fever is the most common symptom (>70%). Other common symptoms are cough, weight loss, and fatigue. Night sweats are classic and unique. Chest pain, shortness of breath, and bloody cough are also reported in one-quarter to one-third of patients. Weight loss and wasting (consumption) are classic features described in the literary sense but are less common end findings.

After the primary infection, 90% of individuals keep their immunity intact, stopping the spread of the disease, which may then clear up or enter the latent phase.[3] The person remains asymptomatic, but latent disease has the potential to become active at any time. Reactivation occurs more frequently in those with compromised immunity and has been classically described in people with HIV/AIDS, chronic kidney failure, and poorly controlled diabetes and in those receiving immunosuppressive medications (including transplant recipients), young children (before the age of 5), and older adults. The remaining 10% of individuals develop progressive primary disease with TB pneumonia and the expansion of "lung bugs" at the site of the initial seeding. Folks with lung involvement may also present with disease at more distant sites, commonly with lymph node, brain, or heart involvement.

Epidemiology

TB is the quintessential airborne disease, classically spread through coughing or sneezing. It is also the leading cause of death from a single infectious agent. Wow. This is probably the most prolific disease in literature over the ages—from Egyptian mummies to the Greeks and Romans, to the Middle Ages, to after the time we finally understood what it was (famously described by Robert Koch), to the era of British colonialism, to the Industrial Revolution, and to today, where it still remains the number-one infectious cause of death. According to the WHO, 10 million new infections occurred in 2018, with approximately 1.5 million dying. And even though it's curable and preventable, it's still in the top-10 causes of death worldwide.[4]

Let's quantify this further. More than 1.7 billion people (or 22% of the global population) are estimated to be infected with *Mycobacterium tuberculosis* (the bacterial agent that causes TB).[5] The global incidence of TB peaked around 2003 and appears to be declining slowly (figure 6.2). The highest rates (300 per 100,000 or higher) are observed in sub-Saharan Africa (SSA), India, and the islands of Southeast Asia and Micronesia. Intermediate rates of TB (26–300 cases per 100,000) occur in China, Central and South America, Eastern Europe, and northern Africa. Low rates (<25 cases per 100,000 inhabitants) occur in the Global North.[6]

Fortunately, as a mycobacterium it can be treated with antibiotics, which is unique from most of the pandemics we've discussed, which have been viral (plague and cholera were also bacterial exceptions). Here's a little trivia for you: The term "antibiotic" can be broken down from its Latin roots to "against life." Antibiotics have no effect on viruses, which are not alive. When antibiotics are not used appropriately, however, very serious consequences occur. This is now the case with TB, where we have multidrug resistance or extensive-drug resistance,

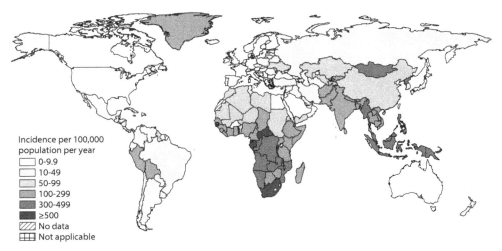

FIGURE 6.2. Estimated tuberculosis incidence rates. *Source:* World Health Organization, *Global Tuberculosis Report 2022*, October 27, 2022, https://www.who.int/teams/global-tuberculosis -programme/tb-reports/global-tuberculosis-report-2022/.

respectively. This is very bad. Treatment for these strains is incredibly complex and expensive, which is a particularly challenging issue, as TB more often develops in the most resource-poor settings in the world without robust public health systems in place. Antimicrobial resistance is increasingly becoming the most formidable challenge in public health.

Sociopolitical Determinants

TB is the quintessential socially driven infectious disease from time immemorial. Poverty, HIV, and drug resistance are major contributors to the resurging global TB epidemic.[7,8] Approximately 95% of TB cases occur in resource-limited countries. And in more resourced areas, we see cases nearly exclusively limited to the most historically marginalized communities—that is, prisoners, people experiencing homelessness (PEH), and migrants. One in every dozen new TB cases occurs in individuals infected with HIV (though many of these are actually reactivated but previously undiagnosed); 74% of these HIV-coinfected persons reside in SSA. Socioeconomic development and access to quality health services appear to be at least as important as any specific TB control measure. The likelihood of successful TB control efforts is strongly linked to socioeconomic indicators, including gross domestic product gross domestic product per capita, the mortality of children <5, access to clean water, and adequate sanitation and health expenditure per capita.[9]

Hargreaves et al. describe the structural determinants of TB epidemiology to include global socioeconomic inequalities, high levels of population mobility, and rapid urbanization and population growth.[10] These conditions give rise to unequal distributions of key social determinants of TB, including food insecurity and malnutrition, poor housing and environmental conditions, and financial, geographic, and cultural barriers to health care access. In turn, the population distribution of TB reflects the distribution of these social determinants, which influence the four stages of TB pathogenesis: exposure to infection, progression to disease, late or inappropriate diagnosis and treatment, and poor treatment adherence and success (figure 6.3).[11]

Thinking back to our unpacking of the core understanding of the social determinants of health (SDoH) in chapter 2, TB can be explained on every level. For example, poor ventilation and overcrowding in homes, workplaces, and communities increase the likelihood of uninfected individuals being exposed to TB transmission.[12,13,14] Poverty, malnutrition, and hunger may increase susceptibility to further progression and severe disease.[15] Symptomatic patients with a persistent cough often face significant social and economic barriers that delay their contact with health systems in which an appropriate diagnosis might be made, including difficulties in transport to health facilities, fear of stigmatization if they seek a TB diagnosis, and a lack of social support to seek care when they fall sick.[16,17] Finally, because of the close relationship between HIV and TB in many settings (notably SSA), which has caused a collision of the two most formidable public health challenges

EXPOSURE	INFECTION	DISEASE	ACCESS TO TB CARE AND CLINICAL OUTCOME
· Being male	· Being male	· Being male	· Being female
· Age of source of infection	· Increased age	· Increase age	· Geographic barriers
· Community TB prevalence	· Race/ethnic group	· Race/ethnic group	· Economic barriers
· High population density	· Contact with source case	· Poverty	· Cultural barriers
· Crowding	· Poverty	· Malnutrition	· Weak health care system
· Urban residence	· Malnutrition	· Lack of BCG	· Stigma
· Poor ventilation at home	· Lack of BCG	· Smoking, alochol/drug abuse	· Lack of social protection
· Indoor pollution	· HIV	· HIV	· MDR-TB
	· Urban residence	· Diabetes, cancer, silicosis	· HIV
		· Other immune-suppresive conditions	· Malnutrition
		· Migration	· Other immune-suppresive conditions
		· Urban residence	

FIGURE 6.3. Social determinants of tuberculosis epidemiology. *Source:* Graphic by author.

in modern medicine, the key structural and social determinants of HIV infection as described in chapter 5 also act as indirect determinants of TB risk.[18]

Malaria

Clinical Manifestations

The initial symptoms of malaria are nonspecific and most commonly include fever, chills, rapid heart and breathing rates, malaise, fatigue, sweating, headache, cough, poor appetite, nausea, vomiting, abdominal pain, diarrhea, and joint and muscle pain.[19] In certain tropical areas, malaria may be as prevalent as the common cold is in other climates and does not cause too much alarm. Our greatest concern is for pregnant women and young children, who can experience more severe manifestations, such as seizures, altered consciousness, severe anemia, low blood sugar, respiratory distress or acute respiratory distress syndrome, severe blood-clotting issues, severe acid-base disturbances, circulatory collapse, renal and liver failure, and, finally, cerebral malaria. Cerebral malaria affects the brain and causes impaired consciousness, delirium, and/or seizures. Cerebral malaria is also one of the most challenging conditions to observe, as it can be so prevalent in certain areas of the tropics and so quickly transition from mild to a more fulminant form overnight without the appropriate resources.[20]

Fortunately, population prevention programs that are relatively straightforward to scale are available, but resources and political stability are essential determinants. When I worked in the most eastern region of Sierra Leone during the Ebola epidemic, cases were improving, and I frankly could not sit still. I would attend the local morning rounds and hear of multiple children crashing in the middle of the night. This was an abhorrent and unacceptable reality coming from the United States, where one overnight death of a child under five would be a freak rarity. I paid attention, I studied the issue, I spoke with the stakeholders, and I saw what I could do.

The problem was threefold. First, they lacked a systematic screening and treatment protocol. Second, they lacked the most effective antimalarial treatment. Third, they were using blood transfusions as a way to "cure" the issue, which was scientifically wrong (and there may have been a side racket perpetuating this practice, albeit unconfirmed). A group of us did what we could. We incorporated new protocols and associated training, introduced new medications (sustainability was a concern), and addressed the blood transfusion myth (as best as we could). Seemingly overnight the rate of childhood mortality precipitously declined. That cacophony of the number of young children dying overnight went from an average of 5–10 to nearly 0. While this experience felt like a victory, I soon realized that it was merely a drop in the ocean and that unless we scale efforts like this, these successes have very minimal impact. Of course, others feel differently, and I love them for that.

Epidemiology

Malaria is endemic throughout most of the tropics, with ongoing transmission taking place in 85 countries and territories.[21] The WHO reported 241 million cases and 627,000 deaths from malaria in 2020, which was a slight increase from the previous year. The malaria parasite is transmitted most frequently via the bite of a female mosquito (*Anopheles*), which occurs mainly between dusk and dawn.[22,23] Other rare mechanisms for transmission include congenitally acquired disease, blood transfusion, sharing of contaminated needles, organ transplantation, and health care associated transmission.[24,25] Malaria is caused by a parasite that we refer to as a plasmodium. There are multiple types. In terms of the prevalence of infections, the *Plasmodium* distribution can be broken down according to the subtypes, with *falciparum*, *vivax*, and *ovale* causing approximately >70%, 10%, and 5% of infections, respectively.[26]

While *Plasmodium vivax* is much more common in the Americas and the western Pacific (figure 6.4), over 95% of the *P. falciparum* burden occurs in SSA, followed by 2% each in the Southeast Asian and Eastern Mediterranean regions, respectively, with the American and Western Pacific regions contributing the remainder. Twenty-nine countries account for 96% of cases (figure 6.5), with a handful of nations representing the vast majority of the burden of disease: Nigeria is responsible for 27%, the DRC for 12%, Uganda for 5%, Mozambique for 4%, and Angola and Burkina Faso each for 3.4%. What do all these nations have in common? They are all either ranked poorest or lowest in the human development indices (ranking as the "unhappiest") in the world.[27]

While the increase in malaria is alarming, with malaria elimination and controlling efforts (very different approaches, which we'll discuss below) the numbers are reportedly decreasing at a substantial rate. As

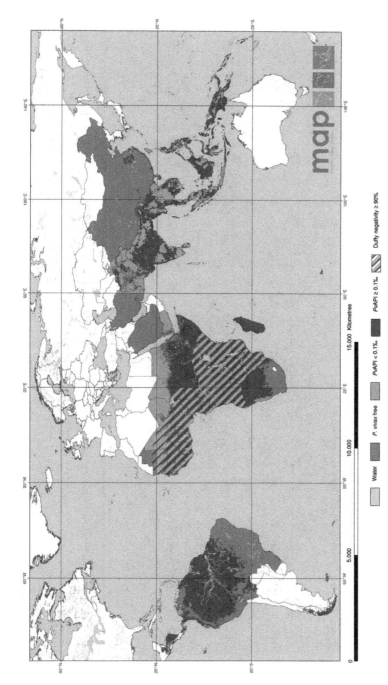

Water P. vivax free PvAPI < 0.1‰ PvAPI ≥ 0.1‰ Duffy negativity ≥ 90%

FIGURE 6.4. Areas at risk of *Plasmodium vivax* malaria. *Source*: Malaria Atlas Project.

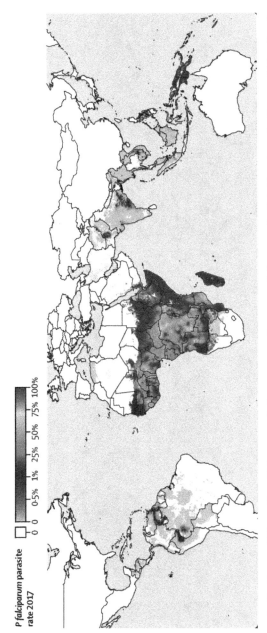

FIGURE 6.5. Incidence of *Plasmodium falciparum* malaria. *Source:* Daniel J. Weiss et al., "Mapping the Global Prevalence, Incidence, and Mortality of *Plasmodium falciparum*, 2000–17: A Spatial and Temporal Modeling Study," *Lancet* 394, no. 10195 (2019): 322–331, https://doi.org/10.1016/s0140-6736(19)31097-9.

a case in point, the Institute for Health Metrics and Epidemiology reported 1.82 million and 1.24 million deaths, respectively, in 2004 and 2010 (a reduction of one-third in just 6 years).[28] Unfortunately, the vast majority of deaths continue to occur mainly among African children <5 years of age.[29,30] In 2018 there were 1,823 confirmed cases in the United States—with 85% of those from Africa and, specifically, 70% from West Africa (figure 6.6).

Sociopolitical Determinants

One could argue that malaria has a higher inequality in distribution than any other disease of public health importance. Malaria is frequently referred to as a disease of the poor, with 58% of malaria deaths occurring among the poorest 20% of the world.[31] Social and livelihood activities are key factors in malaria transmission and control strategies. Several studies suggest that low socioeconomic status is associated with higher malaria prevalence.[32] Moreover, household responses to illness are known to be influenced by socioeconomic and cultural factors, including beliefs about causes and effective cures as well as accessibility to health care sources.[33] Cultural beliefs or inappropriate behavior and practices are known to interfere with the effectiveness of control measures, including health care–seeking patterns.[34]

Endemic malaria results in tremendous economic losses annually and is a central element of the vicious cycle of poverty in many low-income nations (figure 6.7).[35,36] Therefore, any attempt to organize effective control or elimination programs must be focused on strengthening systems that address the SDoH.[37] Malaria-associated morbidity and the cost of treatment create barriers to effective and sustainable social and economic development.

As discussed above, malaria control and elimination have technical delineations, with the latter aimed at a steady reduction to near zero cases (or what the WHO describes as an interruption in local transmission of cases in a defined geographic area). Nations heavily afflicted with a substantial disease burden are confronted with the choice of

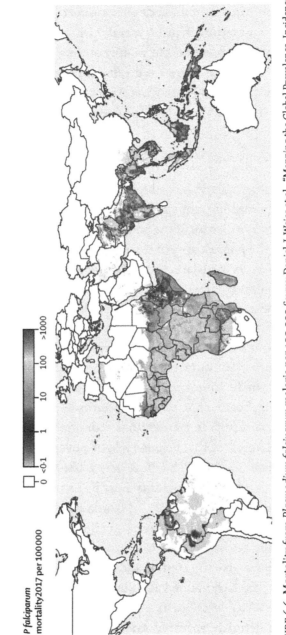

FIGURE 6.6. Mortality from *Plasmodium falciparum* malaria per 100,000 *Source:* Daniel J. Weiss et al., "Mapping the Global Prevalence, Incidence, and Mortality of *Plasmodium falciparum*, 2000–17: A Spatial and Temporal Modeling Study," *Lancet* 394, no. 10195 (2019): 322–331, https://doi.org/10.1016 /s0140-6736(19)31097-9.

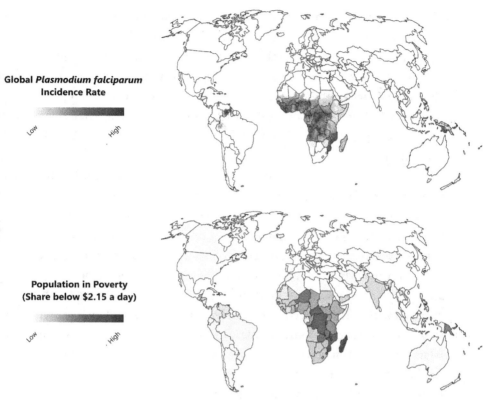

Global *Plasmodium falciparum*
Incidence Rate

Low   High

Population in Poverty
(Share below $2.15 a day)

Low   High

FIGURE 6.7. Relationship between the burden of malaria worldwide and estimated poverty levels in the world. *Source:* Graphic by author.

continuing control activities indefinitely to keep malaria at very low levels or actively pursuing elimination. Malaria elimination is feasible if the technical, operational, and financial challenges to permanently stop malaria's transmission can be overcome.[38] In other words, elimination is possible if control methods can be deployed at a sufficiently high level and length of time to stop transmission and eliminate all malaria parasites circulating locally. The problem is, however, that a public health infrastructure and sociopolitical stability are essential criteria to develop an effective elimination program. Clearly, the instability and incivility of nations like the DRC and Nigeria make these outcomes highly challenging. The operational challenges are clearly defined in terms of the human capital, national infrastructure, and the political commitment needed by nations to reach their elimination goals. This choice is complex, and in the absence of clear guidance, the decision to pursue malaria elimination might be made on a political basis without careful and rigorous assessment of the operational feasibility. Unfortunately, the communities (especially the children dying at an unforgiving rate) most at risk are noticeably absent from these sociopolitical decisions.[39]

The good news is that hope is on the proverbial horizon. During 2000–2009, the overall number of malaria cases was reduced by 23% in 105 countries and the number of deaths by 38%, with 43 countries (11 of them in Africa) cutting malaria cases or deaths by 50% or more.[40] All these successes have been achieved in part by large increases in funding for malaria, from about $100 million to $1.5 billion from 2003–2010. These successes notwithstanding, any celebration needs to be tempered with caution. A comprehensive report published by *The Lancet* in 2010 warns that some countries have not yet begun to scale-up malaria interventions, while others are struggling to sustain their success. Resistance to drugs and insecticides are further threatening gains. The best we can hope for is cautious optimism at this point.[38]

Meningitis

Clinical Manifestations

Meningitis is an inflammatory disease of the leptomeninges (basically, it is the "Saran wrap" around the brain and spinal cord keeping all the tissues and cells in place; figure 6.8).[40] The meninges consist of three parts: the pia, arachnoid, and dura maters. Meningitis can either be viral or bacterial. Bacterial (again, somewhat unique from most of the viral pandemics described in chapter 5 and what we are mostly describing here) meningitis reflects infection of the arachnoid (middle) mater and the cerebrospinal fluid in both the subarachnoid space and the cerebral ventricles.

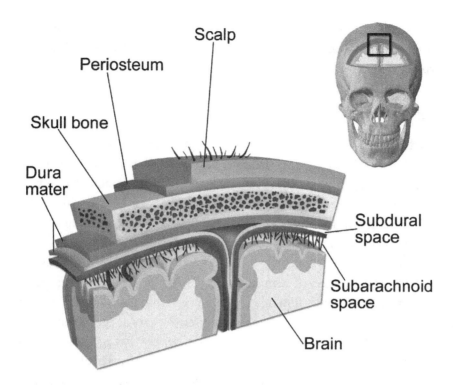

Scalp

Periosteum

Skull bone

Dura
mater

Subdural
space

Subarachnoid
space

Brain

Layers covering the Brain

FIGURE 6.8. Meningeal layers of the brain and spinal cord. *Source:* "Medical Gallery of Blausen Medical 2014," *WikiJournal of Medicine,* https://doi.org/10.15347/wjm/2014.010.

The classic triad of acute bacterial meningitis, which occurs in 41% of patients, consists of fever, stiff neck, and a change in mental status, usually of sudden onset.[41] The most common clinical features include a severe headache (84%), fever greater than 38°C (74%), stiff neck (74%), obtunded (71%), and nausea (62%).[42] In addition to the classic findings, less common manifestations are seizures (23%), aphasia (affected speech) or some form of paralysis (22%), and coma (13%).[43] Co-occurring infections may include a sinus or ear infection (34%) and pneumonia (9%). Other causes of meningitis (known as *aseptic*, which is mostly viral but can have other infectious causes, including fungal) often present with the classic triad but may also exhibit photophobia (pain/discomfort when exposed to light). In contrast to bacterial meningitis, patients do not present with altered mental status, and the onset may be less acute.[44]

Epidemiology

As discussed, the most common causes of aseptic meningitis are viruses (e.g., enteroviruses, arboviruses, herpes). This term also includes more than 100 other causes, however, such as other infections (e.g., mycobacteria, fungi, spirochetes), medications, and cancer. We will mostly cover bacterial meningitis here, which can either be community acquired (meaning anywhere outside of a medical setting) or health care associated.

The major causes of community-acquired bacterial meningitis in adults in developed countries are *Streptococcus pneumoniae*, *Neisseria meningitidis*, and, primarily in patients over 50 years of age or those who are immunocompromised, *Listeria monocytogenes*.[45] In the United States and other nations of the Global North, following the institution of routine infant immunizations with *Hemophilus influenzae* type b (*Hib*) in 1990, *S. pneumoniae* (pneumococcus) (*Sp*) in 2000, and the pneumococcal vaccine in 2010, bacterial meningitis has decreased in frequency, and the peak incidence of bacterial meningitis (*Nm*) has shifted from children under 5 years to adults.[46,47]

In other parts of the globe, *S. pneumoniae* remains the most common cause, accounting for approximately 25–41% of cases.[48] The distribution of pathogens depends upon the region of the world. As a case in point, large epidemics of meningitis due to *N. meningitidis* serogroup A used to occur in SSA, although the implementation of the meningococcal group A conjugate vaccine has virtually eliminated meningococcal group A. Epidemics due to non–group A meningococcal and other meningeal pathogens continue to occur. *S. suis* is an emerging zoonosis that causes meningitis in Asia and has been linked to exposure to pigs. It is the most frequent cause of bacterial meningitis in adults in South Vietnam and has caused outbreaks in China.[49]

While bacterial meningitis affects all countries of the world, the most formidable concern is in SSA, especially in a famed location referred to as the meningitis belt, which extends from Senegal near the Atlantic Coast to Ethiopia and Somalia on the shores of the Red Sea and the Indian Ocean, specifically including the following nations: Ethiopia, The Gambia, Benin, Cameroon, Burkina Faso, Chad, Ghana, Niger, Mali, Senegal, Nigeria, and Sudan (figure 6.9). Apart from epidemics, at least 1.2 million cases of bacterial meningitis are estimated to occur every year, 135,000 of which are fatal.[50] Even when the disease is diagnosed early and adequate treatment is started, 8–15% of patients may die, often within one to two days after the onset of symptoms, or it may result in brain damage, hearing loss, or disability in 10–20% of survivors.[51]

Within the traditional meningitis belt, major epidemics occur every 5–12 years.[52] A strong seasonal pattern influences the scale of these

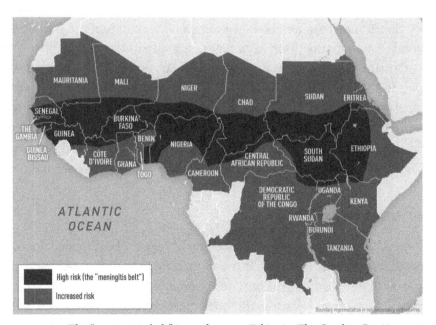

FIGURE 6.9. The "meningitis belt" extends across Ethiopia, The Gambia, Benin, Cameroon, Burkina Faso, Chad, Ghana, Niger, Mali, Senegal, Nigeria, and Sudan.
Source: Map 5-01, of meningitis belt and other areas at risk for meningococcal meningitis epidemics, World Health Organization, International Travel and Health, 2015, https://wwwnc .cdc.gov/travel/yellowbook/2024/infections-diseases/meningococcal-disease.

epidemics during the relatively dry season from January to April, mainly at a specific latitude around Africa. Vaccination efforts are critical for protection, and campaigns have been a great success, particularly in Burkina Faso, Mali, and Niger in 2010, where nearly 20 million people aged 1–29 years were vaccinated.[53] Some epidemics have been shown to occur with irregular cycles within some countries of the belt, suggesting that vaccine campaigns may be operationally complex but are absolutely necessary for population prevention.[54,55]

At the same time, several other African countries located outside the meningitis belt have faced sporadic but significant epidemics of meningitis.[56,57,58] Epidemics occurred toward the end of the 1980s and early 1990s in Burundi, the Central African Republic, Kenya, Rwanda, Uganda, Tanzania, and Zimbabwe, all countries where the disease spread outside the usual boundaries. A possible extension of the African meningitis belt to other African territories has raised the possibility that it may become necessary to extend vaccination programs beyond the previously prioritized targeted countries.[59]

Outside of population prevention efforts, antibiotics can be effective. In the preantibiotic era, bacterial meningitis due to *Sp* and *Hib* was virtually 100% fatal. With the advent of antibiotics, however, the mortality for *Hib* and *Nm* infections decreased to <10%, and that of *Sp* to an impressive 30%. Mortality due to *Sp* meningitis in high-income countries has further decreased with the use of adjunctive steroids.[60]

Sociopolitical Determinants

Generally speaking, studies consistently suggest that low socioeconomic conditions increase the risk of meningococcal disease.[61] Several other studies have shown consistent evidence that meningococcal disease has a direct relationship with poor housing conditions and household overcrowding, which is one of the most compelling social determinants.[62] In one study researchers found that the incidence risk for all cases was about 2.4 times greater in the areas that have poor housing conditions.[63] A "first world" corollary is that all US colleges and universities require that dormitory residents be vaccinated. Another example would be men who have sex with men or transgender females with multiple partners in certain venues, who would be at high risk (because of spit exchange) during certain outbreaks and would be recommended to be vaccinated (I led one of these mass vaccine efforts in Hollywood, California, in 2015). Sadly, much like malaria the nations most at risk are the very ones that lack the resources and sociopolitical stability to scale effective public health interventions (e.g., vaccinations, education) in order to prevent these outbreaks from taking place.

Measles

Clinical Manifestations

Measles is a highly contagious (one of the most contagious, in fact) viral infection with widespread global distribution. The infection is characterized by fever, malaise, cough, a runny nose, and a superficial eye infection (conjunctivitis), followed by rash.[64] Following exposure, approximately 90% of susceptible individuals will develop measles because, again, it is so infectious. The incubation period for measles is 6–21 days (median, 13 days).[65]

The period of contagiousness begins approximately 5 days before the appearance of the rash to 4 days afterward. The illness may be transmitted in public spaces, even in the absence of person-to-person contact.[66] Measles is associated with a number of other comorbidities and vitamin deficiencies (especially A) and can also lead to a depressed immune system in patients who are dealing with prolonged recoveries.[67]

Epidemiology

Measles occurs worldwide and remains a leading cause of mortality, especially among children five years of age or less.[68,69,70] Before the introduction of the measles vaccine, over 2 million deaths occurred annually. The availability of measles vaccination beginning in the 1960s

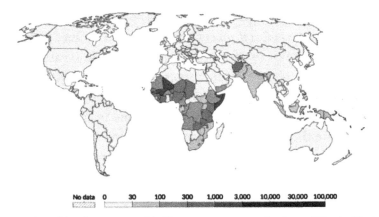

FIGURE 6.10. Measles cases worldwide per 100,000 people. *Source:* "Measles Vaccine Coverage vs. Measles Cases Worldwide, 2021," Our World in Data, https://ourworldindata.org/grapher/measles-coverage-vs-cases-worldwide?tab=map&time=2021.

immediately impacted disease incidence, reduced associated mortality rates, and altered the global distribution. Measles occurs predominantly in areas with low vaccination rates, especially in resource-limited settings (figure 6.10).[71]

Measles is highly contagious; the attack rate in a susceptible individual exposed to measles is 90%.[72,73] This means that 90% of people exposed to measles will be infected (if you recall, this is very different from influenza). Transmission occurs via person-to-person contact as well as airborne (like TB) spread. Infectious droplets from the respiratory secretions of a patient with measles can remain airborne for up to two hours.[74] Therefore, the illness may be transmitted in public spaces, even in the absence of person-to-person contact. Measles is well described during airline travel and mass gathering events.[75]

The Expanded Program on Immunization in the 1970s, a WHO program that expanded childhood vaccination coverage to include measles immunizations, together with the efforts of the United Nations International Children's Emergency Fund (UNICEF), caused the number of global measles deaths to decline from 2.6 million in 1980 to approximately 700,000 in 1990—a 73% reduction.[76] Following this, in addition to the establishment of the Millennium Development Goals (MDGs) along with the assistance of The Global Alliance for Vaccines and Immunizations (GAVI), the Vaccine Alliance, and the Bill & Melinda Gates Foundation, measles deaths declined even further, from approximately 500,000 in 2000 to approximately 100,000 in 2017, according to the Global Burden of Disease Study.[77,78] This was a major feat. I was one of those often in the field in places like South Sudan, where I would be rolling out mass immunizations. Knowing that I was contributing to these audacious goals (measles elimination) was exhilarating. In fact, experiences like these prepared me for my work on COVID-19 mass immunizations in the United States

Remarkable progress has been made toward reducing the contribution of measles to childhood morbidity and mortality worldwide, largely through the commitment to achieve two-dose immunization strategies against measles in all regions of the world.[79] The estimated global coverage with the measles-containing vaccine second dose nearly quadrupled between 2000 and 2019 (from 18% to 71%), largely due to an 86% increase in the number of countries providing a two-dose strategy (from 95 to 177 countries between 2000 and 2019; figure 6.11).

We were so close. Between 2000 and 2017, measles vaccinations prevented approximately 20.4 million deaths. Despite these remarkable feats, since 2017 the amount of effective global coverage has started to migrate in a very different direction for a number of reasons, and more than 140,000 died from measles in 2018 and over 207,000 died in 2019, the highest number reported in over 20 years.[80] Unfortunately, Peter Hotez explains that most of the increase in active cases has been in the poorest and most sociopolitically unstable nations in SSA and South Asia.[81]

As you can see, incivility and conflicts are largely to blame for this abrupt reverse course. The rise in mortality was associated with large outbreaks in several countries; however, all WHO regions reported an increase in cases starting in 2019, attributed to lower vaccine rates. As a result, the number of measles cases increased 556% between 2016 and 2019, from 132,490 to 869,770 (the most reported cases since 1996).[82] Moreover, in Europe more than 80,000 measles cases occurred in 2018

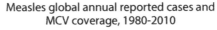

Measles global annual reported cases and
MCV coverage, 1980-2010

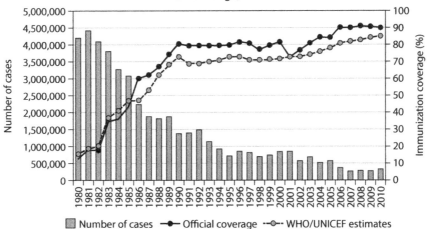

■ Number of cases   ——●—— Official coverage   --◌-- WHO/UNICEF estimates

FIGURE 6.11. Measles cases and vaccine coverage worldwide. *Source:* "Invest in Childhood Vaccination Programs," Center for High Impact Philanthropy, University of Pennsylvania, August 24, 2017, https://www.impact.upenn.edu/child-survival-guidance-for-donors/invest-in -childhood-vaccination-programs/.

(the highest number in more than a decade), while in 2019 more than 90,000 cases sprang up in the first six months. In the Americas, measles returned to Venezuela and neighboring Brazil and Colombia, while more than 1,200 cases of measles occurred in the United States in 2019, the highest number in more than two decades—mostly among certain religious groups in Brooklyn and Rockland County, New York. To add insult to injury, following the onset of the COVID-19 pandemic, a record number of children missed at least one measles vaccine dose.[83] In 2021 alone, nearly 40 million children missed one dose, and an estimated 9 million cases and 128,000 deaths occurred worldwide, with 22 countries experiencing large outbreaks.[84] Heartbreaking.

Sociopolitical Determinants

Measles has been targeted for eradication, given the favorable biological characteristic that humans are the only reservoir. Due to sociopo-

The estimated annual number of deaths caused by several vaccine-preventable diseases, based on statistical modeling. Estimates come with wide uncertainties, especially for countries with poor vital registration.

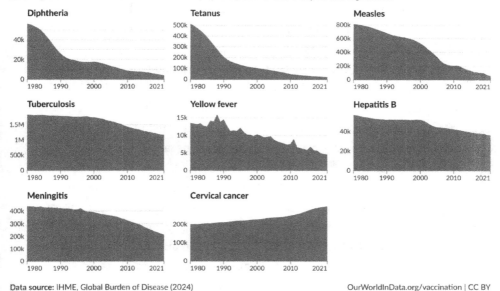

Data source: IHME, Global Burden of Disease (2024)   OurWorldInData.org/vaccination | CC BY

FIGURE 6.12. Deaths caused by vaccine-preventable diseases worldwide.
Source: "Deaths Caused by Vaccine-Preventable Diseases, World," Our World in Data, 2024, https://ourworldindata.org/grapher/deaths-caused-by-vaccine-preventable-diseases-over-time.

litical factors and high transmissibility, however, elimination has been achieved in very few areas of the world.[85] Because of its high transmissibility, the virus is often the first vaccine-preventable disease to return in association with gaps in vaccination, and it serves as a sentinel indicator for vaccine interruptions (figure 6.12).

Unfortunately, there is nothing new here. Much like all pandemics or PHEICs examined since 1899, war and political conflict remains a driving force in terms of epidemic production. In 2019 the WHO and UNICEF reported that roughly 20 million children lack access to life-saving vaccines, including the measles or measles-mumps-rubella (this is the combined format that it is often packaged in) vaccines. These unvaccinated children live disproportionately in 16 countries beset by conflict or fragile states, with limited resources to manage all but the most extraordinary needs—especially in the DRC, where more than 5,000 measles deaths were reported by the end of 2019 (a number now exceeding the deaths from their Ebola virus experience, if you recall the description above).[85] Similarly, measles mortality can also be viewed as a proxy for public health failures in many war-torn nations, including Central African Republic, Chad, Ethiopia, Mali, Niger, Sudan, and South Sudan, as well as in Somalia; Taliban-occupied areas of Afghanistan and Pakistan; and in Iraq, Syria, and Yemen on the Arabian Peninsula. In these nations, ongoing conflicts and hostilities collapse both health systems and vaccine delivery infrastructures.

In addition, vaccine health systems can collapse even in the absence of overt war and violence. For example, in Venezuela, economic failures have halted vaccination programs, leading to the return of measles, which in turn has spread into Brazil and Colombia due to a Venezuelan emigration.[86] In Venezuela, as well as in Syria and Iraq, high temperatures, prolonged drought, and desertification have caused significant crop failures, forcing populations to flee into urban centers. These physical determinants further destabilize nations and contribute to the decline in vaccine coverage by weakening the public health infrastructure. Moreover, as described in chapter 4, key communities lack access to health care systems, and the Indigenous are classically described.

Finally, the systemic issues described in both parts I and II regarding vaccine hesitancy (especially among COVID-19) have played a formidable role with measles, as well. In fact, the term has been more historically described among childhood vaccinations (where parents were the obstructionists). Curiously, that form of childhood vaccine hesitancy has morphed into another more complex and intractable version in the most recent COVID-19 experience. As described above, this issue is far greater than just an American one. In 2019 the WHO listed vaccine hesitancy as one of our top-10 global health threats. This book aims to address it.

Diarrheal Diseases

Clinical Manifestations

This one will be pretty easy for our readers. We've all experienced it. We need no fancy scientifically complex descriptions of it. Let's be clear—this is not just about some mild discomfort. This is one of the biggest infectious killers globally—especially for children under five years. So, it seems necessary to clinically define it.

Diarrhea is technically the passage of loose or watery stools, typically at least three times in a 24-hour period.[87] Acute diarrhea is defined as diarrhea of ≤14 days in duration, in contrast to persistent (>14 days and ≤30 days) or chronic (>30 days). Invasive diarrhea, or dysentery, is defined as diarrhea with visible blood, in contrast to watery diarrhea, which is also commonly associated with fever and abdominal pain.[88]

Diarrhea is usually the result of inflammation of one of many layers of the gut. In low-and middle-income countries (LMICs), much of this can be explained by infections (a wide spectrum of bacterial, viral, and parasitic organisms). The source of these infections can either be water or foodborne, or person-to-person as a result of poor hygiene.

In an outbreak setting, these clinical features are important because they can be used to distinguish cholera (watery diarrhea) from epidemic dysentery due to *shigella* (for example) as the distinction has important therapeutic and public health implications. While we covered cholera earlier in chapter 5, as a refresher it can often be distinguished by the appearance of "rice-water" stool flecked with mucus (figure 6.13). Furthermore, it may present very suddenly with vomiting and abdominal cramping. Fever is uncommon in cholera. In contrast, shigellosis is typically characterized by the frequent passage of small liquid stools that contain visible blood, with or without mucus.[89] Abdominal cramps and tenesmus (feeling like you need to defecate) are common, along with fever and loss of appetite. In practice, it's never really that easy. I have seen my share of poop, and it is often challenging to make a clinical distinction unless we're speaking about two causes—cholera or

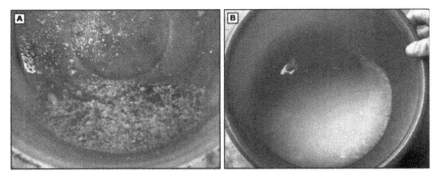

FIGURE 6.13. Images distinguishing different types of acute watery diarrhea.
(**A**) Green-colored stool, often seen in rotavirus gastroenteritis. (**B**) White-colored
stool characteristic of severe cholera. *Source:* Regina LaRocque et al., "Approach to the
Adult with Acute Diarrhea in Resource-Limited Settings," UpToDate, last updated August 10,
2023, https://www.uptodate.com/contents/approach-to-the-adult-with-acute-diarrhea-in
-resource-limited-settings.

Clostridium difficile (C. diff). These two causes are very clear. I saw the
former in plenty of settings in Haiti and South Sudan. It literally looks
like rice water. C. diff (otherwise known as antibiotic-associated diarrhea), has a very distinct odor that you can never unlearn.

Okay, so we've reviewed loose stools, but it's not quite that simple.
The consequences can be quite severe. Severe volume depletion is the
most important systemic complication and can lead to death. Various
clinical features can be helpful in determining the severity of hypovolemia, with sunken eyes, dry mouth and tongue, thirst, and decreased
skin tightness seen with moderate volume depletion and decreased
consciousness / coma, inability to drink, and a weak pulse seen in more
severe stages.[87] Volume depletion and accompanying electrolyte imbal-
ances are the most important complications of cholera (because it is
literally coming out like buckets). Persistent diarrhea (>14 days) is often associated with chronic gut issues, with impaired gut healing and
diminished digestive and absorptive capacity, resulting in malabsorp-
tion or maldigestion. Although less common than acute diarrhea in
resource-limited settings, these prolonged episodes are important

because of their association with chronic complications, including malnutrition and increased risk of death.[89,90] Got it? Okay, let's move on.

Epidemiology

Diarrheal diseases are one of the leading causes of death globally and the second leading cause of death in children under five. They are also entirely preventable and treatable. Most cases of diarrhea are associated with contaminated food and water sources, and more than 2 billion people globally have no access to basic sanitation. The Global Burden of Disease Study found that in 2019, diarrhea contributed to over 1.5 million deaths around the world and was a leading cause of morbidity and mortality in children younger than five years (around 525,000 per year).[91] Moreover, diarrheal illness contributed to the loss of 45.5 million disability-adjusted life years (or years spent when you felt disabled or poorly) and caused 10% of deaths total in this age group.[92] And while death rates from diarrhea have declined with improvements in sanitation and more widespread use of oral rehydration solution, nearly 7 billion cases (including nearly 1.7 billion childhood cases) of diarrheal disease still occur worldwide each year.[93]

Diarrheal illness occurs at such a high baseline frequency in LMICs that our analysis must be taken into context. The extent to which diarrhea episodes become persistent (>14 days) is highly variable and only happens less than 10% of the time. So what factors lead from acute to persistent diarrhea? It's complicated but involves a number of sociopolitical determinants, including nutritional status, geographical location, and other socioeconomic conditions (discussed below).[94,95] It is estimated that diarrhea lasting more than 14 days occurs in up to 3–5% of the infant population worldwide.[96] As discussed above, epidemics are generally due to *Shigella* and cholera, but *E. coli* (serotype O157:H7) can also be responsible for diarrheal outbreaks in LMICs. Major outbreaks due to shigella have occurred in Africa, South Asia, and Central America. In 1994 an explosive outbreak among Rwandan refugees in Zaire (now the DRC) caused approximately 20,000 deaths during the first month alone.[97] Similarly, epidemics due to cholera have had widespread global distribution throughout Africa, Asia, the Middle East, South and Central America, and the Caribbean.[98]

Children who are malnourished or have impaired immunity as well as people living with HIV are most at risk of life-threatening diarrhea. Of course, in the areas where diarrheal illnesses are most prevalent, HIV is often present. Consequently, diarrhea-related morbidity and mortality may be worsened for these patients. In addition, HIV/AIDS increases the spectrum of GI bugs that can cause illness as immune systems are severely compromised. Coinfection with other HIV opportunistic infections may also occur—especially salmonella.

Sociopolitical Determinants

Worldwide, 780 million individuals lack access to potable drinking water, and 2.5 billion (more than one-third of the globe) lack adequate sanitation.[99] Individuals in refugee camps and unplanned urban settlements, with limited access to water and sanitation facilities, are at particular risk of diarrheal epidemics. The SSA region is the most affected in the world, where diarrheal disease accounts for 10–15% of deaths among children under five.[100]

Childhood diarrhea is the result of a host of sociopolitical drivers, including health literacy of the family, occupational status of parents, housing conditions, nutritional status, stressors (e.g., relative poverty), access to adequate water and environmental sanitation, and lack of health care access.[101,102,103] With cholera being the most serious of the diarrhea-associated epidemic spectrum, the WHO wrote the following in its recent report on cholera:[104]

> Cholera is a stark indicator of inequality and lack of social and economic development as it disproportionately affects the world's poorest and most vulnerable populations. . . . Cholera transmission is closely linked to inadequate access to clean water and sanitation facilities. . . . Most of

the counties that reported locally transmitted cholera cases to WHO during the period 2011–2015 were those in which only a low proportion of the population had access to basic drinking water and sanitation services.

Primary prevention strategies such as water, sanitation, and hygiene interventions can reduce the risks and incidences of diarrhea among children.[105] This includes providing adequate safer water infrastructure and administering the rotavirus vaccine.[106] These recommendations have a global consensus and are written squarely into the UN Sustainable Development Goals (this was the 2.0 version of the MDGs). Children infected with diarrhea can be treated via numerous methods (such as oral rehydration solutions, antibiotic treatments, immunization, and feeding practices) to prevent high mortalities and morbidities.[107] These costs can be as little as a few US dollars. Unfortunately, at scale certain resource-limited countries do not even have access to that. Each episode of diarrhea deprives the child of the nutrition necessary for growth. As a result, diarrhea is also the major cause of malnutrition, and malnourished children are, in turn, more likely to fall ill from diarrhea. This narrative of the heartbreaking cycle of poverty is one that I know all too well.

The following is what I wrote one night between tears in a South Sudanese tent in 2014 when I was the medical lead for a pediatric malnutrition hospital and responsible for over 29,000 internally displaced persons (IDPs; figures 6.14a–b).

But I must let go. . . . I cannot "cure" everyone. . . . Surely there will be patients whom I touch who will not survive. This inescapable reality penetrated my awareness one fateful afternoon two weeks following my arrival. We all have experienced loss and tragedy to an extent. . . . We have all cried. . . . We have all suffered. . . . I certainly have had my share of universal (and first world) adversity . . . but I would never wish the despondency of hopelessness and perceived impotence from having a 6 year old child you were treating die in your arms . . . the screams that preceded the death of this cachexic innocent soul. . . . I could not communicate. . . . I could not follow the child's labs (all I have is hemoglobin, which is 4.3 today).... He clearly needs a transfusion (but we don't have a scale to use it).... He was being treated for 2 months ... severely malnourished with Kala-Azar.... He did not respond to treatment.

His desperate mother presented daily.... He started to clinically improve ... until one day, I could envisage the look of death trapped ominously in his eyes.... We rushed him to the local hospital (a dilapidated six room shack with a doctor who wouldn't even move out of her chair to help).... There was also one of our nurses and medical directors there.... No one knew what to do.... No one even tried (was this due to incompetence or knowledge of the futility of intervention ... ? unclear).... I realized I was alone ... with his defecation poured over my clothes.... I rushed him to the larger regional hospital ... 15 minutes later, he stopped breathing ... eyes sank back into his head ... a cacophony of distressing sounds dominated by the desperate screaming of his mother (a sound which will haunt me for years).... I cannot palpate a pulse ... but is this a corollary of the dirt roads ... ? My instinct is to perform CPR.... I start chest compressions with my two fingers.... I breathe into his mouth of a faint fruity odor.... I inject epinephrine.... I am still 45 minutes away from the hospital ... and the reality hits me ... I am completely powerless.... I cannot save this child.... He is gone. We continue to the hospital so that a doctor more familiar with the context can direct me. There is no ambulance there ... perhaps a white sheet ... ? There is nothing. They tie the child's hands and feet ... and I ride over an hour with a dead child fully exposed (with nothing but a small scarf to cover his face) ... and I drop them at their hut within their IDP camp.... When they woke that morning ... the child was walking.... This is the quintessence of impotence.... I had failed.

But this reality cannot be avoided. We are not a hospital ... but merely a clinic with limited resources. We are currently building an inpatient department with a focus on inpatient therapeutic feeding for severely malnourished ... but can extend treatment to anyone requiring 24-hour observation ... potentially 25–30 beds ... more importantly, without a dirt floor. We are awaiting more clinical personnel ... but everything with MSF (Doctors Without Borders) takes place at a snail's pace. Until then, we have very limited resources. I admit that perhaps I overextended my perceived capability ... but with such poor alternatives, it is difficult to let go. There have been other deaths that I know of ... but did not witness their demise. I can only speculate on what went wrong.

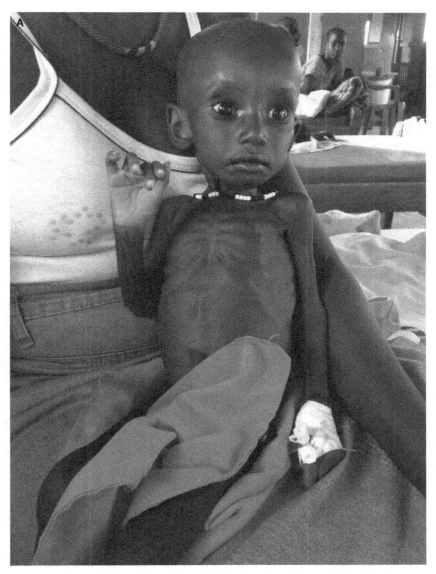

FIGURES 6.14. A–B Photos of a malnourished pediatric patient in Mellut, South Sudan, 2013. *Source:* Photos by author.

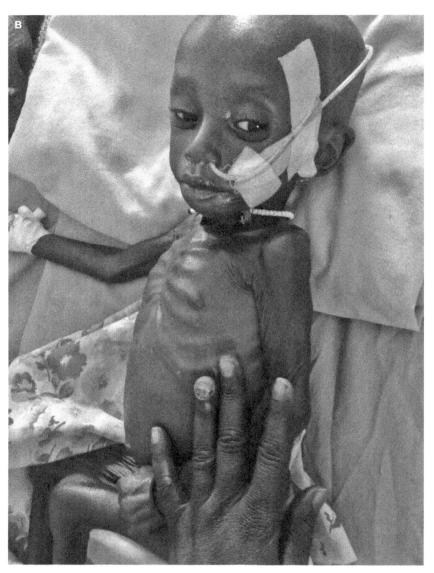

FIGURES 6.14. (Continued)

All of this ... these tragedies ... this frustration ... was rather ironical today as I tuned into a brief portal to America ... and on this little television, my colleague turns on *The Doctors*, with their panel of hair and make-up embellished attractive pseudo-academics discussing the desperation women encounter with PMS ... complemented by (of course) commentary regarding tips on "how to shave your love handles." I was shocked by these parallel universes that were adjoined by time ... merely separated by space.... They would probably never coincide ... for if they did, the western existence of excess and topical obsessions would come undone.

The bureaucracy here shocks me. Taking months to receive medications (which are subpar to begin with) ... unclear agendas poorly articulated by management ... constant bureaucratic interference ... idiosyncratic organizational leadership (my "superiors" are seemingly children in their 20s who have done a few missions with MSF, thereby making them somehow "experienced." I am told that many of these ineptitudes are a corollary of the poor financial support and organizational knowhow of the Spanish division of MSF ... though some issues are experienced universally. Notwithstanding these frustrations (in an environment where I feel more burden than support) ... we are perceived with profound respect ... by all. Our trucks roll down the dirt road in a regal cavalcade of white MSF banners further vandalized by the "no weapons" pictorials.... I walk onto the UNMISS compound ... and the cache of Indian and Nepalese military adorned with their smart blue helmets all pan salute the "big man" with the white vest and stethoscope. Quite a triumphant feeling ...

It is on this compound where I treat the 1,100 Nuer IDPs seeking refuge from the palisade of Dinka archenemies that swarm outside the perimeter of this compound. We have created a mobile clinic here ... just an MSF tent with a few plastic tables and chairs.... Hundreds swarm here twice a week ... awaiting their "plumpy nut" (ready to use therapeutic food that tastes much like peanut butter) and Tylenol (because the majority have very topical issues). It is a Nuer urgent care. They will not move from this compound ... even if their children are in critical condition, which makes health care delivery seriously challenging.

But when I ponder on the demonstrable impact of our presence (not just MSF in Mellut ... but the general humanitarian presence in South Sudan) ... I remain uncertain. These people have been killing each other systematically since 1956 (with a brief 11-year reprieve in the 1970s) in the most catastrophic internecine conflict that has ever hit Africa. This historical deep tribal animosity between Dinka, Nuer, Shilluk, etc. . . . was merely (temporarily) displaced by an even greater abhorrence for a common enemy . . . the Muslim north. Once this was resolved with the referendum and ensuing separation in 2011, these historical hatreds were able to emerge once again.

This is what they know. . . . This is all they know . . . to fight . . . to run . . . itinerant warriors . . . whose actions have been decorated by a rather salient presence of non-African faces . . . the humanitarian presence. The Sudanese have equated their actions with humanitarian aid. . . . The more they fight . . . the more aid comes pouring in. All of this has led to a state of dependence, which has bled into this ridiculous notion of entitlement. The American experience reproduced . . . in South Sudan? This is not the Africa I have known in the past . . . full of convivial spirit and overwhelming appreciation. Many of the Sudanese, so laconic in expression, very rarely demonstrate any appreciation for our efforts . . . for the food that the World Food Programme supplies . . . the security the UN provides . . . the medicine and sanitation that all cluster NGOs offer. This was what I was led to believe anyhow . . . but . . . once in a while . . . you will have that special case . . . where you have clearly helped a mother's child to walk again . . . to breathe easier . . . and these bright African eyes shine like the most incandescent stars . . . and you reflect . . . and it hits you at that very moment . . . that I just made a difference. And I will continue to do so.

I was but one doc on one night dealing with these emotions. We have hundreds of thousands of medical humanitarians dealing with this daily. It's important that our readers understand how these emotions tear us apart. We just try to do the right thing with what we have (which too often is not enough). We must do better.

Summary of the Sociopolitical Determinants of Current Infectious Disease Killers

Let's zoom back out. I hope that the common thread among all these top-five infectious disease killers today, even though not all meet the

Top infectious disease causes of death today: Rubric for determining the sociopolitical determinants of pandemics and PHEICs

	Sociopolitical determinant-linked questionnaire	Yes	No
1	Is there a sociopolitical link to the original spread of disease?	☐	☐
2	Was there a lack of public and community health infrastructure at the time?	☐	☐
3	If yes, did the lack of infrastructure at the time of spread precipitate more widespread distribution?	☐	☐
4	Was the lack of infrastructure at the time linked to a sociopolitical root cause?	☐	☐
5	Is it treatable? In other words, would building more effective sociopolitical infrastructure mitigate the risk of spread?	☐	☐

criteria of pandemic or PHEIC distribution, is now clear. We have covered the scale of these tragedies and the potential prevention and mitigation of much of this global burden of disease. The deterministic factors that have led to these epidemics and PHEICs all connect to current times. There is no difference. And while there have been vast improvements in scientific advancements and biomedical technology, the fallout from these infectious diseases has mostly remained unchanged. If improvements have been made, we see the benefit largely concentrated among the privileged.

The vast disparities we saw of late with COVID-19 are a quintessential example. That's why I wrote this book. In fact, even when it came to discussing measles, while there have been profound advancements in terms of mass vaccine coverage and, in turn, dramatically fewer cases, the collection of sociopolitical determinants are now reversing many of those improvements. So let's visit the rubric one last time and think of Shakespeare's famous words "What's past is prologue."

PART III

HOW CAN WE DO BETTER?

So where do we go from here? We've started with a primer on social medicine in order to better understand the concept of the sociopolitical determinants of health. We then discussed how this concept contributed to every pandemic or PHEIC for over 100 years and ended with how the same phenomena continue today. This is the problem—or rather, the constellation of problems. These seemingly intractable problems notwithstanding, I wouldn't be writing this book unless I had some solutions in mind. Therefore, this closing section provides a road map of what the future of infectious disease (or rather a collision of infectious diseases, which I will call *syndemics*) surveillance and management should look like in order to prevent or mitigate future pandemics or PHEICs.

Unfortunately, at the time of the final editing stage of this book, we have entered a second Trump administration that has made unprecedented cuts to the necessary infrastructure needed in order to help prevent and mitigate the effects of emerging infectious diseases—namely on the most historically marginalized. While the intention of this book is to depoliticize public health, I would be remiss if I did not flag the scale of destruction these actions will have both in the short and long term. The only way forward that helps to protect the interests of the common good (in the same way that law enforcement or a fire service might) is to double down on detection of and response to emerging communicable diseases as well as the systems intended to strengthen the safety net. Taking these steps will ensure that the inequities seen chronically in certain communities do not lead to future population stress, which thereby creates the perfect storm for pandemic production (which ultimately affects all of us). Remember that microbes are blind to partisan politics. In a system that bans the use of the word "inequities," we will struggle to advance toward a future state where all communities are protected. I remain hopeful that people reading this book (and related messaging) will precipitate a rapid reversal of the proverbial pendulum, and we will continue to move toward a state as ideally described in this book. The "pandemics, poverty and politics" cookbook will follow a strict cadence as described below. Please bring your appetite.

First, I'll discuss how any effective solution to pandemic detection and management requires a syndemic approach. I'll focus on how any solution must be framed to address the cascading impacts of chronic vulnerabilities in population health as well as how other conditions (including environmental health) will interact and potentiate these outcomes. I'll describe a number of policy initiatives (either recent, current, or in the pipeline) that are intended to address the SDoH and provide more equitable access to health care both within the United States and abroad, as well as make a number of recommendations to policymakers. I will end with a call to action and opportunities for citizens, community stakeholders, and cultural influencers to effect change—whether by individual behavior or collective advocacy or lobbying.

This book explains how the health, social, and economic impacts of COVID-19 have vastly unequal consequences on the SDoH and how the equally stark preexisting inequalities in the world have amplified death, illness, and suffering from COVID-19. Before this pandemic the evidence clearly showed that overall development was unjust and that inequality was steadily on the rise. COVID-19 has affected people unequally because of disparities in preexisting health and living and working conditions, which means they have unequal exposure and vulnerability to the virus. Disadvantaged population groups have therefore borne the greatest burden of this pandemic, which has exacerbated poverty, deprivation, and discrimination. COVID-19 has also had unequal and potentially much longer-lasting social and economic impacts. Together, these trends mean that COVID-19 is having significant negative impacts on health equity—and the pandemic is far from over at the time of this writing (despite the rhetoric we often hear).

There is a strong case for increased recognition of the significant impact of the SDoH on equity in the response to COVID-19. We must prioritize equity in rebuilding SDoH infrastructures, which will lead to communities that are prepared for future pandemics at all levels. Evidence has shown that people with improved living and working conditions, higher levels of education, more social capital, and better access to health services have been able to implement containment measures more efficiently. Progressive, universal health and welfare systems have been better equipped to mitigate the negative consequences of the pandemic.

There is both a strong moral and practical imperative for prioritizing the SDoH in pandemic prevention and preparedness. COVID-19 has shown the simple truth that no one is protected unless everyone is protected. The concentration of infections in disadvantaged populations, combined with their inability to adhere to public health and social measures and the egregiously inequitable access to vaccines, mean that the pandemic will continue for longer, with greater chances of the emergence of new viral variants. The health systems (whether existing on a local or national level) with the weakest SDoH infrastructures will continue to remain the most vulnerable to infectious disease outbreaks. They must be protected. Politics are irrelevant. This is what public health is—the greater good. It's better for your family and your community, no matter how rich or how poor. A collective approach is required that reaches across health, social, and economic sectors, across communities and countries, with health and social justice at its core, to build a fairer, safer world. Otherwise, the pandemics will continue to widen preexisting social and economic divides, further exacerbating health inequities and the pandemic itself. We cannot allow that. Let's approach these solutions systematically. Ready to close this out?

CHAPTER 7

The Future of Syndemic Management

The reasonable man adapts himself to the world. The unreasonable one persists in trying to adapt the world to himself. Therefore all progress depends on the unreasonable man.

—GEORGE BERNARD SHAW

This book has described in detail how social and political factors (population stress) over time have caused chronic and infectious diseases to interact and amplify their deleterious effects on public health systems, crippling them and leading to the production of pandemics or public health emergencies of international concern (PHEICs). If we can accept this explanation, our next step is to better understand how to address it. The syndemic approach gives us an effective framework to translate these theoretical explanations into effective policy-based and practice-oriented interventions.

Elements of a Syndemic Approach

- Cascading impacts
- Infectious diseases

- Natural disasters and infectious disease (environmental determinants)
- War, conflict, and pandemics

Before we move forward, let's define syndemic theory in more detail.

Merrill Singer (a medical anthropologist originally focusing on HIV interactions in the northeastern United States) first described this theoretical framework in 1996, when he postulated that syndemics are stitched together by three rules: two or more diseases *cluster* together in time or space (*disease concentration*); these diseases *interact* in meaningful ways, often amplifying their individual effects, whether social, psychological, or biological (*disease interaction*); and harmful *social conditions* (social determinants) drive these interactions.[1] Mendenhall et al. recently wrote an excellent paper in which they further refine Singer's original theory through three similar characteristics, as follows:[2]

1. Two or more epidemics must co-occur within certain contexts (disease concentration).
2. They must interact in meaningful ways, often through biological processes but potentially through social or psychological processes (disease interaction).
3. They must share one or more upstream factors driving their co-occurrence and interaction, which may include dynamics that are structural, social, cultural, ecological, and economic in nature [sociopolitical determinants].

At its core, Mendenhall explains, syndemic theory is concerned with how critical structures and experiential dimensions affect the *how*, the *where*, and the *why* people get sick.[3] This approach really allows us to take the principles that we discussed in part I (the sociopolitical drivers of health, or number 3 listed above), combine them with our theory on population stress, also in part I (or disease interaction as discussed in number 2 listed above), and identify how that final cascading impact, in this case a communicable disease, especially a novel one (listed as number 1 above in the disease concentration criteria) drives the proverbial nail through to produce a pandemic or PHEIC. By translating these principles and understanding how they interactively operate, we can create effective public health interventions—at not just the clinical level but the policy level and hopefully address further fundamental or root causes.

The syndemic approach to understanding public health events, Mendenhall explains, recognizes that the "dynamics of an outbreak are shaped and amplified by social, biological, and even political factors, including systemic racism, preexisting health disparities, xenophobia, and misinformation."[4] Clearly, this perspective aligns perfectly with the core tenets of this book.

Recognizing a syndemic requires a rubric very similar to our own. Mendenhall presents three steps to identifying one that boils down to "clustering, interactions, and drivers."[5]

Let's unpack this a bit more. The first necessitates a data map—namely, that we recognize the coclustering of disease states. This relies on epidemiological studies of comorbidities. As a case in point, with COVID-19 we saw a co-clustering of people with diabetes mellitus type 2, obesity, COPD, mental health issues, and more.[6] Another example is HIV, in which we classically see a coclustering with other diseases (e.g., mental health, substance use, other sexually transmitted infections [STIs], hepatitis C).[7] Also know that this coclustering does not just apply to infectious diseases, and we'll explain that further below. Once clustered disease states are identified and localized, the second step is recognizing critical adverse interactions (many of which are measurable) at the levels of biology, psychology, and social relationships. Take the example of the stigma around co-occurring depression that prevents someone from getting tested for chronic or infectious disease, which then worsens, as they did not receive effective primary care or clinical prevention services at a relatively early stage. That's at the individual level. Now scale it. The final step is identifying the sociopolitical drivers that precipitate the degree of disease clustering (e.g., systemic racism or historical trauma), which, as we've discussed extensively, need to be examined by our six domains:

- Economic stability
- Education access and quality
- Health care access and quality (health equity)
- Neighborhood and built environment
- Social and community context
- Political determinants

Connecting the macro to the micro for both policymakers and clinicians can be challenging and is where much of this potential traction comes apart. Social scientists can explain this in detail, and it may make complete sense, but translating this into action is essential (which is where we will spend much of our focus in chapter 8). Clinicians may feel that attending to issues outside the narrow frame of the clinical encounter (e.g., the social determinants of health [SDoH]) may be beyond their scope. Let's be honest—they're right.

Most American community health physicians (or medical providers) will get 15 minutes to manage the multiple complexities or comorbidities of certain communities (if they show up), along with their coexisting social concerns (homelessness, intimate partner violence, etc.). For us to address their underlying SDoH is impractical. Although we can (there are tools for this) and should, it is just not efficient, as the system is not set up for success. Countries with systems set up without any safety networks at all (an out-of-pocket system) are even worse. As described above, I was often the only doctor for tens of thousands of people, seeing hundreds of people a day. In a setting like this, the clinicians are not empowered to make effective changes, yet this is the reality in much of the Global South. Consequently, deep structural and systemic changes are needed so that research scientists (including social scientists), on-the-ground clinicians, influencers, and policymakers are allowed to interact in order to change the practice of public health both in the United States and beyond.

For the clinician, understanding how structural and contextual factors drive and influence that clinical encounter is paramount. Syndemic thinking is cross-disciplinary, actionable, and able to avoid oversimplifying conceptions of disease. It lays the groundwork for integrated, people-centered clinical care and community-based interventions that can mitigate disease interactions.[8] Intervention in the setting of a syndemic will require public health officials and clinicians to consider the clinical and/or upstream interventions that prove most effective for a given set of patients. Although clinicians may lack the economic, political, or administrative training to implement interventions to address social and structural drivers of disease, recognizing how and why certain clustered epidemics emerge is important for thinking through the complexity of intervention packages needed to improve outcomes at the individual level.[741] Without it, the experience will likely lack traction—almost definitely from a sustainable standpoint.

The currently dominant biomedical model incorporates capitalist economic assumptions about health resulting from individually chosen lifestyles. It leaves little scope for understanding how behaviors are related to social conditions or how communities shape the lives of their members. Deciphering how these broader problems fuel interactions in the clinical encounter is essential for thinking about who needs psychotherapy, financial assistance, legal assistance, assistance with medication access, and other clinically relevant needs. And if we are able to implement these changes systematically, we can automate interventions that do not require clinicians to spend too much time identifying who needs what intersecting support system. Make sense?

As discussed above, we need to understand that not all public health emergencies revolve around infectious diseases. While this book focuses on the sociopolitical determinants of pandemics, it is important to note that the first part of the syndemic framework allows a number of other factors to replace an infectious disease. In other words, we can plug and play these cascading impacts. This precipitating factor may very well be an environmental or other political determinant (e.g., war or conflict) that causes the second and third levels of our framework to amplify the impact of these cascading factors. Alternatively, these environmental or political determinants may be long-standing issues and be a part of the second or third characteristics described above, thereby allowing an infectious or noncommunicable disease to tip the scale and activate that population stress threshold. Syndemic frameworks emphasize the disease interactions that underlie multiple convergent public health issues such as obesity, substance use disorder (SUD), mental health, poverty, structural racism, sexual and gender-based violence, and a number of environmental health concerns.[9]

Of course, some of these synergies were noted in part II when I described the meningitis belt or diarrheal diseases. Obviously, malaria and other vector-borne diseases are highly impacted by environmental conditions.[10] Certainly, our current climate crisis is precipitating a number of emerging communicable diseases that we would never see in more environmentally stable conditions. Our constant encroachment into natural habitats that have protected a certain ecological cycle from time immemorial is disturbing them at an alarming rate, and we are experiencing the result of that in the world of infectious diseases.

Mendenhall et al. has proposed the following transdisciplinary agenda for better integrating a syndemic approach into practice, and it is one that I agree that we follow.[11]

1. Work to change the old guard thinking on disease paradigms (those that are heavily focused on the biomedical causes and solutions).
2. Create a multisectoral consortium (e.g., mental health, social sciences, environmental health, public policy).
3. Cultivate a comprehensive view of syndemics.
4. Work to transform models from ethnography to epidemiology to provide evidence for public health practice-based tools.
5. Develop further methods to identify and test syndemic concentrations and interactions (characteristics 1 and 2).

6. Raise further awareness about and develop methods to incorporate biological, psychological, and social interactions in quantitative analysis (characteristic 2).

The political, economic, environmental, and social dimensions of our world are all interconnected, and in turn our public health systems must be able to work within and among them. If not, these common factors that exist across borders will become inflamed and activate the syndemic framework, causing a rapid escalation from epidemic→ syndemic→pandemic. The last 123 years of pandemic history have demonstrated that. While the ingredients may have changed slightly, the end result is very similar.

Consequently, our approach to preventing or mitigating pandemics in the future must look at the individual levels and address them interactively. The more we approach the root causes of disease as separate factors, the more we will miss the target, leading to increasingly more silos. We must apply an integrated "system-oriented" approach on a grander scale, which equally considers the multifactorial models of disease—including not only the biological, psychological, and social but also the political, economic, and environmental. While biomedical interventions are obviously necessary for pandemic response, if we do not factor in the sociopolitical determinants, we will miss the mark, and the variable outcomes that we experienced with the COVID-19 pandemic will be reproduced. COVID-19, HIV/AIDS, and Ebola should provide us with contemporary reminders that we have not liberated ourselves from the constraints of living in a complex web of biological and social relationships. Viruses (much like bacteria) have for countless generations shared our planet and bodies. The human condition seems to continue to forget this inescapable reality.

Rudolf Virchow (a well-known 19th-century German medical anthropologist and physician) once wrote that "medicine is a social science, and politics nothing else but medicine on a large scale."[12] Nearly two centuries later, we still seem to struggle with this concept. Why? When it comes to public and population health, we must treat the system as the patient. If we accept that health (or the absence thereof) and disease are indicators of the moral and material character of the society in which they transpire and the United States had the highest combined rates of COVID-19 morbidity and mortality, then our patient (the United States and interconnected health systems) is sick and needs to convalesce and strengthen.

We cannot be confused when it comes to pandemic response. There is no room for "alternative facts" or "fake news" when it comes to public health. *This is science. End stop.* Without the bench scientist, we would have no understanding of the mechanism underlying the microbiological manifestations of HIV/AIDS, COVID-19, Ebola, and tuberculosis (TB). But it is not enough. These diseases are complex on so many levels and reflect an environment-sensitive, interactive quality that reveals the need to understand the human, organizational, and cultural contexts in which they thrive. The more we come to comprehend that effective disease modeling is multidimensional, the more we comprehend that our interaction with it requires a complex multipolar, multicultural, and universal perspective.

Public Health Emergency Preparedness and Resilience

- Workforce development
- Standardized infection prevention and control (IPC) models
- SDoH data modernization
- Global emerging communicable disease analytics and surveillance
  - Centers for Disease Control and Prevention (CDC) Division of Preparedness and Emerging Infections (DPEI)
  - Center for Strategic and International Studies
  - TropNet
  - GeoSentinel
  - One Health

Effective public health emergency preparedness (PHEP) and resilience programs are absolutely essential to the future of effective syndemic and pandemic prevention and control. Nelson and coauthors define PHEP as the capability of the public health and health care systems, communities, and individuals to prevent, protect against, quickly respond to, and recover from health emergencies, particularly those whose scale, timing, or unpredictability threatens to overwhelm routine capabilities.[13] The US Federal Emergency Management Agency (FEMA) continues, stating that preparedness involves a coordinated and continuous process of planning and implementation that relies on measuring performance and taking corrective action and specifically describes a National Preparedness Goal of five mission areas—prevention, protection, mitigation, response, and recovery. Being able to implement these programs during "blue skies" (the absence of emergencies) is key and often lacking in the United States. While many public health agencies may have had these plans theoretically in place, we were not ready.

Most importantly, we were not prepared to respond to the underlying structural issues and inequities that have such profound potential to amplify any cracks in the preparedness and response systems. During any public health disaster, such glaring disparities are brought to the fore and instigate a resounding public cry to respond accordingly. Underlying issues that predispose certain populations to disproportionate suffering in times of crisis are not caused by the crisis itself, however; they are, conversely, long-standing, structural problems that cannot be quickly rectified and are likely to require a fundamental reevaluation of health equity and long-term investment. This is exactly the reason to invest in this now—as opposed to in the future when we do not have the luxury of time to test our response. Systems must be in place, tested, and interconnected with related government systems, health systems (clinical delivery), and communities in order to be truly effective in addressing the five dimensions of national preparedness goals.

One of the key elements of PHEP is a prepared and sufficient workforce. Unfortunately, public health and the related clinical specialties (e.g., infectious diseases) are critically subpar, and we face an impending apocalypse of both the US and related global public health systems if we do not address these fundamentally and immediately. Here are some key facts that may help animate these concerns.

In the United States, only 56% of infectious disease fellowship programs filled their slots in 2022, compared to 90–95% of other subspecialty programs. In addition, 47% of the current US public health jobs across cities, counties, and states are currently vacant or unfilled. I'll say this again. Approximately half of the US public health system is vacant. This is a crisis. We must do better.

The federal public health workforce is classically described as the CDC, but the reality is that many other agencies exist, including FEMA, the Agency for Strategic Preparedness and Response (ASPR), the Office of Refugee Resettlement (ORR), the Indian Health Service, the Health Resources and Services Administration, the Agency for Health-Care Research and Quality, the US Preventive Services Task Force, the Substance Abuse and Mental Health Services Administration, and the National Institute of Allergy and Infectious Diseases, in addition to multiple other related branches of the National Institutes of Health, the Veterans Administration, the Commissioned Corps of the US Public Health Service (USPHS), and the Office of the Surgeon General. We could also argue that the US Food and Drug Administration and the Centers for Medicare and Medicaid Services (CMS) play a role in this broader infrastructure.

While this alphabet soup of federal agencies is impressive, we know that there are large gaps between the federal, state, local (e.g., county or city), and community levels. While multiple agencies attempt to strengthen capacity through coordinated action and response (e.g., the National Association of City and County Health Officials (NACCHO), Association for State and Territorial health Officials (ASTHO), and the Big Cities Health Coalition), we are still far from building out a sufficient and robust nationwide health care and public health workforce in both the United States and other nations. It is absolutely essential to build this workforce of infectious diseases experts in both health care and public health settings. We can do this a few ways, some of which we are currently advocating for with the HIV Medicine Association

(HIVMA), representing over 12,000 HIV medical providers (I sit on the board), and their sibling organization, the Infectious Diseases Society of America (IDSA).

First, we need to fund workforce student loan repayment programs in the United States—especially for physicians. The average US medical school loan debt is over $200,000.[14] Isn't that wild? What kind of physician do you think this recruits? Typically, those with privilege or access to repay such a loan. I was, personally, very fortunate. As my elder family members died before I reached the age of 22, I needed to cover my undergraduate and graduate studies (17 years of education in total) and came out of my training owing >$600,000. Once interest was added on, my debt added up to over $800,000. Fortunately, I was aware of programs to help cancel my debt through public service, but many young students (especially from Black, Indigenous, and people of color [BIPOC] communities) do not. Moreover, the specialties that are well paid in the United States (mostly surgical specialties and other boutique practices like dermatology) are the furthest you can possibly get from intersecting with the most historically marginalized communities in the fields of primary care or public health. In fact, infectious diseases have historically been one of the lowest-paid specialties of all. Fortunately, the COVID-19 pandemic is now starting to demonstrate our value, and our salaries are starting to rise. Alas, there is much room to grow.

Second, we should continue to invest in our fellowship epidemic surveillance programs (recall the Epidemic Intelligence Service "disease detective" program and the like) to better train medical epidemiologists. Third, we should expand and diversify workforce recruitment, retention, training, and development programs across the nation. One of the most formidable challenges (especially in the public health space) is our inability to quickly and nimbly hire competent public health professionals in the United States—mostly because of the US government apparatus that makes it very difficult to approve and recruit these individuals (it's not all funding). By the time we get these positions approved, the emergency can literally be over. Consequently, we often have to rely on emergency management agencies to hire emergency personnel, as well as depend on voluntary staff. Much of this voluntary staff are retired physicians and nurses (many of whom have not touched patients for years). What happens is that these folks (while good natured and mission driven, representing the altruistic spirit of volunteerism) are not well trained or cannot commit to multiple or sustainable shifts, which seriously compromises quality.

When I oversaw COVID-19 operations in New York City or the Bay Area, I often needed to rely on the Medical Reserve Corps, which was far from an efficient and sustainable process, and factors such as this led to our clumsy emergency response. In addition to the need for an appropriate and effective workforce during "gray skies" (emergency response), we also need sufficient workers during "peace time" (or blue skies) to ensure that public health infrastructure and clinical systems (e.g., community health) are properly aligned.

This is where the Beveridge model health system that we saw with the UK National Health Service was so effective with the COVID-19 pandemic response (after some initial challenges). Both public health and clinical systems were unified. In nations or regions where these systems are disconnected and lacking the surge clinicians to do the work, we will continue to have issues in which they cannot effectively communicate with one another to respond to public health emergencies. In this case it matters little how many PHEP drills or training that system may have. Once push comes to shove, they will be unable to handle the work. When I was brought on as the first chief medical officer (CMO) in New York City, it was because New York's Department of Health and Mental Hygiene (one of the largest in the world) was politically demobilized from responding to the immediate clinical needs of the pandemic, and the other health system that received the contracts (NYC Health and Hospitals [H&H]) had no effective PHEP programs in place. In a perfect world, these two agencies should be uniform or, at the least, have effective connectivity between them. Unfortunately, this was not remotely the case. This caused significant delays (months) when my team (Office of Emergency Management) took over, and things were far from streamlined. This is in a city like New York, where we should have had the very best PHEP in place. The barriers were politics and an effective workforce. We will do better next time.

Many of the public health thought leaders believe that the only effective way to streamline an interdisciplinary system with a strong PHEP component with Bismarck or National Health Insurance models (where there is a hybrid payor mix) is through public-private partnerships. The United States, of course, is a classic example. If the public sector is lacking the sustainable funding and nimble apparatus to hire clinicians or other necessary personnel (especially during gray skies), then we must rely on the private sector to respond quickly to public sector needs in order to activate (and mobilize) contingency clinical service teams. This requires a more diverse, equitable, inclusive, and accessible process of recruitment, retention, training, and engagement. In order to do so, we need to have these PHEP staffing models and contracts already in place to ensure we can easily activate the prevention and protection elements.

Also, to be clear, we are not just in need of clinicians. We must continue to recruit (and retain) new staff with innovative skill sets and abilities in key areas, such as data analytics / visualization (we'll discuss this more in a bit), technology and systems engineering, informatics, behavioral sciences, human-centered design, policy development, and public communications. In addition to this more highly trained workforce, we must also activate alternative workforces that can help to strengthen the highly professionalized ones.

This list is long, but at the top of it are community health workers (CHWs). The COVID-19 pandemic has highlighted the stark workforce disparities among BIPOC communities in several areas, and these communities are often lacking, making it challenging to connect with communities that look, speak, and act like those at risk for disease. We need to do better. One of the ways to fill that gap is to train and recruit more CHWs in key fields (like behavioral health). Wellness Equity Alliance (WEA) tends to focus on CHWs who have "lived experience," meaning that while they may not necessarily have an Ivy League university education, what they do have is "Ivy League" training and experience in empathy and an understanding of the issues that the community they are serving may be struggling with—whether it be homelessness, incarceration, immigration, or substance use. The umbrella term "CHW" is also known by other references, including *promotores* (in Spanish, meaning to promote, referring to implicitly health care here), community ambassadors, and peer navigators or specialists (to name a few).

For example, when we vaccinated communities of adults with access and functional needs (AFN), we were lauded for providing a "practice" vaccination day (put on by staff from our organization in partnership with Disability Voices United and the Friendship Foundation) to facilitate their actual vaccination day several weeks later. CHWs of lived experience led this. In south central Los Angeles, we worked with Homeboy Industries and Sean Penn's Community Organized Relief Effort to target African American communities there, which coordinated with faith-based organizations trained by clinical educators to provide appropriate messaging in relatable language. Moreover, we worked with the University of Southern California (USC) Annenberg School of Journalism to provide videos tailored to BIPOC communities to address the salient issue of vaccine hesitancy.

One novel approach to delivering evidence-based information to low-resourced or underserved communities that we executed during the COVID-19 pandemic was derived from community organizing principles in voter registration referred to as *vax tripling*. Using this approach, we would ask those getting vaccinated to "pledge" to get two other friends, family members, or community members vaccinated. The approach was so effective that we saw an exponential increase in vaccine demand shortly after launching this campaign in challenging areas throughout California.

We remain committed to finding novel ways to educate and engage populations who typically lack access or eschew care as a result of the SDoH. Despite the clear value of CHW models in treating chronic conditions, diabetes, mental health, infectious diseases, and other related illnesses, however, sustainable funding sources continue to remain a persistent issue for providers, who often have difficulty seeking reimbursement for particular services (e.g., home visits and behavioral health). More advocacy is needed.

Understanding the importance of gaining the trust and faith of the local community is critical. Recognizing the barrier of historical mistrust that many minority groups harbor toward the medical system for a number of reasons (as we have discussed at length throughout this book) is essential. Therefore, we engage and coordinate outreach services within a consortium of respective faith-based leaders, community health providers (including local federally qualified health centers), and corresponding public health agencies. Our organization is supporting CHWs in the same way that they have been supremely effective in nations across the world—notably in South Africa in the HIV space, where we do not have close to enough clinically trained personnel to engage with all of the rural communities throughout. Working with CHWs in South Africa in the 1990s and early 2000s is what converted my perspective.

CHWs are but one example of the innovative workforces necessary for effective syndemic management. Another example is community paramedics working within what is referred to as mobile integrated health (MIH). MIH provides clinical extensions of brick-and-mortar facilities. These approaches can help deliver health care to some of the most historically marginalized and remote communities and thereby help mitigate both acute and chronic health disparities—especially clusters of infectious disease outbreaks. Importantly, community paramedics can work in concert with CHWs and respond to acute needs for a number of reasons, thereby keeping patients out of hospitals by working with physicians and medical providers. This is particularly effective in settings where the nearest community hospital may be over 200 miles away (let alone an academic medical center) and emergency medical services (EMS) need to be conserved (especially during a pandemic or PHEIC). Moreover, this model actually engages these folks directly with a local primary care medical home in comparison to sending them to some far-off hospital (often unnecessarily) where they will never be connected with a sustainable primary care physician (PCP). Does it make sense to transport someone in an ambulance hundreds of miles for a few scrapes or bruises, just to be seen by an EMS provider for a few minutes and be discharged without a ride home or a follow-up plan?

All this innovation in terms of recruitment, activation, and retention is incredibly important, but just hiring them is not enough. We will need to work diligently on the appropriate training and activation response to ensure these PHEP teams are truly prepared. First, both the private and public sectors contracted as contingency emergency response staff will need to be engaged in these positions for 6-month to 1-year deployments (rather than 30-to-60-day assignments). As we saw with the COVID-19 pandemic, 30–60 days did not cut it, and we kept needing more replacements. Second, we will need redundancy models for this emergency staffing (i.e., backup or colead staff in all key positions) in order to prevent response burnout and assure continuity in operations. Third, these rapid-response teams will need to quickly address real-time public health emergency science, policy, and communication needs and respond to feedback from various internal and external stakeholders. Fourth, according to true PHEP needs, we will need to conduct emergency drills and scenarios across public health agencies on a routine basis, preparing for a variety of different emergency events and sharing results and lessons learned with agency staff (otherwise known as after-action reviews). Fifth, we will need to maintain, strengthen, and develop new agencywide emergency response data and management information systems and platforms for use in future emergencies and ensure that we have the performance measurement tools and instruments to effectively assess and improve response training and deployment readiness for internal and/or external assignments.

Finally, in addition to PHEP staffing, public health and community health systems require more effective interconnectivity in order to respond to blue sky public health needs (e.g., behavioral health, including substance use, and communicable diseases, including HIV and

STDs/STIs) so these communities are kept safe without these issues snowballing into emergencies. For example, we continue to respond to the needs of those who inject drugs (especially methamphetamine and opioids, where synthetic opioids, especially fentanyl, is one of the most formidable public health challenges we're currently dealing with). While this issue has been officially labeled a federal emergency, we often lack a sufficient workforce to respond. Sadly, it continues to worsen. As a result, more and more people are in crisis, without homes, and the syndemic cofactors (e.g., HIV, COVID-19, hepatitis C) continue to scale unabated. Creating workforce strategies that can respond to this with WEA is a big focus of mine as I write this book.

Moving on from workforce development (I can't underscore the importance of that one), we will need to standardize and streamline our IPC models across the world. This is science. This needs to be universal. We should not be entitled to our opinions.

When I was working in New York City at the beginning of the COVID-19 pandemic in 2020, I was taken back by so many alternative perspectives and associated policies and procedures around IPC. Now, recall that I had worked on the Ebola response twice—both in Sierra Leone in 2015 and the DRC in 2019. We had a very defined and standardized IPC response to Ebola. Our models were not generalizable for two reasons, however. First, they had only been applied to mostly rural sub-Saharan African settings. Second, they focused on the most conservative understanding of Ebola IPC, where there was no room for error in the setting of an anemic emergency response. None of them had truly been tested.

Once the COVID-19 emergency response was activated, we continued to use the Ebola IPC models in the beginning because we had so little information and needed to be as safe as possible (I was one of the proponents, simply leveraging the playbooks from the Ebola treatment units). So there we were—at these large-scale COVID-19 field hospitals at the Billie Jean King Center (where the US Open was played. I'll tell you, I'll never look at tennis the same) or the Javits Center (the largest convention center in New York City) "donning" (putting on personal protective equipment [PPE]) and "doffing" (removing PPE) these hazmat (Tyvek) suits and all of the associated embellishments in an attempt to simply reproduce the Ebola playbooks. While many of us were quite proud of the "temperature"-oriented ("hot" zones), stratified, and seemingly scientific responses we put in place, the reality was that much of it was overblown and completely unnecessary. Of course, as usually happens when rubrics are largely made up (we were doing our best), even more creative (dis)-order emerged, and we had folks wearing two to three pairs of gloves at the same time or using N95s (the masks that are classically used for airborne diseases such as TB, which need to actually be fit tested for the appropriate size or they lose their effectiveness) in cars by themselves or in open fields, and so forth. We quickly entered the world of pseudoscience.

Actually, we eventually realized that we were implementing different permutations of IPC models at each of our representatives' institutions in New York City at the time (and we were all subject-matter experts). Therefore, we decided to create a task force of all the top IPC clinicians across New York City that could deconflict these diverging perspectives on IPC. We ultimately formed the New York City IPC Task Force, which was made up of IPC leads from NYC H&H, the New York City Department of Health and Mental Hygiene, Doctors Without Borders, the CDC, and the New York City Mayor's Office / Office of Emergency Management (me). In time we all came together to create a uniform playbook on what IPC (e.g., PPE, handwashing, social distancing, etc.) would look like across the city. Of course, we now have these playbooks firmly in place across the world for COVID-19, but we must have a similar playbook in place for all potential emerging communicable diseases so we are prepared to respond in uniform to the next big one.

A key component of these IPC models are uniform accurate and efficient diagnostics. A challenge during one of the subsequent "waves" (what we called them in New York City) of the COVID-19 pandemic was not having access to uniform tests and interpreting them with the same understanding. If you recall, we had (and still have) polymerase chain reaction (PCR) tests that represented the gold standard "molecular-based test." But PCR tests often led to confusion among clinicians as to whether or not that presence actually represented infectious material (what we would describe as replication competent). When it came to rolling out rapid antigen tests, interpretation was also a concern because of these concepts of sensitivity and specificity.

Here is a crash course in epidemiology: Sensitivity is a concept used to rule out diseases, and specificity is used to rule them in. Therefore, the antigen test was very specific and a good test for emergency response, as it was, importantly, rapid (and often could display a result within 15 minutes). Because the genetic material (DNA) takes time to code to RNA and then protein (antigen), however, these tests were not great in the beginning of an infectious course and would (erroneously) rule out disease, which is a problem in infectious diseases, as you want to be as conservative as possible. This makes sensitivity more important as a screening tool for diseases like COVID-19, and certainly HIV. With these concerns in mind, we really need standardization and collaboration across public health laboratories across the nation and beyond in order to effectively respond to emerging communicable diseases and protect and prevent them from becoming pandemics. We need robust partnerships between the World Health Organization (WHO), federal, state, academic, and commercial laboratories across the world in order to have functional working relationships in place for transitions before / after / between outbreaks.

As part of these partnerships, we must work together to codify improving communications between these clinical labs in health care facilities and clinicians to help clinicians interpret test results across the United States and beyond. The CDC's Laboratory Response Network is such a platform. As a part of this, we must build out more standardized electronic automated reporting of testing across infectious diseases (especially for people crossing borders). In addition, we must go back to the workforce development piece, as laboratory scientists (especially in public health) are few and far between—especially in the United States. We must expand the clinical laboratory workforce, including training clinical laboratory staff at the CDC, in state and local public health laboratories, and at academic clinical laboratories and health care facilities. Finally, these efforts must be collaborative across disciplines in order to avoid silos. Lab scientists can be tribal and speak an esoteric dialogue (I love them, but they can be a bit nerdy). As such, we need to ensure that we create collaborative partnerships with external partners, including medical societies and other professional associations, opportunities to review and provide input on testing protocols.

We'll next discuss the important task of building out effective PHEP systems using data modernization—especially around the SDoH. As the core of this book focuses on how pandemics and PHEICs are sociopolitically determined, naturally the only effective way for us to implement sustainable change is for us to map them, right? The real value in the syndemic model, Mendenhall explains, lies in how it can change the ways we think about, measure, and respond to disease. Measuring this is key. We must not go with feelings. Our decisions must be driven by hard data, and in order to do this, we will need data modernization—especially around the SDoH.

During emerging communicable diseases (as we experienced both with COVID-19 and monkeypox), ready access to accurate, complete demographic data on patients who are infected was critical to making decisions about where to target resources and evaluating the impact of those interventions. This importance notwithstanding, our analytic capacity is not just about finding humans in general because when it comes to infectious disease risk, not all humans are the same. Based on humans' seemingly infinite series of choices and associated resources in life (many of which are involuntary and sociopolitically determined, as we discussed in extensive detail in part I, mostly chapter 2), it is helpful to visualize how those choices and access barriers lead to risk and where exactly that risk is concentrated. From a syndemic standpoint, that risk concentration depends on a host of other factors (including other co-occurring infectious diseases and noncommunicable diseases, including behavioral health). If we can take these factors into consideration and zoom in as much as possible (in the United States, we often look at zip codes as a unit of measurement) but with more powerful data analytic technology, we can get this down to the census tract (and in certain cases the census block in certain densely populated urban environments) (figure 7.1). Not only are we able to increase the granularity of our search but we can actually track human movement in real time and make our clinical interventions accordingly.

WEA currently works with over 100 data sets on the SDoH, which leverages public- facing data sets and layers on additional proprietary data sets (from pharmacies and other relevant metrics, for example). We're able to perform 360-degree community health needs assessments using a data-science technique that consolidates all these SDoH data sets, focusing on social vulnerability as well as the other syndemic cascading impacts of risk, coupled with geographic information system (GIS)-guided anonymized cell phone data. Our group will evaluate this data overlaid on GIS to determine the hot spots where alternative medical services (e.g., infectious disease strike forces) should be deployed in order to achieve maximal impact (see figure 7.1). These data-driven decisions enhance our coordination with chief business officers (CBOs) and other community stakeholders involved in identifying sites (folks often know what's in their backyard, but they may definitely not know what they don't know). With this in mind, we coordinate with local partners in the planning and operational stage to better understand local needs and incorporate their opinions and points of view into the needs assessment of the emergency response.

Leveraging all these syndemic risk factors, we are able to identify, score, and rank specific neighborhoods with much greater granularity based on how many of these specific risk factors they have and how they interact with other syndemic factors placing them at higher risk of adverse outcomes.

As a case in point, we worked with a group during the COVID-19 pandemic that created an Urban Health Vulnerability Index in which risk was color coded from green (i.e., Low) to red (High). Clearly,

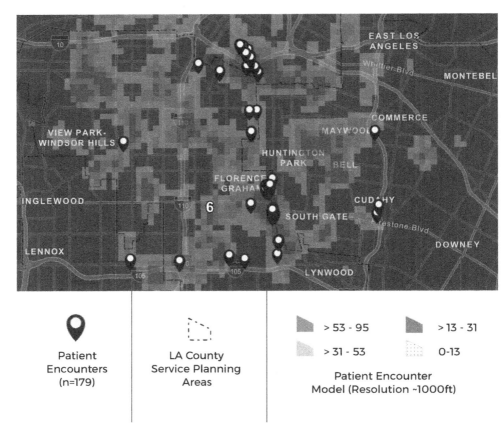

Patient Encounters (n=179)	LA County Service Planning Areas	> 53 - 95	> 13 - 31
		> 31 - 53	0-13
		Patient Encounter Model (Resolution ~1000ft)	

FIGURE 7.1. Geographic Information System (GIS)-coded heat map of the social drivers of HIV transmission risk in South Los Angeles layered with areas where our Wellness Equity Alliance (WEA) HIV street medicine team is operating based on those drivers. *Source:* ESRI.

examining a wider data set enables us to gain a more granular understanding of the community health ecosystem to advise how best to leverage resources to target specific communities. For example, performing a deeper dive of the southeast area with highest "urban health vulnerability" (i.e., darkest red), we can better understand that the residents tend to be largely under the age of 65, with an uninsured rate of 25%. Moreover, we can analyze the most prevalent chronic health conditions and associated health behaviors in certain areas to strategically plan our community health outreach and interventions.

In addition, when we superimpose anonymized cell phone movement data (see figure 7.1), we can better understand where people are spending their time. The information seen in figure 7.1 is from our current work in South Los Angeles, and it provides both a graphical representation of movement patterns of a population of interest within a specific area and data regarding dwell time and numbers of unique visitors. Data like this can be analyzed to identify specific places, days of the week, and times of day to reach out to these residents. This data can also be used to identify movement patterns and behaviors to help inform strategy, such as how often residents visit health centers, childcare facilities, and other locations (e.g., fast food restaurants, liquor establishments, churches, grocery stores, etc.). Having a data-informed strategy to manage equitable distribution of resources, close gaps in access, and meet patients and residents "where they are at" with targeted interventions based on information rather than anecdotes is key to success and is a major differentiator in how we design our population health programs.

While much of the US public health discourse is currently focused on data modernization, we need to ensure it is collaborative, scalable, and centered around the SDoH if we are really going to have an effect from a syndemic standpoint. Here is how we can do that. First, we must automate data collection / sharing to the fullest extent possible to reduce the burden on providers, health care systems, labs, and public health agencies. Public health agencies need resources to automate their data monitoring and reporting systems and better access to patient-level data and demographic info to ensure equitable response and planning. Health information technology (HIT) systems need to be in place in addition to regulatory levers to ensure information is shared without barriers such as cumbersome individual data use agreements, which can grind effective clinical responses to a halt. This is often the case with electronic medical records (EMRs) when we are unable to access multiple EMR systems to get the full clinical picture of one patient—let alone an entire community. I can't explain how many times I have been working in one place where I literally could not read records from another department in the same system or hospital. As discussed above, health information exchanges with data-sharing agreements in place are key to accessible HIT, but we must go beyond this if we want GIS-guided maps. Public health agencies must have barriers reduced in order to access commercial (proprietary) data.

Next, the WHO and leading federal and independent agencies should be given the coordination authority, capacity, and resources to collect accurate global and nationwide data (including patient-level data on subpopulations) and share it with local communities, including provincial, state, and local public health departments, in a timely manner to help inform and strengthen local responses. Moreover, these agencies must ensure that this ongoing data surveillance and collection inform the research and development of medical countermeasures and vaccines in real time to achieve the greatest public health impacts and build in systems to ensure equitable access to new therapeutics.

Fortunately, an increasing number of US-based and global organizations are enhancing the connectivity between multisectoral surveillance and response. The CDC has two programs that I believe have the chops to respond to many public health needs of the future and are worth sharing. The first is the CDC DPEI, which serves a number of functions and objectives, from developing infectious disease surveillance and laboratory and capacity-building activities to collaborating with international partners on bioterrorism, emerging infections, and other public health emergencies.

The CDC also has the One Health Office,[15] which technically started in 2009 but has recently received an infusion of additional funding and attention in order to strengthen its capacity. The One Health Office works within the United States and with other countries and regions to take a strategic, targeted approach to control and prevent zoonotic (animal→human) and emerging infectious diseases and other related issues. From a syndemic standpoint, ensuring an agency is also tracking and responding to these diseases within an ecological framework is absolutely essential.

In addition to the CDC are some other important coordinating and surveillance agencies that serve to strengthen the PHEP global infrastructure. GeoSentinel (which I actually used be a leading member of and coinvestigator), with funding from the CDC, the Canadian Public Health Agency, and the International Society of Travel Medicine, engages an incredibly impressive network of travel and tropical medicine doctors across the world in order to focus on syndromic surveillance (identifying patterns of clusters of symptoms of certain diseases across the world), sometimes before they're even officially recognized by the respective regional public health authority.[16]

Organizations like GeoSentinel have a great deal of potential but, as per usual, lack appropriate funding (and staffing, as most of the investigators are volunteers) to work at their full capacity. Other organizations aim to serve similar objectives, including TropNet, which is basically the European counterpart to GeoSentinel. The International Society for Infectious Diseases is another great (US-based) organization that connects clinicians across the world in the infectious disease space with a number of helpful tools, including ProMed (Program for Monitoring Emerging Diseases), which is a very cool email program that shares any outbreaks taking place across the world (assuming they have been detected). Again, its capacity is limited by its historical funding support mechanisms, and I hope that the COVID-19 pandemic and books like this can help increase funding and support for such programs and organizations. These are necessary for the future of effective syndemic surveillance and management.

Community and Multisectoral Partnerships

- Effective leadership
- Coherent and collective strategies
- Trusted messengers

The COVID-19 pandemic clearly demonstrated the formidable issues involved when it came to coherent and collective strategies led by global and national leaders in science, medicine, and public health. Again, science should be the equalizer of global messaging, and the world should have been sending and receiving the same universal messages. Anyone who had access to the media between 2020 and 2023 knows that this was anything but true.

In early 2023 I participated in a committee of infectious disease and public health leaders to recommend general cultural and workforce reform and changes for the CDC and related federal emergency response agencies (e.g., ASPR). I've included here some key recommendations we offered:

> The CDC would benefit from being nimbler and more flexible. CDC must upskill and train toward a response-capable agency while maintaining the core public health work that is critical to the health of the nation. Throughout its history, the CDC has effectively responded to disease outbreaks, which have been relatively small in terms of size and scope as compared to recent public health emergencies (e.g., Ebola,[17] Zika,[18] EVALI,[19] COVID-19,[20] and Mpox[21]). Over the past decade, outbreaks and their resultant responses have grown larger and more complex—and the agency has not had the capacity to keep pace. The agency needs a new approach to preparedness from top to bottom, including structure, function, budget, staffing, and authorities. CDC needs to be fast-paced and response-oriented and needs to move agency culture towards integrating preparedness and response into every activity, including defining roles and responsibilities for CIOs and employees. CDC should elevate response-related activities and better integrate cross-cutting preparedness and response elements across the organization. With budget flexibility, and a change to how the agency can execute its budget to support response work, CDC should develop a response-ready cadre of staff trained for preparedness and response activities. This would enable rapid assignment of staff to an emergency response or other urgent public health crisis for the duration of the response.

The CDC is not some magical organization. It is one organization of just a little over 10,000 staff (2018)[22] with some senior management, some of whom are placed without the support or grooming to lead this organization. They are not set up for success. This is what happened with Rochelle Walensky. Rochelle and I served on the same HIVMA board the day that she was appointed (I'll always remember her expression on Zoom). Rochelle is a brilliant and dedicated physician, but she was not set up for success. Almost no one would have been during the height of the COVID-19 pandemic. The politics involved with the public health response cost thousands of lives. Our response needs to be science-driven, with multiple stakeholder buy-in on all levels to ensure a rapid and effective response. We must do better. We must create development courses that focus on adaptive leadership rather than technical skills. We should initiate a formal succession planning effort that supports promotions and advancements for both technical experts and executive leaders / managers (not just at the CDC but at all levels of public health leadership). We should expand programs to embed staff (including front-line, leadership, and data staff) who are more diverse, equitable, and inclusive in state and local health departments, representing the tenets of the communities they serve.

To begin with, the WHO and all leading federal public health agencies should foster durable partnerships between public health and health care professionals across the spectrum on a routine basis to ensure strong relationships are in place before a public health emergency takes place. We must ensure that there is sufficient workforce capacity in both public health and health care as a key first step, and these conversations can serve as a primer to discover any major inequities in communications in certain parts of the world. In addition, joint training, clear and regular bidirectional communication channels, and clear roles and responsibilities that include protected time and compensation can all help build stronger bridges between health care and public health and allow more effective and efficient emergency response. While they were a bit delayed, during the COVID-19 pandemic both the CDC and IDSA ended up creating joint clinician calls on the weekends to ensure the US health care workforce was updated on scientific developments, especially around newly available therapeutics, vaccines, or diagnostics. This was important for a number of reasons. It not only engaged the local communities of clinicians but created collaborative partnerships with subject matter experts and key stakeholders (in this case, infectious disease specialists) to provide medical guidance in the development phase, especially during public health emergencies, and to ensure such guidance reflected on-the-ground needs and capacities.

The reality is that many infectious disease specialists (including myself) often disagree with the CDC, and that's okay. It's important to note that many CDC personnel are not trained in infectious diseases or even human medicine at all. Many of them are veterinarians, which is, of course, a critical field given the role of zoonotic infections in pandemic preparedness and response, but this training must be contextualized with clinicians who understand and support human populations. The CDC often receives feedback that its reports or guidance may lack context, may be too conservative in perspective, and may be at odds (and not optimally collaborating) with its European, African, and Asian colleagues. When this happens and consensus is not reached, the entire scientific community (globally, as we're all connected) fails. Listening to the infectious disease, community health, and public health leaders, especially those from disproportionately impacted populations (many of whom are nongovernment messengers), before new guidance is released to the public is key so they are prepared to implement it and respond to questions locally. In other words, the US CDC needs more forums where they can listen more effectively to stakeholders from different communities.

A variety of different stakeholders and partners rely on the CDC (and its European and Asian counterparts) for the latest scientific information and data to inform their actions and decision-making. State and local health officials, employers, providers, other researchers, the American public, and the global public health community often turn to the CDC for its expertise and knowledge. During a crisis, the need for this type of information is frequently time sensitive and urgent. At the same time, we found that the latest scientific information or data were often incomplete and half-baked. If the CDC does not share the latest information in a timely or understandable manner, people and organizations will have to make decisions without the benefit of the agency's scientific expertise and knowledge.

So how do we guarantee effective multisectoral communications worldwide from SME organizations around the world, like the CDC? First, we need to release scientific findings and data more quickly (prior to formal publication) in response to the need for information and action and be as transparent as possible about the emerging science. During a public health emergency, we simply cannot wait for peer-reviewed journals. We need to act in real time and contextualize our findings (perhaps with standardized levels of scientific confidence, which we currently use when we look at data—for example, on prevention), disclosing when we lack facts. The beauty of science is that it can (and should) change as evidence continues to emerge. The US public really fixated on this during the COVID-19 pandemic. "You said this . . . Dr. Fauci said that." Stop. They shared the science as best as they could at the time, and that's okay. It doesn't mean that it was wrong.

We need to ensure that we have a protected space for this. We can establish a new mechanism (or add this component to an existing scientific or data release mechanism) to share real-time scientific information and data that clearly differs from current CDC (or WHO) scientific publications (i.e., *Morbidity and Mortality Weekly Reports*, *Science Briefs*, and *Vital Signs*). While creating a dynamic forum of information is incredibly important, we still need to strengthen and expedite the process by which we publish results (including laboratory data) in peer-reviewed journals during public health emergencies (perhaps by engaging outside reviewers and reducing the number of internal review layers and personnel involved). Next, we need to establish priority areas of scientific focus based on emerging public health emergency trends and needs rather than relying on individual / center priorities (which may be static by virtue of their bureaucratic oversight).

The science and policy implications must also be easy to follow. Not all local health departments across the world will have the scientific acumen to distill a complex scientific paper. We need to get to the point and take scientific literacy into consideration when it comes to access, especially during a pandemic or PHEIC (especially for smaller local health jurisdictions). During the COVID-19 crisis, the CDC produced a large number of policy guidance documents specific to the implementation needs of various stakeholders. These documents were often long and overly complex, with a large number of caveats and footnotes. As a result, their central message became obscured or misinterpreted by the public, media, or other stakeholders. In certain circumstances, the accompanying science brief or scientific background was published after the initial release of the guidance document.

In addition, without the up-front involvement of key stakeholders these guidance documents did not always reflect the reality on the ground, which was needed to effectively implement the policy or communicate its importance. In order to address this, we should develop and implement a standardized policy development process for implementation guidance documents. This process should simply and frankly include the following key steps:

- Document the latest scientific facts available (i.e., what do we know or not know?).
- Speak in plain language with clear public talking points and central messages.
- Apply these facts over multiple settings (e.g., high-density congregate settings) and situations to reduce the number and length of guidance documents.
- Build infrastructure to integrate communications across CDC agencies and the state and local health jurisdictions (LHJs) to ensure the science and its dissemination are as seamless as possible.
- Support a forum modeled after the National Prevention Council to coordinate and lead infectious disease prevention efforts across the federal government, including enhancing public health literacy skills to recognize mis/disinformation.

- Determine whether to develop an implementation guidance and review its priority status according to whether it responds to a major emerging public health issue (e.g., guidance needed for upcoming school year) identified by grantees, partners, agency staff (e.g., front-line responders), and/or the public. Decide whether the latest scientific or data release already provides sufficient implementation support or guidance for decision-makers/key implementers, including the public.
- Develop a set of options (a minimum of two) to implement the latest scientific information; each implementation option should include a set of pros and cons and a discussion of its practical feasibility, net benefit/harm, alignment with current official public health emergency guidance, goals and objectives (e.g., low/no transmission, reduced hospitalizations and deaths, addressing needs of populations at higher risk, community mitigation, self-protection), and impact on all populations.
- Share proposed options with key internal (including public communications staff) and external stakeholders (e.g., through town halls, listening sessions, forums, meetings) for reactions, comments, and suggestions, including the opportunity to introduce new options.
- Finalize options with pros and cons and provide a policy recommendation for the decision-maker(s).
- Develop the implementation guidance and expedite its clearance for publication.
- Provide dashboards for health care and public health professionals with real-time, accurate data that can be shared with policymakers and the public.
- Use FAQs to address unique or changing circumstances not covered by the implementation guidance; these FAQs should accompany the implementation guidance and be actively managed to assure that the latest relevant information is shared and out-of-date material is archived.

- Establish a feedback loop to quickly assess the effectiveness of the implementation guidance by engaging key stakeholders on its clarity, ease of implementation, timeliness, and resultant outcomes.

Public health agencies have multiple audiences for their scientific knowledge and implementation guidance documents, including state/local/territorial health officials, local clinicians, researchers, employers, policymakers, media, and the public. Given the need for a credible source of public health information and communication, however, agencies like the CDC need to prioritize and strengthen their public-facing health communication practices and staff expertise.

During the public health emergency, the lack of regular communications and consistent channels/methods for sharing information also impacted the CDC's ability to effectively communicate internally and externally. I can't recall how many times I was in a restaurant or some other public facility in 2020 in New York City and had some media-advised "epidemiologist" tell me what the CDC "requires" (even after I identified myself). Because organizations like the CDC have a duty to report their findings to so many varying public-facing entities, we need to do better when it comes to streamlining and stratifying the right message to the right people. In order to do so, we need to focus our efforts on the general public first, with additional messages tailored to key partners. Moreover, we must employ a risk-communication strategy and speak with a unified voice throughout a public health emergency response—communicating regularly about what is known and what is not known. Again, we must disseminate the messages in plain language with taglines or prefaces, such as "bottom-line up-front" headlines (including visual representations) in all scientific publications, with more detailed information available for health professionals, policymakers, researchers, and others in the body of the documents. We must also ensure that this layered content is available for those with AFN, especially those who struggle with literacy (including digital literacy). Websites should be appropriately accessible for all (and include multiple languages).

In addition to messaging that is nimble, dynamic, bite-sized, accessible, and digestible, we also need to be clear that not all public health messaging can come from public health professionals—much of it needs to come from trusted messengers relative to the observer. This obviously means something very different to different target communities. The information and resources must travel through strategic and effective distribution channels. Therefore, the United States and other related nations should establish an effective and nimble incident command system (ICS) that allows federal, state, and LHJs to work effectively with one another across state lines and under one leader. An ICS structure, used in emergency management mechanisms, creates a new organizational chart based on the needs of the given emergency. For example, someone may be the head of noncommunicable diseases, but once a public health emergency is activated, that person may take on an entirely different role and report to others for the first time in order to specifically respond to the critical emergent needs. The US Public Health Service (USPHS) Commissioned Corps would be ideal to activate in a national ICS coordinate response and can be further governed by the Office of the Surgeon General (who oversees all USPHS Commissioned Corps), who reports directly to the White House. This uniform and coordinated command is necessary during a public health emergency in order to get the right information and resources to communities in a rapid and efficient manner.

Also, let's be clear. During emergencies, public health leaders do not have time to have an opinion. We must simply act in the best interest of the communities we serve. And because we are all connected, I strongly recommend that an ICS structure actually be set up across the country (and even possibly regionally or globally). The WHO should be given centralized coordinating oversight during public health emergencies so it can determine and govern the response of the large CDC agencies (e.g., United States, China, Europe), which then work collaboratively with other federal emergency response agencies (e.g., CMS, ASPR) to expand access to outpatient therapeutics and treatments in hospital and home health settings (e.g., COVID-19 therapeutics). The federal/national agencies then oversee state or provincial health departments (possibly through the help of third-party coordinating organizations—e.g., ASTHO or NACCHO), which further govern LHJs.

Beyond this, we should coordinate effective communications between LHJs and local community hospitals, CBOs, and stakeholders to deliver messages effectively to high-priority communities from trusted messengers. When it comes to risk communication from a syndemic standpoint, community engagement is one of the most important categories of intervention. History has repeatedly demonstrated that when national and local authorities partner with communities, results are seen faster than when outsiders alone impose exogenous health strategies on a community. Intersectoral collaboration, teamwork, and empowerment are all key concepts for effective public health intervention and are often missing from effective pandemic responses (certainly those that I have worked on). If we want to centralize these messages early on to key communities, we should actually engage CHW task forces that are primed by the relevant public health SMEs.

Beyond gray skies, and similar to what the CDC DPEI is now coordinating in theory, the United States and related nations should have a multiagency performance-based feedback loop framework for operations and programs focused on key agency goals and results, timeliness and quality of products/services, customer/grantee satisfaction (as measured through a new annual grantee survey), and staff satisfaction. If the DPEI is able to pull this off, we should be monitoring the quality of implementation of new agencywide initiatives (e.g., Public Health Workforce, Data Modernization, Lab Capacity, Global Health, Emergency Response, Health Equity) with dedicated resources and cross-agency leadership, established outcomes and time frames for deliverables, and regular feedback/updates to senior leadership. We should accelerate new ways of doing internal operations by supporting process reengineering initiatives on key agency priorities or improvement areas (e.g., streamlined clearance processes, lab capabilities, data platforms, etc.)—utilizing both program staff and innovation experts. Moreover, we need to work more in partnership with others in and outside of government to turn science into public health action and results. We should engage CDC senior leadership and decision-makers in ongoing forums to receive feedback on issues and concerns from key stakeholders: state / local / territorial health officials, providers, researchers, employers, CBOs, policymakers, and the public.

In addition, we should adopt a partnership approach in grants and cooperative agreement management, focusing on achieving key results together using internal and external performance dashboards, promoting the use of evidence practices and peer-based technical assistance, and reducing administrative / prescriptive implementation procedures and requirements. In the spirit of the public-private partnership, we should invite private-sector entrepreneurs to help with accelerating key CDC DPEI priorities such as data modernization, lab capabilities, predictive analytics, communications, and more. We should also invest in and incentivize the private sector to push innovation and new partnership models through the use of prize challenges and other resources. Clinicians from key organizations (e.g., IDSA, HIVMA) should continue to serve as key advisors to the CDC and related agencies on infectious diseases, especially syndemic policy decision-making. As the CDC implements new agencywide initiatives (e.g., DPEI), it should continue support for crosscutting initiatives that address critical needs, including the Antibiotic Resistance Solutions Initiative (again, one of the most formidable public health challenges we are currently facing).

Health Equity in Practice

- Innovative clinical service delivery models
- Diverse, equitable, and inclusive workforce
- Policy initiatives
    - Centers for Medicare and Medicaid Services' model called Realizing Equity, Access, and Community Health (REACH)

- Healthy People 2030
- CalAIM
- EuroHealthNet

We discussed some innovative workforce development models above, such as CHWs and MIH (or community paramedicine). Innovation is essential when it comes to the clinical delivery models we operate in order to reach certain key communities. The reality is that the conventional models we use in clinical medicine in the United States and abroad do not work for everyone. Times are changing and we must allow the new guard to lead the way. Somewhere between one-third and one-half of the residents of the United States (and arguably the world) does not engage in health care as they should, either because they do not know how to or because they lack the resources to do so. In other words, their access is severely limited—whether that is real or perceived.

We discussed this in extensive detail in the first part. Now I will discuss what we are going to do about it. This is the direction my life has taken. How do we create equitable policies and clinical models that speak to the communities in need by opening up critical access? Many folks (especially youths) do not want to be "sick." They do not want to seek out the conventional Western biomedical clinical model (i.e., white coat, exam room, and judgment). They want to consume health care their own way. Even if they know how to, they choose a different path. Others, of course, do not know how to. We need to adapt models to them that respect and contextualize what they find important. I'll be discussing some models that take these key challenges into consideration and go the extra mile (or kilometer) to meet folks where they are.

The differentiated service delivery (DSD) model is one that is patient-centered and simplifies and adapts the intensity, frequency, and location of clinical services depending on the needs and preferences of patients.[23] DSD models are used to tailor services to patient needs and to efficiently deploy resources.[24] In the Global South (particularly in sub-Saharan Africa in countries like Uganda, Nigeria, Zambia, and Tanzania), the DSD has primarily been used to streamline services for stable patients and offer low-barrier HIV care delivery to meet their needs and preferences while preserving the resources needed for higher-acuity patients. In the United States this model has been similarly used to create more resource allocation efficiencies, with programs tailoring more intensive services for patients with greater needs and less intensive services for patients who want or need fewer clinical touchpoints.[25] In Seattle, for instance, the DSD model has been geared toward two different clinic systems. The Max Clinic offers more intensive services to higher-acuity patients, while the Mod Clinic is able to offer tailored services to patients whose needs are fewer.[26] These models have shown considerable success in helping clients achieve viral suppression (i.e., control their HIV).

The key to service delivery in a DSD model is to ratchet the interventions offered up or down based on patients' needs and preferences. For low-intensity services, this could mean fewer clinic appointments for patients who are virally suppressed and stable in treatment. It could also include the use of telehealth and remote care technology (e.g., self-testing for STIs). For higher-intensity services, the model optimizes the offerings discussed above, with more touchpoints, service offerings, and patient incentives. In one program in Iowa, case management services are broken into distinct tiers that are aligned with patient acuity, starting with more intensive interventions and moving to what the program refers to as "brokering" services designed to provide a lighter touch for patients with fewer needs. A key element of the DSD model is the ability to identify the appropriate service needs for each patient through an acuity scale or other intake/assessment procedures. This approach is clearly patient centered and empowers patients to work collaboratively with their care team.

We should be doing this for all community health models (e.g., complexity-based tailoring) far beyond HIV, but certain communities using it thrive more than others. In other words, the 63-year-old with 12 complex comorbidities and other social barriers should certainly not spend the same amount of time with their PCP or specialist as the

23-year-old with a urinary tract infection. This makes no sense and is easily addressed. Low-barrier DSD interventions may allow easier access to services through walk-in availability and expanded hours. The model was important both in the United States and globally as a way to tailor service delivery during the COVID-19 pandemic.[27] Allowing for fewer touchpoints based on patient need and social-distancing guidelines allowed clinics to not only deliver care and treatment safely during the pandemic but to conserve resources, particularly as clinics and health centers grappled with severe resource and capacity strains.

Street medicine is yet another quintessential example of an innovative clinical service delivery model. It was developed by Jim Withers, an internist in the 1980s, in the streets of Pittsburgh in order to deliver clinical care (mostly primary care) to the unsheltered homeless. Dr. Withers (a friend) describes street medicine as a "radical commitment" to the reality of people who are living on the street and a tool to address both the "immediate and social justice needs of people."[27] The model acknowledges and lifts up the strength and dignity of the unstably housed individuals being served and requires providers to approach care delivery with trust building, humility, and solidarity.

The model, which is being implemented primarily in urban settings all over the country (especially in California), involves meeting would-be patients exactly where they are (there's that term again; recognize the pattern?)—on the street. This means leaving the four walls of a clinic; carrying supplies in backpacks; and dispensing medications, performing electrocardiograms, and drawing blood for labs outside on the street.[27] The distinction between this model and, for instance, mobile care units (cars or vans) may be subtle, but it is important. Some interpretations of street medicine do not make this distinction. Our models that we use in California engage a combination of people on foot (especially helpful for encampments) and vehicles. Providing care on the street, where people live, flips the power dynamic in favor of unstably housed individuals in a world where the power dynamic is often skewed against them. Street medicine requires a recognition of the trauma that survivors may have experienced in medical institutions and a commitment to take services directly to where people are on the street. This shift can be transformative, facilitating the engagement of patients who were not being reached through traditional models.

The street medicine model can be broken down into three categories:

1. Providing direct clinical service delivery to people on the streets (including for HIV, hepatitis C, COVID-19, primary care, and behavioral health services)
2. Providing temporizing clinical services with the intent to connect individuals with ambulatory brick-and-mortar facilities or mobile care units
3. Engaging individuals on the street and connecting more medically and socially complex populations with inpatient services

The model requires health systems and providers to be as responsive as possible to the needs of the community. This necessitates cross-disciplinary care teams that are nimble and able to cover a lot of ground. The team includes a mix of clinicians and nonclinician providers, which could be a physician or other medical provider, a CHW, a social worker, a behavioral health therapist, and possibly even a paramedic. We (WEA) along with the USC Keck School of Medicine (where I am on the faculty) typically include a CHW, nurse, and medical provider.

As the name implies, street medicine is designed to bring care and services to people on the street. While the model can include people who are in and out of shelters or other housing, including refugees, the focus of the model is to specifically reach an unsheltered homeless population. Street medicine models have typically been deployed in urban settings, mostly due to the greater availability of resources in those settings. The model, however, can be adapted to suburban or rural settings—including migrant farmworkers. Successfully reaching unstably housed individuals in rural areas simply requires transforming the model from the streets to the woods and other rural encampment locations.[27] It has also been successfully deployed in a number of international settings.

An inflection point for me in my career came after my position as the CMO for New York City ended. I came back to California and ultimately ended up leading an organization (Curative Medical) with >60 physician leaders (many of whom were former state, county, or city public health officials) and >2,000 nurses in which we administered more than 2 million COVID-19 vaccinations in the most precarious locations. We were delivering upward of 14,000 shots a day in a baseball stadium and a host of other venues: churches, mosques, ferry terminals, bus stations, libraries. We did it with scale, style, and equity. In the beginning of the COVID-19 pandemic, we used to jokingly describe most of the communities we were serving as the three C's (Caucasians with cars and computers). We needed to change that, and we successfully did. We were able to operationalize that public-private partnership to extend beyond the capacity of public health agencies and scale the work of thousands of seasoned clinicians and public health professionals. At that point I saw the world differently. I could not allow conventional thinking to get in the way of scaling-up models that would serve large communities in settings convenient and familiar to them.

Street medicine leverages this same thinking, but there are many other models. Fortunately, innovations in health care technology and generative artificial intelligence (AI) can also be aligned with these clinical service delivery models geared toward historically marginalized communities. I often spend my time thinking about this, and we will now be leading a working group at the famed Open AI on how to leverage the "powers" of generative AI to meet the needs of those at risk. One silver lining of COVID-19 has been innovative technologies, including new mobile health technologies, that can be incorporated into routine health care.

We should also discuss school-based health centers (SBHCs). Based on how adverse childhood experiences influence the future health status of large communities (as discussed in chapter 2), it is critical to engage our youths early (especially those who are most at risk). SBHCs provide that direct intervention in the place where the young are at— schools. We are currently managing a program in New Mexico (one of the poorest states with some of the lowest graduation rates in the country). The model is similar to street medicine (focusing mostly on mental health, substance use, sexual health, and family planning). We will activate school buses and medical providers and behavioral health therapists in alternative settings to bring health care to students in the hope of addressing the intersectional social covariates—including improving graduation rates.

In addition to creating innovative clinical service delivery models, we must think deeply to ensure our staff represent the attributes reflected in the communities served (including sexual orientation and gender identity, especially those of transgender/nonbinary experience). We must diversify the CDC, related agencies, and nongovernment clinicians on the ground, as well as encourage cross-center and cross-department integration and collaboration between centers, branches, and divisions of the CDC and related agencies. Our goal must be to advance health equity and address inequities, embedding health equity in every branch or division and coordinating with other federal agencies. Fortunately, some divisions now have a health equity component. We must continue to use data regarding, and input from, historically marginalized populations in developing guidance and make additional equity recommendations for these populations where appropriate.

Fortunately, we do have a number of health equity policy initiatives either currently in place or in the pipeline that will provide either a proverbial carrot or a stick when it comes to deploying equitable programs that focus both on access and workforce. We'll focus on four—three of which are United States based, two on the federal level, and the other from the state level. The CMS recently launched the REACH model for accountable care organizations (ACOs) to start off with. What is an ACO? As a refresher, they are groups of doctors, hospitals, and other health care providers (e.g., insurance companies) who come together voluntarily to give coordinated high-quality care to the Medicare patients they serve (typically folks over >65 years, which is different from Medicaid). This is an important policy in the population health management system space. Coordinated care helps ensure that patients (especially the chronically ill and the most historically marginalized) get the right care at the appropriate time, with the goal of avoiding unnecessary duplication of services and preventing medical errors. In other words, it's a quality improvement–oriented model that, if metrics are achieved, provides savings for all members through the CMS's incentive modeling.

The ACO REACH model effectively created the previous Medicare payment model (the Global and Professional Direct Contracting [GPDC] model)[28] with serious, tangible health equity requirements. Importantly, it is the first model launched by the CMS that puts a strong emphasis on health equity. All participating ACOs must develop a plan for how they will identify health disparities in their respective communities and then take specific actions to address those disparities. This requirement is truly the first of its kind at the CMS. ACOs must then collect patients' demographic and SDoH data, which is another requirement that did not previously exist at Medicare. In future years, ACOs may receive a downward adjustment (stick) on the total quality score for incomplete reporting of these demographic data. As part of the application process, the CMS will consider applicants' demonstrated ability to provide high-quality care to historically marginalized communities.

Probably of greatest significance is the introduction of a health equity benchmark adjustment. ACOs' financial spending targets will be higher and easier to achieve if they serve the most socially and economically at-risk patients. Conversely, ACOs that serve the least at-risk patients will have their benchmarks slightly lowered. Questions have arisen about the budget-neutral approach to these adjustments and whether there are better ways to incentivize medical providers to treat more historically marginalized patients. In any event, it's a promising start to the CMS system and should certainly protect many (older) communities at risk.

Healthy People 2030 is the new iteration of the ongoing Healthy People series started by the US Department of Health and Human Services in 2000.[29] It provides 10-year measurable public health objectives within a comprehensive, nationwide health promotion and disease prevention agenda originally containing 467 objectives (organized into 28 focus areas) to serve as a framework for improving the health of the United States.[30] The newest version is focused on health equity and closely tied to objectives of health literacy and addressing the SDoH.[31] While measuring health disparities has been a core driver of the Healthy People series, Healthy People 2030 has disregarded many of the objectives to focus more on addressing disparities to advance health equity.[32]

On the state level, 1115 Medicaid Waivers (from Section 1115 of the Social Security Act) authorize the US Department of Health and Human Services to approve experimental demonstration projects for state Medicaid programs, which are important to test state-specific policies to better serve their intended (poorer) populations. This flexibility for state programs allows them to contextualize the needs of some of their most historically marginalized populations. In California, CalAIM is a novel 1115 Medicaid Waiver (an opportunity for a state to explore pilot or experimental changes) program, run by the California Department of Healthcare Services (DHCS), that provides Medicaid-managed care plans (insurance companies) with funding to serve the needs of the most historically marginalized. It's also incredibly complicated, given its incredible scope and reach and the fragmented system that it strives to improve. Starting in 2022, and over a span of five years, CalAIM has introduced a host of new programs and making important reforms to many existing programs.[33] To be clear, it is not entirely novel. It builds on a number of prior DHCS initiatives (e.g., the Whole Person Care pilots, Health Homes program, Drug Medi-Cal Organized Delivery System, and Coordinated Care Initiative), some of which have struggled to find an acceptable level of effectiveness.[34] CalAIM has multiple objectives (from its website), including the following:[35]

- Make services more standardized and more equitable across the state, bringing consistency to the current patchwork of programs that vary by county ($n = 58$ in California).
- Ensure that the Californians who need the most help and support actually get it—by emphasizing proactive outreach to bring people with complex needs into care and offering a "no wrong door" approach to people seeking help.

- Enable Medicaid managed care plans to couple clinical care with a range of new non-medical services, including housing supports, medical respite (for people experiencing homelessness [PEH]), personal care, medically tailored meals, and peer supports.
- Require plans and incentivize public health systems to be more responsive, equitable, and outcome focused by:
  - Focusing on population health equity
  - Implementing payment reform to lay the foundation for paying physical and behavioral health providers based on outcomes rather than services.
  - Ensuring greater accountability for Medicaid managed care plans by requiring them to coordinate access to services provided by counties and CBOs.

As a public health leader, I do appreciate CalAIM's focus on communities, which are those with the most complex needs, including the following:[35]

- People with significant behavioral health needs (including SUD)
- Seniors and people living with AFN and disabilities
- People experiencing homelessness
- Justice-impacted communities
- Children with complex medical conditions, such as cancer, epilepsy, or congenital heart disease
- Children and youth in foster care

How do they do so? They have a number of innovative programs with deep pockets in order to support the work sustainably, including the following:[36]

- *Enhanced care management (ECM):* In response to the highly fragmented Medicaid system, ECM simplifies care coordination for highly complex individuals (the folks discussed extensively throughout the book).
- *Community supports:* This benefit provides additional support for patients to thrive beyond conventional medical services. To

illustrate, a PEH who is diagnosed with cancer may not be able to tolerate chemotherapy if they don't have a safe place to stay, rest, and recover from treatment. Traditionally, Medicaid has not covered that safe place to recuperate, instead only covering a nursing home or hospital, which is more than what is needed. This will change that.

- *Housing supports:* These include housing transition navigation services (e.g., assistance applying for and finding housing, signing a lease, securing resources for setup, utilities, moving in), housing deposits, and housing tenancy and sustaining services.
- *Short-term recovery supports:* These include short-term, posthospitalization housing, recuperative care (medical respite for PEH), respite services for caregivers (such as those caring for people with dementia or children with disabilities) who need short-term relief, and sobering centers (harm reduction—focused centers that extend beyond the short-term detox facility focus).
- *Independent living supports,* including the following:
  - Day rehabilitation programs (e.g., training on independent living skills like cooking, cleaning, and shopping)
  - Nursing facility transition / diversion to assisted living facilities, such as residential care facilities for the elderly and adult residential facilities
  - Community transition services / nursing facility transition to a home
  - Personal care and homemaker services
  - Environmental accessibility adaptations (home modifications)
  - Medically tailored meals / medically supportive food
  - Asthma remediation
- *Prerelease / in-reach care for people who are incarcerated:* However you feel about folks who are being released from carceral settings (e.g., jails and prisons), those transitioning from

incarceration face increased risk of adverse health events, including death. Research shows that former prisoners are 129 times more likely than the general public to die of a drug-involved overdose in the 2 weeks after release[1] and are also at higher risk for suicide after release.[2] As part of CalAIM, DHCS is seeking federal authority to expand coverage for key Medicaid services in the 90 days prior to release from jail or prison to ensure adequate planning for a smooth transition. Services while incarcerated would include care management / care coordination, physical and behavioral health consultation services, and medication for substance use.

- *Providing access and transforming Health:* The PATH initiative assists in expanding access to medical providers who have not historically accessed Medicaid, with some key areas of focus on workforce development and staff training.
- *Population health management:* DHCS will require managed care plans to develop programs that prioritize prevention and wellness in the following ways:
  - Assessing member risk consistently and equitably
  - Ensuring effective care coordination to safeguard members during transitions across settings and systems
  - Ensuring that plans provide services to address social risk factors (e.g., housing, nutrition) and to meet needs outside the managed care delivery system (e.g., behavioral and oral health)
- *Behavioral health system reforms:* The Medi-Cal (California's version of Medicaid) behavioral health system today is divided three ways, with SUD services and specialty mental health services administered by counties, often across different departments or agencies, and nonspecialty mental health services for people with mild to moderate illness administered by managed care plans. These divisions, and the different rules for payment and documentation surrounding them, make it incredibly difficult for patients to effectively navigate services and for providers to respond in a patient-centered way. Conse-

quently, the DHCS has implemented reform to ensure that patients can get treatment wherever they seek care ("no wrong door") and to clarify the division of responsibility for mental health services between managed care plans and county mental health plans. The DHCS is also working on streamlining clinical documentation requirements for specialty mental health and SUD treatment services, with the goal of mitigating administrative burden and supporting clinicians to focus more on patient care. Finally, CalAIM is seeking to facilitate the integration of specialty mental health and SUD services at the county level into one behavioral health managed care program and proposes a new benefit (i.e., contingency management) for people using methamphetamines.

- *Aligned incentives and integrated care for seniors and people with disabilities:* While much of the care provided to older adults is funded by Medicare, Medicaid can also help to fill the gap for a number of services, including nursing home care and personal care attendants. Under CalAIM, the DHCS proposes reforms and managed care plans to make it easier for seniors and people with disabilities to stay in their homes and communities rather than move to nursing homes. It would require these plans to provide aligned Medicare and Medi-Cal plans for people eligible for both programs, thereby supporting better integration and coordination of services.

While much of the health equity policy initiatives we've discussed have focused on the United States, it's helpful to provide some examples of promising policies that address the needs of historically marginalized communities in other parts of the globe. One example is Euro-HealthNet, which is a collaboration between the WHO, the European Union, and the associated agencies and supporting laws working to contribute to a healthier Europe by promoting equitable policies around universal insurance coverage between and within European countries in order to reduce the risk of future public health emergencies.[37]

Founded in 1996, EuroHealthNet seeks to address the factors that shape health and social inequalities, building the evidence base for public health and health-related policies and health promotion interventions, addressing the SDoH in particular. Its main areas of focus (much like US-based policies) are as follows:[38]

- Health equity
- Chronic diseases
- Mental health
- Childhood development
- Health literacy
- Aging
- Sustainable lifestyles
- Evidence-based policymaking
- HIV/AIDS
- Social protection
- Vaccinations (especially vaccine hesitancy)

As you can see, there is a lot of concordance in these policies and programs, which is where we need to be. The creation and sustainability of more policies and organizations that focus on core equitable outcomes are essential to maintaining a global health framework that mitigates the risk of further syndemic collisions. These policies, when coupled with innovative clinical operations and a diverse and uniquely tailored workforce to deliver the appropriate care to the populations most at risk, is how we can continue to protect them from infectious disease outbreaks that have the predilection to scale and lead to public health emergencies.

So, that's it. This is the recipe. We need to first find global consensus when it comes to the recipe for pandemic potential. As we've discussed, the syndemic rubric should be our guiding North Star. Once we agree on what we should be looking for, we need to implement effective PHEP programs that prioritize workforce, data modernization, and standardized IPC models. In a highly pluralistic and multipolar world, we must do all we can to ensure that our planning and response is collaborative and multisectoral and led by effective leadership but explained through trusted messengers to get from the cockpit of decision-making to the communities with uniform and evidence-based messages. Finally, we need to ensure that our public, population, and community health programs are interconnected and innovative and meet communities where they are—especially the most historically marginalized.

CHAPTER 8

A Call to Action

Never doubt that a small group of thoughtful, committed citizens can change the world. It's the only thing that ever has.
　　—MARGARET MEAD

In chapter 7 we covered what changes are necessary for the future of effective infectious disease (syndemic) management. While those changes are no short order, I truly believe that if we follow many of these directions (ideas that most public health leaders seem to agree with today), we will experience a world where infectious disease outbreaks are managed and controlled at early stages and greatly contain their potential to disproportionately impact the most historically marginalized (especially the poorest). In order to achieve these goals, *the reality is that we need your help.*

Let me be clear. I did not write this book for academic purposes. I also did not write it just to tell a story (or a collection of narratives). I wrote it to make an impact. I realized a while back that, as a physician, I may have the capacity to help thousands, but as a leader and writer, I can help millions. The proverbial pen is mighty. And it's time. I am tired. I am tired of viewing poverty and disease through the same seemingly infinite loop I have looked through my entire career (as have the tens of thousands of dedicated public health professionals before me). The COVID-19 pandemic was hopefully a wake-up call for thousands of us out there. After being at the forefront of operations in the city to experience the greatest death toll in contemporary history, I knew that my career needed to change. I knew I needed to think differently and influence others to work together with me in order to do the same. My passion notwithstanding, I also knew that to effect true change, I needed to tell a story that was compelling enough for a sufficient number of people to heed a call to action and want to make a difference.

As I wrote in the preface, this book is not necessarily intended for clinicians or health care professionals. This book is meant for a large audience that wants to better understand why infectious diseases have such deleterious effects on certain communities and why those communities are predisposed to that risk. This book is targeted at those who have enough compassion and agency to make a difference for those communities. It aims to reach people's hearts and souls and help them understand that while we are entitled to our own politics, we are not entitled to opinions that hurt other communities lacking the agency to effectively express themselves. The objective of public health is to protect communities from macroscopic risk factors—whether they be infectious or environmental in nature.

Through centuries of study and ensuing evidence, we've identified that infectious disease and environmental health outcomes do not exist in vacuums. They are influenced by underlying factors that collide and interact with one another in order to potentiate impact on certain communities in time and space. We have the tools now to make a difference. Public health is not about individual decisions.[1] It is focused on the utilitarian argument of promoting the greatest good.[2] Therefore, public health should not be politicized. It is a necessary public resource as essential as a fire brigade or law enforcement. It's here to save lives.

Throughout history many felt relatively protected from most public health dangers. The COVID-19 pandemic changed all that, and we can now see the importance of protecting the most vulnerable. It is important not necessarily because of a moral obligation to individuals but because if we fail to do so collectively, then everyone suffers. When we have profound system inequities in place once an emergency is activated, the outcome is polarizing and generates enough population stress to buckle the system so that all humans are affected. If you feel that people who are homeless or undocumented do not have the same rights as your suburban neighbors, you are entitled to that opinion. Once the next public health emergency is activated and we have done nothing to protect these folks from a primary care or population prevention standpoint, however, then your wife or dad having a heart attack or stroke will be unable to see a doctor because all the hospital beds will be full. We are all connected, and public health is the system that aims to promote that universal principle.

The first place this sense of awareness needs to be awakened is at the local level. Local communities need to understand that while they may not love seeing dirty needles on the ground used by certain folks, if they do not allow their local public health agencies to do their job and try to clean the needles, their communities will remain at elevated risk. When I was the chief medical officer for Santa Cruz County, much of my time was focused on syringe exchange programs. Much of the county (despite its ostensibly progressive surf town feel) was very conservative about homelessness and exhibited a great deal of nimbyism ("not in my backyard"). We needed to reassure them regarding the syringe exchange programs. They were intended to reduce the harm from infectious diseases (e.g., HIV and hepatitis C) from dirty needles—that's all. But this group saw something entirely different—they believed that the public health leaders were somehow condoning or enabling homelessness and drug use. Unfortunately, they were missing the point. They allowed their politics to play into the county's legal requirement to protect the public health from harm. In this case, these were infectious diseases. They created a whole slogan and advocacy group called Take Back Santa Cruz.[3,4] We heard them and what was at the core of this approach. They felt that "drug addicts" were making the streets unsafe and putting their community (including their kids) at risk. They allowed their emotions to impact our requirement to protect the public—whether the elite or the homeless.

Public health should not be about individual emotions. It is about creating a culture of tolerance.[5] We may not support, affirm, or respect other people's lifestyles or choices, but in public health we are not here to judge. We are merely here to protect certain communities in reducing additional harm. As a doctor, am I thrilled about the idea of a few teenagers shooting up heroin or fentanyl? Of course not, and while I am absolutely ready to have a respectful and motivational meeting when they are willing, the science suggests that if folks are not engaged in a stage of change, any encounter to effect such will be useless. My time is best spent ensuring they don't contract an infectious disease that may afflict them for the rest of their lives. To be tolerant is not to be supportive or affirming. It simply means that in this world of polarizing ideas, I cannot assume that my ideas and beliefs will be shared by all. In fact, if they were, I would be pretty bummed, as it would make for a pretty mundane and insipid world.

To be tolerant as a public health professional means to be kind, compassionate, empathetic, nonjudgmental, and medically neutral (despite how difficult that may be at times). Believe me, when I worked in war zones or conflict regions (Palestinian Territories, the Democratic Republic of the Congo, Kosovo, South Sudan), I had opinions about how certain people were treated—especially those who were tortured or gang-raped—but I would lose my objectivity as a doctor if I made decisions that supported one set of behavior over another while I am in the midst of managing medical emergencies. As a human, as a private citizen, that is a different story. I am not impacting the outcomes of a community during an emergency.

There were many illustrative examples of intolerance from various communities in the public health space during the COVID-19 pandemic. I'm not sure if the mechanisms of protection (e.g., vaccines, face masks, stay-at-home orders) mattered as much as the mandate imposed on them to do something. People just don't like being told what to do—especially Americans (New Yorkers particularly). Public health officers and directors of public health agencies across the nation (including my-self) were met with a litany of complaints and protests regarding these measures—some even with death threats (many of whom I knew). These folks were certainly entitled to their opinions and in some way or another were exercising their democratic right to express it. As a result, nearly half of the public health workforce left.

While the voices of communities are essential, an effective and equitable public health system works through speed and uniformity. Opinions matter in the long term, but they have no place in the short term (in the midst of the emergency). Think for a moment: If someone were having a heart attack and a group of doctors and nurses were standing around them, would we stop and ask them about their politics, feelings, or emotions at that moment? Of course not. We respond to the emergency and can deal with that after the fact.

In his seminal book *Rules for Radicals*, Saul Alinsky writes that "self-interest, like power, wears the black shroud of negativism and suspicion.[6] The myth of altruism as a motivating factor in our behavior could arise and survive only in a society bundled in the sterile gauze of New England puritanism and Protestant morality and tied together with the ribbons of Madison Avenue public relations. It is one of the classic American fairy tales."[7] Aristotle wrote in *Politics* that "everyone thinks chiefly of his own, hardly of the public interest."[8] So let's get beyond that. It's fine to have an opinion that is guided by your own self-interest. Just not right now, okay? By the way, we could factor that person's feelings, emotions, and politics about the procedure ahead of time in something called "advance directives," but at that very moment, there is just no room for that.

When it comes to public health (especially emergencies), the same is true, just in aggregate. People need to know that while they may express a particular concern about X, the majority of others in that community may not agree with them, and we, as public health professionals, must optimize the greater good for that community. At a minimum, this should be protection from harm. It's simple. That is our general maxim. Now, these public health officers and directors tend to be accountable to other elected officials. These elected officials can certainly discuss the priorities of the communities they are sworn to govern, and the health officials will have the mandate to follow those directives. Health officials, however, also must report to another (sometimes competing) supervisor. That's the science and the application of it to protect the health of the community they are sworn to serve. That can be a conflict for some, but most of the public health professionals I know will go with the science and health promotion any day. *That's our duty.* It should never be politicized, and we should never be forced to choose.

For the folks who did invoke their sense of self-righteousness, privilege, or set of politics during the COVID-19 pandemic, I ask that you rethink this when it comes to the next big one. How would this differ if we were discussing emergency management for tropical storms in the Gulf of America, or fighting fires throughout Northern California, or responding to a mass shooter in a mall in America? We need to let these experts work in order to keep us safe. We need to let the painters paint. We cannot always assume that our opinion is entitled to be broadcast if that means it could potentially hurt others at the moment. Public health is not political. It is a universal right and driven by science. While the Joe Rogans and Glenn Becks are important to help facilitate the American narrative, please hold your opinions until the emergency has ended and try to help the professionals who are there to save lives. Your opinions are vital, but please express them after the fact and in respectful forums to ensure they are heard with reason and without judgment.

If we can agree to this common code of respect, I think it's time to move on and find ways to empower and activate certain community members to make the sustainable change needed for public health to protect the vulnerable. The voices of doctors, nurses, and other allied health care leaders cannot be the only ones raised. The messages must be heard and amplified by people who have a voice in this world (for better or for worse). I've narrowed this group down to the following:

- Community champions and leaders
- Spiritual interfaith leaders

- Policymakers
- Political activists
- Health care leaders
- Cultural influencers

One does not require a doctorate or advanced degree in health care or scientific theory in order to be effective in this space. Anyone who is reading this and feels an ounce of compulsion to act—you should go with that. *I am hereby writing a physician standing order to act out.* This is a collective call to action and an opportunity for people to effect change, whether through individual behaviors or collective advocacy or lobbying. I am making a case for policymakers, political activists, community leaders, and cultural influencers (globally) to address these social (and political) determinants. While the moral argument may not track with many, the economic argument is certainly compelling for any bipartisan audience. *Once again, public health should not be politicized.*

We have the recipe . . . now it's time to cook. So how do we organize for action? Alinksy argued that the core drivers of change need to be the white middle class. While I fundamentally disagree with this, I do agree that we need a diverse, equitable, inclusive, and collaborative approach (including the white middle class) to effect this sustainable change. Actually, we need the community leaders and champions who are more heavily impacted because of generations of marginalization to be the most vocal. We need to hear what their local issues are, and we need to address them. If any political barriers exist on the local stage, these communities must connect with national and global movements in acts of solidarity to ensure they are properly heard. We must stop suffocating certain opinions and listening to others. No, opinions should not be expressed during times of emergencies, but there is a time and place, and we need to hear them—with respect and tolerance. We need these local voices to connect with their local public health officials and regional academics and scientists to ensure the public health issues they are vocalizing are known and that data are collected.

We need a united front of all classes, races, ethnicities, gender identities, sexual orientations, and immigration statuses to come together to fight for one common goal—the protection of our community's health from "outside invaders." We need to deconstruct the compelling feeling that public health should be driven by political polarities.

We need to hear from our spiritual and interfaith leaders. We need these leaders to not be polarized or triggered about certain scientific or biomedical principles that may not necessarily track with their beliefs. We need them to think about what is best for their communities. In almost any scenario I can imagine, the public's health is in the community's best interests. That is not always the case, however.

Let me be clear: Science is not out there to trick people. There is no alternative science. Science is a process and a set of universal and irreducible principles whereby findings endure a series of observations and experiments, and trained experts make determinations to the best of our abilities.[9] Science is intended to operate outside of bias or outside influence.[10] Science is a system in which outcomes are independent of the observer and are intended to be reproducible.[11]

Faith and spirituality are incredibly important elements of daily life, and I supremely respect the power of this presence in people's lives. That importance notwithstanding, science and faith may not always align. This is why we must connect with the leaders of faith in certain unique circumstances and ask them to listen to the scientists and public health professionals. By doing this, they can communicate what is in their communities' best interests and help deliver that message to the people who trust and believe them.

If the world of public health (led by global and national health authorities) can continue to work on the effective dissemination of content while planning for and responding to public health emergencies, and trusted community leaders can connect to those messages in real time and share that information from trusted scientists, doctors, and nurses to their community, I truly believe that the global response (and associated health behavior) can fundamentally change. We can then mitigate the degree of impact from these future syndemics.

While my plea for a greater trust in science and medicine and the leaders in this space is a core message of this book, I also call upon the political activists, tech leaders, and cultural influencers to connect with the policymakers in order to disrupt and affect needed change—especially for the most historically marginalized communities. We need all the cooks working on the same line for us to achieve the impact we so desire. Our communities need us.

Let me give you an example of how this can work. As an HIV/AIDS doctor, I am always amazed by how the riveting words of the American anthropologist Margaret Mead could be so effective in the HIV/AIDS space: "Never doubt that a small group of thoughtful, committed citizens can change the world. It's the only thing that ever has."[12] That quote has guided many of my decisions throughout my career. It would be difficult to use a more compelling example than the 1980s AIDS advocacy group ACT UP (AIDS Coalition to Unleash Power). ACT UP was formed on March 12, 1987, at the Lesbian and Gay Community Services Center in New York City.[13] Larry Kramer was asked to speak as part of a rotating speaker series, and his well-attended speech focused on action to fight AIDS. Kramer spoke out against the current state of the Gay Men's Health Crisis (GMHC), which he perceived as politically impotent.[14] Kramer had cofounded the GMHC but had resigned from its board of directors in 1983. His new focus was on political action, and 300 people followed him to form this new organization.[15] Alinksy certainly would have approved. At the 2nd National March on Washington for Lesbian and Gay Rights, in October 1987, ACT UP New York made its debut on the national stage, as an active and visible presence in both the march, at the main rally, and during the civil disobedience at the US Supreme Court building the following day.[16,17]

Inspired by this new approach to radical, direct action, other participants in these events returned home to multiple cities and formed local ACT UP chapters in Boston, Chicago, Los Angeles, Rhode Island, San Francisco, Washington, DC, and other locations.[18,19,20] ACT UP spread internationally. In many countries separate movements arose based on the American model. Since that time they have taken on a number of other targets—including Wall Street, the US Food and Drug Administration, and the National Institutes of Health. Kramer and Anthony Fauci (who was the head of the National Institute for Allergy and Infectious Diseases for several decades) would form a long, respectful, and enduring relationship that, moving forward, asserted the effectiveness of the activist-scientist alliance through a number of important medical breakthroughs during the HIV/AIDS pandemic.

Please sear this model into your mind, for we need more of these. The political activists, scientists, public health leaders, community leaders, and policymakers all need to be working in lockstep with one another in order to effect change. A series of successful policies helped fundamentally address the HIV/AIDS response both in the United States and beyond—starting with the formation of UNAIDS (a coordination of a number of United Nations agencies intended to cut through the proverbial red tape and address one of the most formidable global public health emergencies of all time, which ultimately served as the origin of the red ribbon used as a symbol of solidarity for the HIV/AIDS movement), the creation of Ryan White federal legislation to fund HIV treatment, and the US President's Emergency Plan for AIDS Relief, which has funded over $100 billion in programming across the globe). The beauty of all these effective policies is that they were cross-cutting, bipartisan, and uniform in intent and spirit. Still today, HIV/AIDS lobbying (which I continue to do annually on Capitol Hill) is often met with universal empathy and respect.

We must use this example and continue to cut through the silos that separate and identify the ties that unite and bind us. Again, *please hear that this is the intent of this book*. The objective is to touch you and for you to do something about it. Yes, this even means cultural influencers. Get on your X and Instagram and talk about this (or graphically represent it). While this new tribe of changemakers is relatively new for me, I know how important you are in order to change public opinion. I also need for you to do your thing and amplify this message— *public health must be depoliticized* in order to protect and promote the public good. Please don't go out there and send the wrong messages because you are confused or frustrated or simply want to stir up debate.

We have increasingly become so polarizing, adversarial, and contradictory in our messaging because everyone wants to be right. I hear that and I understand it, but public health is that one field where you should just let go with the maxim of protecting your communities. Listen to the experts around you—both on the local and global levels (we will do our best to delineate who those folks are) and help to amplify their messages in order to protect all the communities around you. Politics should not influence these actions. We are all connected through concentric circles in the public health space. Even if people who don't look or think like you don't matter to you, please understand that public health decisions to help them ultimately also help your immediate community (that you do care about).

My life has taken me through so many twists and turns—from being an orphan, a high school dropout, an inmate, and a father at the age of 17 to one of the top public health leaders in the United States. I have sat with so many patients from different communities in my exam rooms (which could have been tents in South Sudan or homeless encampments in the Los Angeles Skid Row) and have seen them suffer. I have given so many talks about this subject to so many communities. The more that I travel and experience the world and engage with the folks embedded in it, the more I realize one simple and universal truth. Despite our diverging beliefs and narratives that we follow and the sometimes confusing way in which we express these core messages— we all ultimately want the same thing. Survival is the first step. More importantly, however, we all ultimately seek health and wellness for ourselves, our families, and our immediate communities. In order to achieve that, we must all do our part to address the social and political determinants that amplify infectious disease outbreaks and related public health emergencies (and believe me, there will be more, almost definitely in your lifetime). I have given you the tools to do so. Now it is up to you to make that difference. Light up the darkness.

ACE	adverse childhood experience
ACO	accountable care organization
AFN	access and functional needs
AIDS	acquired immunodeficiency syndrome
APHA	American Public Health Association
ARDS	acute respiratory distress syndrome
BIPOC	Black, Indigenous, and people of color
BMI	body mass index
CDC	Centers for Disease Control and Prevention
CFR	case fertility rate
CHW	community health worker
CMS	Centers for Medicare & Medicaid Services
COVID-19	coronavirus disease 2019
disease control	When there is a reduction in the number of new infections, the number of people currently infected, and the number of people who become sick or die from that disease in a restricted area.
DRC	Democratic Republic of the Congo

elimination	Stopping the transmission of a disease in a specific geographic area or country but not worldwide.
endemic	Describes a disease distribution that is consistently present in one particular geographical area.
epidemic	When the number of cases exceeds the endemic rate (or that which can normally be expected).
epidemiology	Study of epidemics, but more specifically the study of patterns of disease distribution and the causes that may have contributed to that spread.
eradication	Complete elimination of a disease worldwide, often requiring elimination of the microbe itself. Of the very few examples of this, smallpox was one.
flu	influenza
FPL	federal poverty level
FQHC	federally qualified health center
GI	gastrointestinal
HBV	hepatitis B virus
HIV	human immunodeficiency virus
IDU	injecting drug user
IFR	infection fatality ratio
IPV	intimate partner violence
LGBTQIA+	lesbian, gay, bisexual, transgender, queer or questioning, intersex, asexual, and other related communities
LMICs	low- and middle-income countries
MMR	measles, mumps, rubella
MSM	men who have sex with men
outbreak	A sudden rise in the number of cases, in which the time of onset is important.
pandemic	When an epidemic crosses multiple national borders and its replication rate becomes exponential.
PCP	primary care provider
PEH	people experiencing homelessness

PHEIC	public health emergency of international concern. Where an epidemic has spread in a way that, if not controlled immediately, it will likely lead to a pandemic distribution and so requires a coordinated international response.
PTSD	post-traumatic stress disorder
SDOH	social determinants of health
SES	socioeconomic status
SGBV	sexual and gender-based violence
SOGI	sexual orientation and gender identity
SSA	sub-Saharan Africa
STI	sexually transmitted infection
SUD	substance use disorder
syndemic	Recent and timely term that describes a synergistic epidemic of more than one epidemic colliding and causing an amplified outcome, driven by disparities that are largely socially determined.
TB	tuberculosis
TG/NB	transgender/nonbinary
WHO	World Health Organization

Introduction

1. "Who Was Ryan White?," Health Resources and Services Administration, last modified February 2022, https://ryanwhite.hrsa.gov/about/ryan-white.

2. "How Marin County Changed Its Reputation on Vaccines," *New York Times*, October 11, 2022, https://www.nytimes.com/2022/10/11/us/marin-county-vaccines.html.

3. "Public Charge," California Department of Social Services, accessed September 9, 2022, https://www.cdss.ca.gov/inforesources/cdss-programs/refugees/public-charge.

1. A Primer in Health Systems

1. "Defining Health Systems," Agency for Healthcare Research and Quality, last modified January 2023, https://www.ahrq.gov/chsp/defining-health-systems/index.html.

2. "Defining Health Systems," Agency for Healthcare Research and Quality, last modified January 2023, https://www.ahrq.gov/chsp/defining-health-systems/index.html.

3. "Healthcare Systems—Four Basic Models," Physicians for a National Health Program, accessed September 30, 2023, https://www.pnhp.org/single_payer_resources/health_care_systems_four_basic_models.

4. "Global Healthcare: 4 Major National Models and How They Work," Vera Whole Health, September 10, 2020, https://www.verawholehealth.com/blog/global-healthcare-4-major-national-models-and-how-they-work.

5. G. B. Risse, *Mending Bodies, Saving Souls: A History of Hospitals* (Oxford University Press, 1999).

6. Institute of Medicine (US) Committee on the Changing Market, Managed Care, and the Future Viability of Safety Net Providers, *America's Healthcare Safety Net: Intact but Endangered* (National Academies Press, 2001).

7. Institute of Medicine (US) Committee on the Changing Market, Managed Care, and the Future Viability of Safety Net Providers, *America's Healthcare Safety Net: Intact but Endangered* (National Academies Press, 2001).

8. Mark A. Hall and Janet Weiner, "Healthcare Safety-Net Programs After the Affordable Care Act," Penn LDI, 2019, https://repository.upenn.edu/server/api/core/bitstreams/4cfc8cf9-6aa2-494d-89b5-0cf5ca085abc/content.

9. Sujoy Chakravarty, Kristen Lloyd, Jennifer Farnham, and Susan Brownleem, "Medicaid DSRIP in New Jersey: Trade-Offs Between Broad Hospital Participation and Safety Net Viability," *Journal of Health Politics, Policy and Law* 44, no. 5 (2019), https://doi.org/10.1215/03616878-7611659.

10. Y. Shin, "Proceedings of the Health Welfare Policy Forum," *Korea Institute for Health and Social Affairs*, 2009, 17–28.

11. Elizabeth Hagan and Christine Nguyen, "Healthcare Safety-Net Programs Continue to Serve Most Vulnerable," *Healthcare Access and Coverage* (blog), Penn LDI, October 15, 2019, https://ldi.upenn.edu/our-work/research-updates/health-care-safety-net-programs-continue-to-serve-most-vulnerable.

12. Kathleen M. MacQueen et al., "What Is Community? An Evidence-Based Definition for Participatory Public Health," *American Journal of Public Health*, 2001, https://ajph.aphapublications.org/doi/full/10.2105/AJPH.91.12.1929.

13. "Federally Qualified Health Centers (FQHCs) and the Health Center Program," Rural Health Information Hub, last modified December 13, 2021, https://www.ruralhealthinfo.org/topics/federally-qualified-health-centers.

14. "Community Needs Assessment," Centers for Disease Control and Prevention, 2013, https://www.cdc.gov/globalhealth/healthprotection/fetp/training_modules/15/community-needs_pw_final_9252013.pdf.

15. Meredith Deal, "Future of Community Health Centers Hangs in the Balance as Financial Uncertainty Abounds" *Chartis* (blog), Chartis Top Reads, June 30, 2023, https://www.chartis.com/insights/future-community-health-centers-hangs-balance-financial-uncertainty-abounds.

16. Matthew Newman and James Paci, *California's Healthcare Safety Net: Essential Access for Millions* (California Healthcare Foundation), June 15, 2021, 2, https://www.chcf.org/wp-content/uploads/2021/06/healthcareSafetyNetAlmanac2021.pdf.

17. Matthew Newman and James Paci, *California's Healthcare Safety Net: Essential Access for Millions* (California Healthcare Foundation), June 15, 2021, 16, https://www.chcf.org/wp-content/uploads/2021/06/healthcareSafetyNetAlmanac2021.pdf.

18. Matthew Newman and James Paci, *California's Healthcare Safety Net: Essential Access for Millions* (California Healthcare Foundation), June 15, 2021, 5, https://www.chcf.org/wp-content/uploads/2021/06/healthcareSafetyNetAlmanac2021.pdf.

19. Jessica L. Alpert et al., "Primary Care in the COVID-19 Pandemic," Care Quest, accessed September 30, 2023, https://www.carequest.org/system/files/Primary-Care-in-the-COVID-19-Pandemic-Harvard-Report.pdf#page=209.

20. "The History of Federally Qualified Health Centers (FQHC's)," *Visualutions* (blog), accessed September 30, 2023, https://www.visualutions.com/blog/the-history-of-federally-qualified-health-centers/.

21. "The History of Federally Qualified Health Centers (FQHC's)," *Visualutions* (blog), accessed September 30, 2023, https://www.visualutions.com/blog/the-history-of-federally-qualified-health-centers/.

22. "Introduction to Public Health," Centers for Disease Control and Prevention, accessed September 30, 2023, https://www.cdc.gov/training/publichealth101/public-health.html.

23. "What Is Public Health?," CDC Foundation, accessed September 30, 2023, https://www.cdcfoundation.org/what-public-health.

24. "Population Health," Institute for Healthcare Improvement, accessed September 30, 2023, https://www.ihi.org/Topics/Population-Health/Pages/default.aspx.

25. "Population Health," Institute for Healthcare Improvement, accessed September 30, 2023, https://www.ihi.org/Topics/Population-Health/Pages/default.aspx.

26. Ryan L. Bridge et al., "Examining Primary Healthcare Performance Through a Triple Aim Lens," *Healthcare Policy* 11, no. 3 (2016), https://pubmed.ncbi.nlm.nih.gov/27027790.

27. "Physician Burnout," Agency for Healthcare Research and Quality, July 2017, https://www.ahrq.gov/prevention/clinician/ahrq-works/burnout/index.html.

28. "U.S. Centers for Disease Control and Prevention (CDC)—'Population Health Training' [One Health in Action]," One Health Initiative, January 6, 2019, https://onehealthinitiative.com/u-s-centers-for-disease-control-and-prevention-cdc-population-health-training-one-health-in-action/.

29. Niñon Lewis, "Populations, Population Health, and the Evolution of Population Management: Making Sense of the Terminology in US Health Care Today," Institute for Healthcare Improvement, March 19, 2014, https://www.ihi.org/insights/populations-population-health-and-evolution-population-management-making-sense-terminology.

2. Defining the Social (and Political) Determinants of Health

1. Jo C. Phelan, Brice G. Link, and Parisa Tehranifar, "Social Conditions as Fundamental Causes of Health Inequalities: Theory, Evidence, and Policy Implications," suppl., *Journal of Health and Social Behavior* 51, no. S1 (2010): S28–S40, https://doi.org/10.1177/0022146510383498.

2. James S. House, Ronald C. Kessler, and Regula Herzog, "Age, Socioeconomic Status, and Health," *Milbank Quarterly* 68, no. 3 (1990): 383, https://doi.org/10.2307/3350111.

3. James S. House et al., "The Social Stratification of Aging and Health," *Journal of Health and Social Behavior* 35, no. 3 (1994): 213, https://doi.org/0.2307/2137277.

4. D. Fassin and H. Schneider, "The Politics of AIDS in South Africa: Beyond the Controversies," *BMJ* 326, no. 7387 (2003): 495–497, https://doi.org/10.1136/bmj.326 .7387.495.

5. J. C. Phelan, B. G. Link, and P. Tehranifar, "Social Conditions as Fundamental Causes of Health Inequalities: Theory, Evidence, and Policy Implications," suppl., *Journal of Health and Social Behavior* 51, no. S1 (2010): S28–S40, https://doi.org/10 .1177/0022146510383498.

6. "Economic Stability-Goal: Help People Earn Steady Incomes That Allow Them to Meet Their Health Needs," Healthy People 2030, Office of Disease Prevention and Health Promotion, US Department of Health and Human Services, accessed August 16, 20222, https://health.gov/healthypeople/objectives-and-data/browse -objectives/economic-stability.

7. Francis Fukuyama, "30 Years of World Politics: What Has Changed?," *Journal of Democracy* 31, no. 1 (2020): 11–21, https://www.journalofdemocracy.org/articles/30 -years-of-world-politics-what-has-changed/.

8. Daniel A. Hartley, "Urban Decline in Rust-Belt Cities," *Economic Commentary (Federal Reserve Bank of Cleveland)*, no. 6 (2013): 1, https://doi.org/10.26509/frbc-ec -201306.

9. "Employment," Healthy People 2030, Office of Disease Prevention and Health Promotion, US Department of Health and Human Services, accessed September 2023, https://health.gov/healthypeople/priority-areas/social-determinants -health/literature-summaries/employment#cit1.

10. "Obesity and Overweight," World Health Organization, accessed July 19, 20222, https://www.who.int/news-room/fact-sheets/detail/obesity-and-overweight.

11. C. D. Fryar, M. D. Carroll, and J. Afful, "Prevalence of Overweight, Obesity, and Severe Obesity Among Adults Aged 20 and Over: United States, 1960–1962 Through 2017–2018," National Center for Health Statistics, 2020, https://www.cdc .gov/nchs/data/hestat/obesity-adult-17-18/obesity-adult.htm.

12. F. Siddiqui, R. A. Salam, Z. S. Lassi, and J. K. Das, "The Intertwined Relationship Between Malnutrition and Poverty," *Frontiers in Public Health* 8, no. 453 (2020), https://doi.org/10.3389/fpubh.2020.00453.

13. Alana Rhone, "Food Access Research Atlas," US Department of Agriculture, 2022, https://www.ers.usda.gov/data-products/food-access-research-atlas /documentation.

14. "Diabetes and American Indians/Alaska Natives," US Department of Health and Human Services, accessed August 16, 2022, https://minorityhealth.hhs.gov /diabetes-and-american-indiansalaska-natives.

15. "California Needs to Change Its Homeless Policies, Not Spend More Money," Cal Matters, 2023, https://calmatters.org/commentary/2023/11/change-home lessness-policies-spend-more.

16. *Report of the Special Rapporteur on Adequate Housing as a Component of the Right to an Adequate Standard of Living, and on the Right to Non-Discrimination in This Context*, United Nations, accessed August 26, 2022, https://documents.un.org/doc/undoc/gen/n18/292/50/pdf/n1829250.pdf?token=ZJm4tPJgO9CNYI6vPH&fe=true.

17. "2022 Greater Los Angeles Homeless Count Data," Los Angeles Homeless Services Authority, 2022, https://www.lahsa.org/news?article=893-2022-greater-los-angeles-homeless-count-data.

18. Jason M. Ward, Rick Garvey, and Sarah B. Hunter, *Recent Trends Among the Unsheltered in Three Los Angeles Neighborhoods: An Annual Report from the Los Angeles Longitudinal Enumeration and Demographic Survey (LA LEADS) Project*, RAND Corporation, RR-A1890–2, 2023, accessed June 6, 2024, https://www.rand.org/pubs/research_reports/RRA1890-2.html.

19. "HUD Releases January 2023 Point-in-Time Count Report," US Department of Housing and Urban Development, accessed September 10, 2022, https://www.hud.gov/press/press_releases_media_advisories/hud_no_23_278.

20. "Homelessness Statistics," Urban Vision Alliance, accessed September 11, 2023, https://urbanvisionalliance.org/homelessness-statistics/.

21. "Data Reporter," United Nations Human Settlements Program, accessed September 20, 2022, https://unstats.un.org/sdgs/metadata/files/Metadata-11-01-01.pdf.

22. "Housing Instability," Healthy People 2030, Office of Disease Prevention and Health Promotion, US Department of Health and Human Services, accessed September 19, 2022, https://health.gov/healthypeople/priority-areas/social-determinants-health/literature-summaries/incarceration.

23. "Homeless People Are 16 Times More Likely to Die Suddenly," University of California San Francisco, 2023, https://www.ucsf.edu/news/2023/10/426426/homeless-people-are-16-times-more-likely-die-suddenly.

24. "Measuring Housing Insecurity in the American Housing Survey," Office of Policy Development and Research, US Department of Housing and Urban Development, accessed September 21, 2022, https://www.huduser.gov/portal/pdredge/pdr-edge-frm-asst-sec-111918.html.

25. "World AIDS Day #WorldAIDSDay," HIV.gov, accessed September 20, 2022, https://www.hiv.gov/events/awareness-days/world-aids-day/.

26. D. Royles, "Grassroots AIDS Activists Fought for and Won Affordable HIV Treatments Around the World—but Pepfar Didn't Change Governments and Pharma," *The Conversation*, January 24, 2023, https://theconversation.com/grassroots-aids-activists-fought-for-and-won-affordable-hiv-treatments-around-the-world-but-pepfar-didnt-change-governments-and-pharma-194908.

27. "Behavioral Health Services for People Who Are Homeless," Substance Abuse and Mental Health Services Administration, accessed September 23, 2022, https://store.samhsa.gov/sites/default/files/pep20-06-04-003.pdf.

28. B. F. Henwood, T. Byrne, and B. Scriber, "Examining Mortality Among Formerly Homeless Adults Enrolled In Housing First: An Observational Study," *BMC Public Health* 15, no. 1209 (2015), https://doi.org/10.1186/s12889-015-2552-1.

29. Kendra Cherry, ed., "Maslow's Hierarchy of Needs: Maslow Believed That Physiological and Psychological Needs Motivate our Actions," last modified August 2022, https://www.verywellmind.com/what-is-maslows-hierarchy-of-needs -4136760.

30. Harper Sutherland, Mir M. Ali, and Emily Rosenoff, "Individuals Experiencing Homelessness Are Likely to Have Medical Conditions Associated with Severe Illness from COVID-19," issue brief, Office of the Assistant Secretary for Planning and Evaluation, June 2020, https://aspe.hhs.gov/reports/individuals-experiencing -homelessness-are-likely-have-medical-conditions-associated-severe-illness-0.

31. S. C. Segerstrom and G. E. Miller, "Psychological Stress and the Human Immune System: A Meta-Analytic Study of 30 Years of Inquiry," *Psychological Bulletin* 130, no. 4 (2004): 601–630, https://doi.org/10.1037/0033-2909.130.4.601.

32. "Poverty Rate Second-Highest in 45 Years; Record Numbers Lacked Health Insurance, Lived in Deep Poverty," Center on Budget and Policy Priorities, accessed September 24, 2022, https://www.cbpp.org/research/poverty-rate-second-highest-in -45-years-record-numbers-lacked-health-insurance-lived-in.

33. "UNICEF Innocenti," accessed September 25, 2022, UNICEF, https://www .unicef.org/innocenti/.

34. "Poverty," Healthy People 2030, Office of Disease Prevention and Health Promotion, US Department of Health and Human Services, accessed September 25, 2022, https://health.gov/healthypeople/priority-areas/social-determinants-health /literature-summaries/incarceration.

35. *These Charts Show the Growing Income Inequality Between the World's Richest and Poorest*, World Economic Forum, December 2021, https://www.weforum.org /agenda/2021/12/global-income-inequality-gap-report-rich-poor/.

36. "UNU-WIDER Blog: Global Inequality," *UNU WIDER*, accessed September 25, 2022, https://www.wider.unu.edu/publication/global-inequality-0.

37. "Early Childhood Development and Education," Healthy People 2030, Office of Disease Prevention and Health Promotion, US Department of Health and Human Services, accessed September 15, 2023, https://health.gov/healthypeople/priority -areas/social-determinants-health/literature-summaries/early-childhood -development-and-education#cit2.

38. "Early Childhood Development and Education," Healthy People 2030, Office of Disease Prevention and Health Promotion, US Department of Health and Human Services, accessed September 15, 2023, https://health.gov/healthypeople/priority -areas/social-determinants-health/literature-summaries/early-childhood -development-and-education#cit2.

39. J. Currie, "Health Disparities and Gaps in School Readiness," in *The Future of Children*, 2005, 117–138, https://pubmed.ncbi.nlm.nih.gov/16130544/.

40. L. S. Whitehead and S. D. Buchanan, "Childhood Lead Poisoning: A Perpetual Environmental Justice Issue?," *Journal of Public Health Management and Practice* 25 (2019): S115–S120.

41. N. Zhang, H. W. Baker, M. Tufts, R. E. Raymond, H. Salihu, and M. R. Elliott, "Early Childhood Lead Exposure and Academic Achievement: Evidence from Detroit Public Schools, 2008–2010," *American Journal of Public Health* 103, no. 3 (2013): e72–e77.

42. *High School Graduation Rates*, National Center for Education Statistics, 2024, https://nces.ed.gov/programs/coe/indicator/coi.

43. "On-Time Graduation," National Center for Education Statistics, US Department of Education, Institute of Education Sciences, Equity in Education Dashboard, 2023, https://nces.ed.gov/programs/equity/indicator_c6.asp.

44. M. Arenson, P. J. Hudson, N. Lee, and B. Lai, "The Evidence on School-Based Health Centers: A Review," *Global Pediatric Health* 6 (2019): 2333794X19828745, Phttps://doi.org/10.1177/2333794X19828745.

45. "College Enrollment Rates," National Center for Education Statistics, US Department of Education, 2022, https://nces.ed.gov/programs/coe/pdf/2022/cpb_508.pdf.

46. A. Carnevale, B. Cheah, and E. Wenzinger, "The College Payoff: More Education Doesn't Always Mean More Earnings," Georgetown University Center on Education and the Workforce, 2021, https://cew.georgetown.edu/collegepayoff2021.

47. L. Nielsen-Bohlman, A. M. Panzer, and D. A. Kindig, eds., *Health Literacy: A Prescription to End Confusion* (National Academies Press, 2004).

48. I. S. Kirsch, "The Framework Used in Developing and Interpreting the International Adult Literacy Survey (IALS)," *European Journal of Psychology of Education* 16, no. 3 (2001): 335–361, https://doi.org/10.1007/BF03173187.

49. D. P. Andrulis and C. Brach, "Integrating Literacy, Culture, and Language to Improve Health Care Quality for Diverse Populations," *American Journal of Health Behavior* 31, no. 1 (2007): S122–S133.

50. S. Kripalani, L. E. Henderson, E. Y. Chiu, R. Robertson, P. Kolm, and T. A. Jacobson, "Predictors of Medication Self-Management Skill in a Low-Literacy Population," *Journal of General Internal Medicine* 21, no. 8 (2006): 852–856, https://doi.org/10.1111/j.1525-1497.2006.00536.x.

51. D. A. DeWalt, N. D. Berkman, S. Sheridan, K. N. Lohr, and M. P. Pignone, "Literacy and Health Outcomes," *Journal of General Internal Medicine* 19, no. 12 (2004): 1228–1239, https://doi.org/10.1111/j.1525-1497.2004.40153.x.

52. N. D. Berkman, S. L. Sheridan, K. E. Donahue, D. J. Halpern, A. Viera, K. Crotty, and M. Viswanathan, "Health Literacy Interventions and Outcomes: An Updated Systematic Review," *Evidence Report/Technology Assessment*, no. 199 (2011): 1–941.

53. "Access to Health Services," Healthy People 2030, Office of Disease Prevention and Health Promotion, US Department of Health and Human Services, accessed

October 3, 2022, https://health.gov/healthypeople/priority-areas/social-determinants-health/literature-summaries/incarceration.

54. Institute of Medicine (US) Committee on the Future of Primary Care, M. S. Donaldson, K. D. Yordy, K. N. Lohr, and N. A. Vanselow, eds., *Primary Care: America's Health in a New Era* (National Academies Press, 1996).

55. Mark W. Friedberg, Peter S. Hussey, and Eric C. Schneider, "Primary Care: A Critical Review of the Evidence on Quality and Costs of Health Care," *Health Affairs*, 2010, https://www.healthaffairs.org/doi/full/10.1377/hlthaff.2010.0025.

56. "Mission, Work, and Impact," National Health Service Corps, November 2021, https://nhsc.hrsa.gov/about-us.

57. J. Hadley, "Sicker and Poorer—the Consequences of Being Uninsured: A Review of the Research on the Relationship Between Health Insurance, Medical Care Use, Health, Work, and Income," suppl., *Medical Care Research and Review* 60 (2003): 3S–112S, https://doi.org/10.1177/1077558703254101.

58. K. T. Call, D. D. McAlpine, C. M. Garcia, N. Shippee, T. Beebe, T. C. Adeniyi, and T. Shippee, "Barriers to Care in an Ethnically Diverse Publicly Insured Population: Is Health Care Reform Enough?," *Medical Care* 52, no. 8 (2014): 720–727, https://doi.org/10.1097/MLR.0000000000000172.

59. Jennifer Tolbert, Patrick Drake, and Anthony Damico, "Key Facts About the Uninsured Population," KFF, accessed October 2, 2022, https://www.kff.org/uninsured/issue-brief/key-facts-about-the-uninsured-population/.

60. BBC News, "Ebola Crisis: Sierra Leone Bodies Found Piled Up in Kono," accessed May 12, 2015, http://www.bbc.com/news/world-africa-30429360.

61. M. Kutner, E. Greenburg, Y. Jin, and C. Paulsen, *The Health Literacy of America's Adults: Results from the 2003 National Assessment of Adult Literacy*, NCES 2006–483, Institute of Education Sciences, National Center for Education Statistics, 2006.

62. "Mapping Food Deserts in the United States," Economic Research Service, US Department of Agriculture, 2011, https://www.ers.usda.gov/amber-waves/2011/december/data-feature-mapping-food-deserts-in-the-u-s/.

63. "Food Insecurity in the U.S. by the Numbers," NPR, September 27, 2020, https://www.npr.org/2020/09/27/912486921/food-insecurity-in-the-u-s-by-the-numbers.

64. "Criminology: Theories of Crime and Punishment," Simply Psychology, n.d., https://www.simplypsychology.org/theories/criminology.

65. C. C. Lanfear, R. L. Matsueda, and L. R. Beach, "Broken Windows, Informal Social Control, and Crime: Assessing Causality in Empirical Studies," *Annual Review of Criminology* 3 (2020): 97–120, https://doi.org/10.1146/annurev-criminol-011419-041541.

66. A. Yanuari, N. Soetikno, and R. Sahrani, "Criminality and Antisocial Behavior in Young Adult," *Atlantis Press*, December 2021, https://www.atlantis-press.com/proceedings/ticmih-21/125965093.

67. "Civil Disorder," FindLaw, n.d., https://www.findlaw.com/criminal/criminal -charges/civil-disorder.html.

68. C. Graif, A. S. Gladfelter, and S. A. Matthews, "Urban Poverty and Neighborhood Effects on Crime: Incorporating Spatial and Network Perspectives," *Sociology Compass* 8, no. 9, (2014): 1140–1155, https://doi.org/10.1111/soc4.12199.

69. Darryl Fears, "Redlining Means 45 Million Americans Are Breathing Dirtier Air, 50 Years After It Ended," *Washington Post*, March 9, 2022, https://www .washingtonpost.com/climate-environment/2022/03/09/redlining-pollution -environmental-justice/.

70. Darryl Fears, "Redlining Means 45 Million Americans Are Breathing Dirtier Air, 50 Years After It Ended," *Washington Post*, March 9, 2022, https://www .washingtonpost.com/climate-environment/2022/03/09/redlining-pollution -environmental-justice/.

71. "Discrimination," Healthy People 2030, Office of Disease Prevention and Health Promotion, US Department of Health and Human Services, accessed September 2, 2022, https://health.gov/healthypeople/priority-areas/social -determinants-health/literature-summaries/discrimination.

72. Lauren A. Taylor, "Housing and Health: An Overview of the Literature," *Health Affairs*, June 7, 2018, https://www.healthaffairs.org/do/10.1377/hpb20180313.396577/.

73. David L. Maness and Muneeza Khan, "Care of the Homeless: An Overview," April 15, 2014, https://www.aafp.org/pubs/afp/issues/2014/0415/p634.html.

74. Colette L. Auerswald, Jessica S. Lin, and Andrea Parriott, "Six-Year Mortality in a Street-Recruited Cohort of Homeless Youth in San Francisco, California," PeerJ, April 14, 2016, https://peerj.com/articles/1909/.

75. Toby Schmitt et al., "Traumatic Brain Injury in a Community-Based Cohort of Homeless and Vulnerably Housed Individuals," *Journal of Neurotrauma* 34, no. 23 (2017): 3301–3310, https://doi.org/10.1089/neu.2017.5076.

76. Dorota Szymkowiak et al., "Persistent Super-Utilization of Acute Care Services Among Subgroups of Veterans Experiencing Homelessness," *Medical Care* 55, no. 10 (2017): 893–900, https://doi.org/10.1097/MLR.0000000000000796.

77. L. A. Taylor, "Housing and Health: An Overview of the Literature," Robert Wood Johnson Foundation, June 7, 2018, https://www.rwjf.org/en/insights/our -research/2018/06/housing-and-health--an-overview-of-the-literature.html.

78. K. Saeki, K. Obayashi, and N. Kurumatani, "Short-Term Effects of Instruction in Home Heating on Indoor Temperature and Blood Pressure in Elderly People: A Randomized Controlled Trial," *Journal of Hypertension* 33, no. 11 (2015): 2338–2343, https://doi.org/ 10.1097/HJH.0000000000000729.

79. C. D. Solari and R. D. Mare, "Housing Crowding Effects on Children's Well-being," *Social Science Research* 41, no. 2 (2012): 464–476, https://doi.org/10.1016/j .ssresearch.2011.09.012.

80. P. Whitney, "More Than 42 Million US Households Were Cost Burdened in 2022," *Joint Center for Housing Studies* (blog), accessed September 28, 2022,

https://www.jchs.harvard.edu/blog/more-42-million-us-households-were-cost
-burdened-2022.

81. "Civic Participation," Healthy People 2030, Office of Disease Prevention and Health Promotion, US Department of Health and Human Services, accessed September 28, 2022, https://health.gov/healthypeople/priority-areas/social -determinants-health/literature-summaries/civic-participation.

82. "Discrimination," Healthy People 2030, Office of Disease Prevention and Health Promotion, US Department of Health and Human Services, accessed September 27, 2022, https://health.gov/healthypeople/priority-areas/social -determinants-health/literature-summaries/discrimination.

83. "Discrimination," Healthy People 2030, Office of Disease Prevention and Health Promotion, US Department of Health and Human Services, accessed September 27, 2022, https://health.gov/healthypeople/priority-areas/social -determinants-health/literature-summaries/discrimination.

84. *2019 National Healthcare Quality and Disparities Report*, Agency for Healthcare Research and Quality, 2019, https://www.ahrq.gov/sites/default/files/wysiwyg /research/findings/nhqrdr/2019qdr.pdf.

85. E. K. Pavalko, K. N. Mossakowski, and V. J. Hamilton, "Does Perceived Discrimination Affect Health? Longitudinal Relationships Between Work Discrimi-nation and Women's Physical and Emotional Health," *Journal of Health and Social Behavior* 44, no. 1 (2003): 18–33.

86. "What Is Intersectionality," Center for Intersectional Justice, accessed September 27, 2022, https://www.intersectionaljustice.org/what-is-inter sectionality.

87. "Incarceration," Healthy People 2030, Office of Disease Prevention and Health Promotion, US Department of Health and Human Services, accessed September 27, 2022, https://health.gov/healthypeople/priority-areas/social-determinants-health /literature-summaries/incarceration.

88. "Social Cohesion," Healthy People 2030, Office of Disease Prevention and Health Promotion, US Department of Health and Human Services, accessed September 27, 2022, https://health.gov/healthypeople/priority-areas/social -determinants-health/literature-summaries/social-cohesion.

89. Daniel Dawes, *The Political Determinants of Health* (Johns Hopkins University Press, 2020), https://www.press.jhu.edu/books/title/12075/political-determinants -health.

90. Heidi J. Larson, Emmanuela Gakidou, and Christopher J. L. Murray, "The Vaccine-Hesitant Moment," *New England Journal of Medicine*, July 7, 2022, https:// www.nejm.org/doi/full/10.1056/nejmra2106441.

91. Heidi J. Larson, Emmanuela Gakidou, and Christopher J. L. Murray, "The Vaccine-Hesitant Moment," *New England Journal of Medicine*, July 7, 2022, https:// www.nejm.org/doi/full/10.1056/nejmra2106441.

92. S. Machingaidze and C. S. Wiysonge, "Understanding COVID-19 Vaccine Hesitancy," *Nature Medicine* 27 (2021): 1338–1339, https://doi.org/10.1038 /s41591-021-01459-7.

93. L. Eggertson, "'Lancet' Retracts 12-Year-Old Article Linking Autism to MMR Vaccines," *Canadian Medical Association Journal (Journal de l'Association medicale canadienne)* 182, no. 4 (2010): E199–E200, https://doi.org/10.1503 /cmaj.109-3179.

94. Atwoli Lukoye et al., "Trauma and Posttraumatic Stress Disorder in South Africa: Analysis from the South African Stress and Health Study," *BMJ Psychiatry*, 2013, https://link.springer.com/article/10.1186/1471-244X-13-182.

95. Peter A. Newman, "COVID-19 Vaccine Hesitancy Among Marginalized Populations in the U.S. and Canada: Protocol for a Scoping Review," *PLoS One* 17, no. 3 (2022): e0266120, https://doi.org/10.1371%2Fjournal.pone.0266120.

96. Jim Lee and Yuxia Huang, "COVID-19 Vaccine Hesitancy: The Role of Socioeconomic Factors and Spatial Effects," *Vaccines* 10, no. 3 (2022), https://doi.org /10.3390/vaccines10030352.

97. "Fact Sheet," *New England Journal of Medicine*, accessed October 1, 2023, https://www.nejm.org/media-center/fact-sheet.

98. Heidi J. Larson, Emmanuela Gakidou, and Christopher J. L. Murray, "The Vaccine-Hesitant Moment," *New England Journal of Medicine*, July 7, 2022, https:// www.nejm.org/doi/full/10.1056/nejmra2106441.

99. W. Bruine de Bruin, H. W. Saw, and D. P. Goldman, "Why Conservatives Turned Against Science," *Journal of Risk and Uncertainty*, 2020, https://doi.org /10.1007/s11166-020-09336-3.

100. L. C. Hamilton and T. Safford, "Conservative Media Consumers Less Likely to Wear Masks and Less Worried About COVID-19: Carsey Perspectives," University of New Hampshire, 2020, https://carsey.unh.edu/publication/conservative-media -consumers-views-COVID-19.

101. J. M. Barrios and Y. Hochberg, "Risk Perception Through the Lens of Politics in the Time of COVID-19 Pandemic," National Bureau of Economic Research Working Paper 27008, Cambridge, 2020, https://doi.org/10.3386/w27008.

102. D. P. Calvillo, B. J. Ross, R. J. Garcia, T. J. Smelter, and A. M. Rutchick, "Political Ideology Predicts Perceptions of the Threat of COVID-19 (and Susceptibil- ity to Fake News About It)," *Social Psychological and Personality Science* 11, no. 8 (2020): 1119–1128, https://doi.org/10.1177/1948550620940539.

103. T. Hill, K. E. Gonzalez, and A. Davis, "The Nastiest Question: Does Popula- tion Mobility Vary by State Political Ideology During the Novel Coronavirus (COVID-19) Pandemic?," *Sociological Perspectives* 64, no. 5 (2020): 786–803, https:// doi.org/10.1177/0731121420979700.

104. T. Hill, K. E. Gonzalez, and A. Burdette, "The Blood of Christ Compels Them: State Religiosity and State Population Mobility During the Coronavirus (COVID-19)

Pandemic," *Journal of Religion and Health* 59 (2020): 2229–2240, https://doi.org/10.1007/s10943-020-01058-9.

105. S. L. Perry, A. L. Whitehead, and J. B. Grubbs, "Culture Wars and COVID-19 Conduct: Christian Nationalism, Religiosity, and Americans' Behavior During the Coronavirus Pandemic," *Journal for the Scientific Study of Religion* 59, no. 3 (2020): 405–416, https://doi.org/10.1111/jssr.12677.

106. D. E. Albrecht, "COVID-19 in Rural America: Impacts of Politics and Disadvantage," *Rural Sociology* 87, no. 1 (2022): 94–118, https://doi.org/10.1111/ruso.12404.

107. J. S. Solís Arce, S. S. Warren, and N. F. Meriggi, et al., "COVID-19 Vaccine Acceptance and Hesitancy in Low- and Middle-Income Countries," *Nature Medicine* 27 (2021): 1385–1394, https://doi.org/10.1038/s41591-021-01454-y.

108. J. S. Solís Arce, S. S. Warren, and N. F. Meriggi, et al., "COVID-19 Vaccine Acceptance and Hesitancy in Low- and Middle-Income Countries," *Nature Medicine* 27 (2021): 1385–1394, https://doi.org/10.1038/s41591-021-01454-y.

109. "Majority of Africans Would Take a Safe and Effective COVID-19 Vaccine," Africa Centres for Disease Control and Prevention, December 2020, https://africacdc.org/news-item/majority-of-africans-would-take-a-safe-and-effective-covid-19-vaccine/.

110. R. J. I. Wilson, C. Vergélys, J. Ward, P. Peretti-Watel, and P. Verger, "Vaccine Hesitancy Among General Practitioners in Southern France and Their Reluctant Trust in the Health Authorities," *International Journal of Qualitative Studies on Health and Well-Being* 15, no. 1 (2020): 1757336, https://doi.org/10.1080/17482631.2020.1757336.

111. "Infodemics and Misinformation Negatively Affect People's Health Behaviours, New WHO Review Finds," World Health Organization, September 1, 2022, https://www.who.int/europe/news/item/01-09-2022-infodemics-and-misinformation-negatively-affect-people-s-health-behaviours--new-who-review-finds.

3. Population Stress

1. Lukoye Atwoli et al., "Trauma and Posttraumatic Stress Disorder in South Africa: Analysis from the South African Stress and Health Study," *BMJ Psychiatry*, 2013, https://link.springer.com/article/10.1186/1471-244X-13-182.

2. "2014–2016 Ebola Outbreak in West Africa," Centers for Disease Control and Prevention, March 2019, https://www.cdc.gov/vhf/ebola/history/2014-2016-outbreak/index.html.

3. "2014–2016 Ebola Outbreak in West Africa," Centers for Disease Control and Prevention, March 2019, https://www.cdc.gov/vhf/ebola/history/2014-2016-outbreak/index.html.

4. Ronald Carshon-Marsh et al., "Child, Maternal, and Adult Mortality in Sierra Leone: Nationally Representative Mortality Survey, 2018–20," *Lancet Global Health* 10, no. 1 (2022): e114-e115, https://doi.org/10.1016%2FS2214-109X(21)00459-9.

5. "Missing Dimensions Projects," Oxford Poverty and Human Development Initiative, accessed September 14, 2023, https://ophi.org.uk/research/missing-dimensions/projects/.

6. "Human Development Insights, Human Development Reports," accessed September 28, 2023, https://hdr.undp.org/data-center/country-insights#/ranks.

7. Manny Fernandez and Audra D. S. Burch, "George Floyd from 'I Want to Touch the World' to 'I Can't Breathe,'" *New York Times*, April 20, 2021, https://www.nytimes.com/article/george-floyd-who-is.html.

4. Selected Vulnerable Populations Around the World

1. A. Gu, H. Shafeeq, T. Chen, and P. Gadhoke, "Factors Associated with COVID-19 Infection, Hospitalization and Death in New York City Neighborhoods," *Innovations in Pharmacy* 12, no. 3 (2021), https://doi.org/10.24926/iip.v12i3.3379.

2. K. Ahmad, S. Erqou, N. Shah, U. Nazir, A. R. Morrison, G. Choudhary, and W. C. Wu, "Association of Poor Housing Conditions with COVID-19 Incidence and Mortality Across US Counties," *PloS One* 15, no. 11 (2020): e0241327, https://doi.org/10.1371/journal.pone.0241327.

3. K. Daras, A. Alexiou, T. C. Rose, I. Buchan, D. Taylor-Robinson, and B. Barr, "How Does Vulnerability to COVID-19 Vary Between Communities in England? Developing a Small Area Vulnerability Index (SAVI)," *Journal of Epidemiology and Community Health* 75, no. 8 (2021): 729–734, https://doi.org/10.1136/jech-2020-215227.

4. A. Adiga, S. Chu, S. Eubank, C. J. Kuhlman, B. Lewis, A. Marathe, M. Marathe, E. K. Nordberg, S. Swarup, A. Vullikanti, and M. L. Wilson, "Disparities in Spread and Control of Influenza in Slums of Delhi: Findings from an Agent-Based Modelling Study," *BMJ Open* 8, no. 1 (2018): e017353, https://doi.org/10.1136/bmjopen-2017-017353.

5. S. Selvaraju, M. S. Kumar, J. W. V. Thangaraj, T. Bhatnagar, V. Saravanakumar, C. P. G. Kumar, K. Sekar, E. Ilayaperumal, R. Sabarinathan, M. Jagadeesan, et al. "COVID Sero-Surveillance Team: Population-Based Serosurvey for Severe Acute Respiratory Syndrome Coronavirus 2 Transmission, Chennai, India," *Emerging Infectious Diseases* 27, no. 2 (2021): 586–589, https://doi.org/10.3201/eid2702.203938.

6. Y. Borofsky and I. Günther, "Mobility in Informal Settlements During a Public Lockdown: A Case Study in South Africa," *PloS One* 17, no. 12 (2022): e0277465, https://doi.org/10.1371/journal.pone.0277465.

7. "Chicago: Black People Are 30% of Its Population but 60% of Its Covid-19 Deaths," *Guardian*, May 24, 2020, https://www.theguardian.com/world/2020/may/24/chicago-black-coronavirus-fatalities-us.

8. "ERS Charts of Note," Economic Research Service, US Department of Agriculture, accessed July 19, 2022, https://www.ers.usda.gov/data-products/charts-of-note/charts-of-note/?page=3&topicId=2d26875b-d523-4e2c-bf40-5281a376d38d.

9. Centers for Disease Control & Prevention. "HIV in the South," accessed July 20, 2022, https://www.cdc.gov/hiv/pdf/policies/cdc-hiv-in-the-south-issue-brief.pdf.

10. Centers for Disease Control & Prevention. "HIV in the South," accessed July 20, 2022, https://www.cdc.gov/hiv/pdf/policies/cdc-hiv-in-the-south-issue-brief.pdf

11. R. S. Bono, B. Dahman, L. M. Sabik, L. E. Yerkes, Y. Deng, F. Z. Belgrave, D. E. Nixon, A. G. Rhodes, and A. D. Kimmel, "Human Immunodeficiency Virus—Experienced Clinician Workforce Capacity: Urban-Rural Disparities in the Southern United States," *Clinical Infectious Diseases* 72, no. 9 (2021): 1615–1622, https://doi.org/10.1093/cid/ciaa300.

12. "COVID-19 Cases in Appalachia" ArcGIS, https://www.arcgis.com/home/item.html?id=9862199203d64643ba7f549f21208fd1.

13. S. Fazel, J. R. Geddes, and M. Kushel, "The Health of Homeless People in High-income Countries: Descriptive Epidemiology, Health Consequences, and Clinical and Policy Recommendations," October 25, 2014, https://www.thelancet.com/journals/lancet/article/PIIS0140-6736(14)61132-6/abstract.

14. S. Fazel, J. R. Geddes, and M. Kushel, "The Health of Homeless People in High-income Countries: Descriptive Epidemiology, Health Consequences, and Clinical and Policy Recommendations," October 25, 2014, https://www.thelancet.com/journals/lancet/article/PIIS0140-6736(14)61132-6/abstract.

15. S. E. Kidd, J. A. Grey, E. A. Torrone, and H. S. Weinstock, "Increased Methamphetamine, Injection Drug, and Heroin Use Among Women and Heterosexual Men with Primary and Secondary Syphilis—United States, 2013–2017," *Morbidity and Mortality Weekly Report* 68 (2019):144–148, http://dx.doi.org/10.15585/mmwr.mm6806a4.

16. S. Badiaga, D. Raoult, and P. Brouqui, "Preventing and Controlling Emerging and Reemerging Transmissible Diseases in the Homeless," *Emerging Infectious Diseases* 14, no. 9 (2008): 1353–1359, https://doi.org/10.3201/eid1409.080204.

17. "About Homelessness: Supporting Communities to Prevent and End Homelessness—Infectious Diseases," Homeless Hub, accessed August 17, 20222, https://www.homelesshub.ca/about-homelessness/health/infectious-diseases.

18. Harper Sutherland, Mir M. Ali, and Emily Rosenoff, "Individuals Experiencing Homelessness Are Likely to Have Medical Conditions Associated with Severe Illness from COVID-19," issue brief, Office of the Assistant Secretary for Planning and Evaluation, June 2020, https://aspe.hhs.gov/reports/individuals-experiencing-homelessness-are-likely-have-medical-conditions-associated-severe-illness-0.

19. T. Roederer, B. Mollo, C. Vincent, B. Nikolay A. E. Llosa, and R. Nesbitt, "Seroprevalence and Risk Factors of Exposure to COVID-19 in Homeless People in Paris, France: A Cross-Sectional Study," April 2021, https://www.thelancet.com/journals/lanpub/article/PIIS2468-2667(21)00001-3/fulltext.

20. L. Schrooyen, M. Delforge, F. Lebout, T. Vanbaelen, A. Lecompte, and N. Dauby, "Homeless People Hospitalized with Covid-19 in Brussels," *Clinical Microbiology and Infection* 27, no. 1 (2021): 151–152, https://doi.org/10.1016/j.cmi.2020.08.002.

21. S. L. Li, R. H. M. Pereira, C. A. Prete, A. E. Zarebski Jr., L. Emanuel, P. J. H. Alves, P. S. Peixoto, C. K. V. Braga, A. A. de Souza Santos, W. M. de Souza, et al.

"Higher Risk of Death from COVID-19 in Low-Income and Non-White Populations of São Paulo, Brazil," *BMJ Global Health* 6, no. 4 (2021): e004959, https://doi.org/10.1136/bmjgh-2021-004959.

22. "Indigenous Peoples Rights Are Human Rights," Amnesty International, April 3, 2024, https://www.amnesty.org/en/what-we-do/indigenous-peoples.

23. United Nations, "People Living in Poverty," accessed July 25, 2002, https://www.un.org/en/fight-racism/vulnerable-groups/people-living-in-poverty.

24. *A Bill to Reauthorize the Indian Healthcare Improvement Act and H.R. 2440, Indian Healthcare Improvement Act Amendments of 2003: Joint Hearing Before the Senate Committee on Indian Affairs and the House Resources Committee, Office of Native American and Insular Affairs,* 108th Cong. (2003) (statement of Dr. Charles W. Grim, Director, Indian Health Service).

25. Indian Health Service, "Disparities," accessed August 5, 2022, https://www.ihs.gov/newsroom/factsheets/disparities/.

26. T. Burki, "COVID-19 Among American Indians and Alaska Natives," *Lancet Infectious Diseases* 21, no. 3 (2021): 325–326, https://doi.org/10.1016/S1473-3099(21)00083-9.

27. "COVID-19 Among American Indian and Alaska Native Persons—23 States, January 31–July 3, 2020," *Morbidity and Mortality Weekly Report*, August 27, 2020, https://www.cdc.gov/mmwr/volumes/69/wr/mm6934e1.htm.

28. P. C. Hallal, F. P. Hartwig, B. L. Horta, M. F. Silveira, C. J. Struchiner, L. P. Vidaletti, N. A. Neumann, L. C. Pellanda, O. A. Dellagostin, M. N. Burattini, et al., "SARS-CoV-2 Antibody Prevalence in Brazil: Results from Two Successive Nationwide Serological Household Surveys," *Lancet Global Health* 8, no. 11 (2020): e1390–e1398, https://doi.org/10.1016/S2214-109X(20)30387-9.

29. *Roma Health Report: Health Status of the Roma Population*, European Commission, 2014, accessed November 7, 2015, http://ec.europa.eu/health/social_determinants/docs/2014_roma_health_report_en.pdf.

30. G. Cilla, E. Perez-Trallero, J. M. Marimon, et al., "Prevalence of Hepatitis A Antibody Among Disadvantaged Gypsy Children in Northern Spain," *Epidemiology and Infection* 115 (1995): 157–161, https://doi.org/10.1017/s0950268800058210.

31. J. L. Morales, L. Huber, S. Gallego, et al. "A Seroepidemiologic Study of Hepatitis A in Spanish Children: Relationship of Prevalence to Age and Socio Environmental Factors," *Infection* 20 (1992): 194–196, https://doi.org/10.1007/BF02033057.

32. M. Cruz, A. Dieguez, E. Fos, and F. Hierro, "Epidemiologic Survey on Hepatitis B in Gypsy Women," *European Journal of Epidemiology* 4 (1988): 314–317, https://doi.org/10.1007/BF00148916.

33. P. Pazdiora, V. Nemecek, and O. P. Topolcan, "Initial Results of Monitoring Hepatitis E Virus Antibodies in Selected Population Groups in the West Bohemia Region: Preliminary Report," *Epidemiology, Microbiology, Immunology* 45 (1996): 117–118, https://pubmed.ncbi.nlm.nih.gov/8998603/.

34. Ahmad Jallad, *Al-Jallad: A Manual of the Historical Grammar of Arabic*, Academia.edu, 2020, https://www.academia.edu/38100372/Al_Jallad_A_Manual_of _the_Historical_Grammar_of_Arabic.

35. "A Threshold Crossed," Human Rights Watch, 2021, https://www.hrw.org/sites /default/files/media_2021/04/israel_palestine0421_web_0.pdf.

36. T. Munzel, T. Hori, W. Babisch, and M. Basner, "Cardiovascular Effects of Environmental Noise Exposure," *European Heart Journal* 35, no. 13 (2014): 829–836, https://pmc.ncbi.nlm.nih.gov/articles/PMC3971384/#:~:text=Beyond%20its%20 effects%20on%20the,%2C%20myocardial%20infarction%2C%20and%20stroke.

37. "Concluding Observations of the Committee on Economic, Social and Cultural Rights: Israel," Article 28, December 4, 1998, UN Committee on Economic, Social and Cultural Rights, https://www.refworld.org/policy/polrec/cescr/1998/en/32518.

38. "Off the Map: Land and Housing Rights Violations in Israel's Unrecognized Bedouin Villages," Human Rights Watch, 2008, https://www.hrw.org/report/2008 /03/30/map/land-and-housing-rights-violations-israels-unrecognized-bedouin -villages.

39. O. Almi, *No Man's Land: Health in the Unrecognized Villages in the Negev* (PHR-Israel, 2003).

40. H. Hafeez, M. Zeshan, M. A. Tahir, N. Jahan, and S. Naveed, "Healthcare Disparities Among Lesbian, Gay, Bisexual, and Transgender Youth: A Literature Review," *Cureus* 4, no. 9 (2017): e1184, https://doi.org/10.7759/cureus.1184.

41. Jennifer A. Pellowski, Seth C. Kalichman, Karen A. Matthews, and Nancy Adler, "A Pandemic of the Poor: Social Disadvantage and the U.S. HIV Epidemic," *American Psychologist* 68, no. 4 (2013): 197–209, https://doi.org/10.1037/a0032694.

42. Susan Reif, Brian Wells Pence, Irene Hall, Xiaohong Hu, Kathryn Whetten, and Elena Wilson, "HIV Diagnoses, Prevalence and Outcomes in Nine Southern States," *Journal of Community Health* 40, no. 4 (2015): 642–651, https://doi.org /10.1007/s10900-014-9979-7.

43. *Fatal Violence Against the Transgender Community in 2016*, Human Rights Campaign, n.d., https://www.hrc.org/resources/violence-against-the-transgender -community-in-2016.

44. *Sexual Assault in the Transgender Community: The Numbers*, Office for Victims of Crime, June 2014, https://ovc.ojp.gov/sites/g/files/xyckuh226/files/pubs/forge /sexual_numbers.html.

45. D. M. Tordoff, J. W. Wanta, A. Collin, C. Stepney, D. J. Inwards-Breland, and K. Ahrens, "Mental Health Outcomes in Transgender and Nonbinary Youths Receiving Gender-Affirming Care," *JAMA Network Open* 5, no. 2 (2022): e220978, https://doi.org/10.1001/jamanetworkopen.2022.0978.

46. S. E. Stutterheim, M. van Dijk, H. Wang, and K. J. Jonas, "The Worldwide Burden of HIV in Transgender Individuals: An Updated Systematic Review and Meta-Analysis," *PloS One* 16, no. 12 (2021): e0260063, https://doi.org/10.1371 /journal.pone.0260063.

47. T. Poteat, B. Ackerman, D. Diouf, N. Ceesay, T. Mothopeng, K.-Z. Odette, S. Kouanda, H. G. Ouedraogo, A. Simplice, A. Kouame, et al., "HIV Prevalence and Behavioral and Psychosocial Factors Among Transgender Women and Cisgender Men Who Have Sex with Men in 8 African Countries: A Cross-Sectional Analysis," *PLOS Medicine*, November 7, 2017, https://journals.plos.org/plosmedicine/article?id=10.1371%2Fjournal.pmed.1002422.

48. S. E. Stutterheim, M. van Dijk, H. Wang, and K. J. Jonas, "The Worldwide Burden of HIV in Transgender Individuals: An Updated Systematic Review and Meta-Analysis," *PloS One* 16, no. 12 (2021): e0260063, https://doi.org/10.1371/journal.pone.0260063.

49. P. Parmar, S. Hsu Hnin Mon, and C. Beyrer, "The Rohingya Genocide and Lessons Learned from Myanmar's Spring Revolution," September 10, 2020, https://www.thelancet.com/journals/lancet/article/PIIS0140-6736(22)01651-8/abstract.

50. P. Parmar, S. Hsu Hnin Mon, and C. Beyrer, "The Rohingya Genocide and Lessons Learned from Myanmar's Spring Revolution," September 10, 2020, https://www.thelancet.com/journals/lancet/article/PIIS0140-6736(22)01651-8/abstract.

51. "Chinese Persecution of the Uyghurs," United States Holocaust Memorial Museum, https://www.ushmm.org/genocide-prevention/countries/china/chinese-persecution-of-the-uyghurs.

52. *OHCHR Assessment of Human Rights Concerns in the Xinjiang Uyghur Autonomous Region, People's Republic of China*, United Nations Human Rights Office of the High Commissioner, August 22, 2022, https://www.ohchr.org/sites/default/files/documents/countries/2022-08-31/22-08-31-final-assesment.pdf.

53. *World Migration Report 2022*, Institute of Medicine, 2022, https://worldmigrationreport.iom.int/wmr-2022-interactive/.

54. R. Chicas, N. Xiuhtecutli, M. Houser, S. Glastra, L. Elon, J. M. Sands, L. McCauley, and V. Hertzberg, "COVID-19 and Agricultural Workers: A Descriptive Study," *Journal of Immigrant and Minority Health* 24, no. 1 (2022): 58–64, https://doi.org/10.1007/s10903-021-01290-9.

55. "Global HIV, Hepatitis and STIs Programmes," World Health Organization, accessed August 25, 2022, https://www.who.int/teams/global-hiv-hepatitis-and-stis-programmes/populations/sex-workers.

56. "Protecting the Rights of Sex Workers," UNAIDS, June 2, 2017, https://www.unaids.org/en/resources/presscentre/featurestories/2017/june/20170602_sexwork.

57. S. K. Brooks, S. S. Patel, and N. Greenberg, "Struggling, Forgotten, and Under Pressure: A Scoping Review of Experiences of Sex Workers During the COVID-19 Pandemic," *Archives of Sexual Behavior* 52, no. 5 (2023): 1969–2010, https://doi.org/10.1007/s10508-023-02633-3.

58. "Figures at a Glance: How Many Refugees Are There Around the World?," United Nations High Commissioner for Refugees, accessed August 25, 2022, https://www.unhcr.org/about-unhcr/who-we-are/figures-glance.

59. "Figures at a Glance: How Many Refugees Are There Around the World?," United Nations High Commissioner for Refugees, accessed August 25, 2022, https://www.unhcr.org/about-unhcr/who-we-are/figures-glance.

60. "What Is a Refugee?," United Nations High Commissioner for Refugees, https://www.unhcr.org/what-refugee.

61. "Gender-Based Violence," United Nations High Commissioner for Refugees, accessed September 1, 2022, https://www.unhcr.org/sexual-and-gender-based -violence.html.

62. K. Johnson, J. Scott, B. Rughita, M. Kisielewski, J. Asher, R. Ong, and L. Lawry, "Association of Sexual Violence and Human Rights Violations with Physical and Mental Health in Territories of the Eastern Democratic Republic of the Congo," *JAMA* 304, no. 5 (2010): 553–562, https://doi.org/10.1001/jama.2010.1086.

63. D. van Reybrouck, *Congo: The Epic History of a People* (Harper Collins, 2014), 76–77.

64. C. McGreal, "Congo Conflict Causes 45,000 Deaths a Month: Study," *Guardian*, January 22, 2008, https://www.theguardian.com/world/2008/jan/22/congo .chrismcgreal.

65. K. Johnson, J. Scott, B. Rughita, M. Kisielewski, J. Asher, R. Ong, and L. Lawry, "Association of Sexual Violence and Human Rights Violations with Physical and Mental Health in Territories of the Eastern Democratic Republic of the Congo," *JAMA* 304, no. 5 (2010): 553–562, https://doi.org/10.1001/jama.2010.1086.

66. Sharon G. Smith et al., "The National Intimate Partner and Sexual Violence Survey: 2015 Data Brief—Updated Release," 2018, https://stacks.cdc.gov/view/cdc /60893.

67. S. Saxena, G. Thornicroft, M. Knapp, and H. Whiteford, "Resources for Mental Health: Scarcity, Inequity, and Inefficiency," September 8, 2007, https://www .thelancet.com/journals/lancet/article/PIIS0140-6736(07)61239-2/fulltext.

68. World Health Organization, *Mental Health Atlas 2011*, 2011, http://apps.who .int/iris/bitstream/10665/44697/1/9799241564359_eng.pdf.

69. "Refugee Facts, Statistics and FAQs," International Rescue Committee, September 26, 2023, https://www.rescue.org/article/facts-about-refugees-key-facts -faqs-and-statistics.

70. "Refugees in America," International Rescue Committee. accessed July 25, 2022, https://www.rescue.org/topic/refugees-america.

71. A. C. Miller, L. A. Polgreen, J. E. Cavanaugh, D. B. Hornick, and P. M. Polgreen, "Missed Opportunities to Diagnose Tuberculosis Are Common Among Hospitalized Patients and Patients Seen in Emergency Departments," *Open Forum Infectious Diseases* 2, no. 4 (2015): ofv171, https://doi.org/10.1093/ofid/ofv171.

72. D. Razavi-Shearer, I. Gamkrelidze, C. Q. Pan, K. Razavi-Shearer, S. Blach, C. Estes, E. Mooneyhan, and H. Razavi, "The Impact of Immigration on Hepatitis B Burden in the United States: A Modelling Study," *Lancet Regional Health: Americas* 22 (2023): 100516, https://doi.org/10.1016/j.lana.2023.100516.

73. N. Coppola et al., "Hepatitis B Virus Infection in Immigrant Populations," *World Journal of Hepatology* 7, no. 30 (2015): 2955–2961, https://doi.org/10.4254/wjh.v7.i30.2955.

74. "Guidance for Overseas Presumptive Treatment of Strongyloidiasis, Schistosomiasis, and Soil-Transmitted Helminth Infections for Refugees Resettling to the U.S," US Department of Health and Human Services, Centers for Disease Control and Prevention, National Center for Emerging and Zoonotic Infectious Diseases, Division of Global Migration and Quarantine, 2023, https://www.cdc.gov/immigrantrefugeehealth/pdf/intestinal-parasites-overseas.pdf.

75. K. Johnson, J. Scott, B. Rughita, M. Kisielewski, J. Asher, R. Ong, and L. Lawry, "Association of Sexual Violence and Human Rights Violations with Physical and Mental Health in Territories of the Eastern Democratic Republic of the Congo," *JAMA* 304, no. 5 (2010): 553–562, https://doi.org/10.1001/jama.2010.1086.

76. M. Sudhinaraset, N. Cabanting, and M. Ramos, "The Health Profile of Newly-Arrived Refugee Women and Girls and the Role of Region of Origin: Using a Population-Based Dataset in California Between 2013 and 2017," *International Journal for Equity in Health* 18, no. 1 (2019): 158, https://doi.org/10.1186/s12939-019-1066-3.

77. *World Migration Report 2022*, International Organization for Migration, United Nations Migration, n.d., https://worldmigrationreport.iom.int/wmr-2022-interactive/.

78. H. Hamadah, B. Alahmad, M. Behbehani, S. Al-Youha, S. Almazeedi, M. Al-Haddad, M. H. Jamal, and S. Al-Sabah, "COVID-19 Clinical Outcomes and Nationality: Results from a Nationwide Registry in Kuwait," *BMC Public Health* 20, no. 1 (2020): 1384, https://doi.org/10.1186/s12889-020-09490-y.

79. Wellness Equity Alliance (website), https://www.wellnessequityalliance.com/.

80. Sandro Galea and David Vlahov, "Social Determinants and the Health of Drug Users: Socioeconomic Status, Homelessness, and Incarceration," suppl., *Public Health Reports* 117, no. S1 (2002), https://www.ncbi.nlm.nih.gov/pmc/articles/PMC1913691/pdf/pubhealthrep00207-0140.pdf.

81. T. Dzinamarira and E. Moyo, "The Use of Oral HIV Pre-Exposure Prophylaxis Among People Who Inject Drugs: Barriers and Recommendations," *Frontiers in Public Health* 11 (2023): 1265063, https://doi.org/10.3389/fpubh.2023.1265063.

82. M. Peña-Orellana, A. Hernández-Viver, G. Caraballo-Correa, and C. E. Albizu-García, "Prevalence of HCV Risk Behaviors Among Prison Inmates: Tattooing and Injection Drug Use," *Journal of Health Care for the Poor and Underserved* 22, no. 3 (2011): 962–982, https://doi.org/10.1353/hpu.2011.0084.

83. N. K. Conteh, A. Latona, and O. Mahomed, "Mapping the Effectiveness of Integrating Mental Health in HIV Programs: A Scoping Review," *BMC Health Services Research* 23, no. 1 (2023): 396, https://doi.org/10.1186/s12913-023-09359-x.

84. "Provisional Drug Overdose Death Counts," National Center for Health Statistics, February 15, 2023, https://www.cdc.gov/nchs/nvss/vsrr/drug-overdose-data.htm.

85. "Mass Incarceration: Punishing the Families," University of Illinois Chicago, January 15, 2020, https://socialwork.uic.edu/news-stories/mass-incarceration -punishing-the-families.

86. A. Nellis, "Incarcerated Women and Girls," The Sentencing Project, 2020, https://www.sentencingproject.org/publications/incarcerated-women-and-girls.

87. D. M. Dumont, B. Brockmann, S. Dickman, N. Alexander, and J. D. Rich, "Public Health and the Epidemic of Incarceration," *Annual Review of Public Health* 33 (2012): 325–339, https://doi.org/10.1146/annurev-publhealth-031811-124614.

88. *Economic Perspectives on Incarceration and the Criminal Justice System*, Obama White House, April 2016, https://obamawhitehouse.archives.gov/sites/whitehouse .gov/files/documents/CEA+Criminal+Justice+Report.pdf.

89. "Recidivism," National Institute of Justice, n.d., https://nij.ojp.gov/topics /corrections/recidivism.

90. K. M. Budd, *Private Prisons in the United States*, The Sentencing Project, February 21, 2024, https://www.sentencingproject.org/reports/private-prisons-in -the-united-states/.

91. Kristen M. Budd and Niki Monazzam, *Private Prisons in the U.S.*, The Sentencing Project, June 2023, https://www.sentencingproject.org/reports/private-prisons -in-the-united-states/.

92. J. Bronson and M. Berzofsky, "Indicators of Mental Health Problems Reported by Prisoners and Jail Inmates," US Department of Justice, Bureau of Justice Statistics, 2017, https://www.bjs.gov/content/pub/pdf/imhprpji1112_sum.pdf.

93. S. I. Ranapurwala, M. E. Shanahan, A. A. Alexandridis, S. K. Proescholdbell, R. B. Naumann, and D. Edwards, "Opioid Overdose Mortality Among Former North Carolina Inmates: 2000–2015," *American Journal of Public Health* 108, no. 9 (2018): 1207–1213.

94. I. A. Binswanger, P. M. Krueger, and J. F. Steiner, "Prevalence of Chronic Medical Conditions Among Jail and Prison Inmates in the U.S. Compared with the General Population," *Journal of Epidemiology and Community Health* 63, no. 11 (2009): 912–919.

95. D. M. Dumont, B. Brockmann, S. Dickman, N. Alexander, and J. D. Rich, "Public Health and the Epidemic of Incarceration," *Annual Review of Public Health* 33 (2012): 325–339.

96. Z. G. Restum, "Public Health Implications of Substandard Correctional Healthcare," *American Journal of Public Health* 95, no. 10 (2005): 1689–1691.

97. L. M. Maruschak and R. Beavers, "HIV in Prisons, 2007–08," *Bureau of Justice Statistics Bulletin*, 2009.

98. A. C. Spaulding, R. M. Seals, M. J. Page, A. K. Brzozowski, W. Rhodes, and T. M. Hammett, "HIV/AIDS Among Inmates of and Releases from US Correctional Facilities, 2006: Declining Share of Epidemic but Persistent Public Health Opportunity," *PLoS One* 4, no. 11 (2009), https://pubmed.ncbi.nlm.nih.gov/19907649/.

99. S. S. Covington, "Women and the Criminal Justice System," *Women's Health Issues* 17, no. 4 (2007): 180–182.

100. N. Messina and C. Grella, "Childhood Trauma and Women's Health Outcomes in a California Prison Population," *American Journal of Public Health* 96, no. 10 (2006): 1842–1848.

101. R. L. Braithwaite, H. M. Treadwell, and K. R. J. Arriola, "Health Disparities and Incarcerated Women: A Population Ignored," suppl., *American Journal of Public Health* 98, no. S1 (2008): S173–S175.

102. M. Gal, "The Physical and Mental Health of Older Offenders," *Mental Health* 38, no. 30.8 (2003): 17–22.

103. R. H. Aday, "Golden Years Behind Bars: Special Programs and Facilities for Elderly Inmates," *Federal Probation* 58, no. 2 (1994): 47–54.

104. C. M. Lemieux, T. B. Dyeson, and B. Castiglione, "Revisiting the Literature on Prisoners Who Are Older: Are We Wiser?," *Prison Journal* 82, no. 4 (2002): 440–458.

105. D. E. Merianos, J. W. Marquart, K. Damphousse, and J. L. Hebert, "From the Outside In: Using Public Health Data to Make Inferences About Older Inmates," *Crime & Delinquency* 43, no. 3 (1997): 298–313.

106. S. J. Loeb and A. AbuDagga, "Health-Related Research on Older Inmates: An Integrative Review," *Research in Nursing & Health* 29, no. 6 (2006): 556–565.

107. J. Travis and J. Petersilia, "Reentry Reconsidered: A New Look at an Old Question," *NCCD News* 47, no. 3 (2001): 291–313.

108. S. Stojkovic, "Elderly Prisoners: A Growing and Forgotten Group Within Correctional Systems Vulnerable to Elder Abuse," *Journal of Elder Abuse & Neglect* 19, no. 3–4 (2007): 97–117.

109. Vera Institute, "More Than 5 Million Children Have Had an Incarcerated Parent," accessed July 25, 2022, https://www.vera.org/news/more-than-5-million-children-have-had-an-incarcerated-parent

110. C. Wildeman, "Parental Incarceration, Child Homelessness, and the Invisible Consequences of Mass Imprisonment," *Annals of the American Academy of Political and Social Science* 651, no. 1 (2014): 74–96.

111. D. Murphey and P. M. Cooper, "Parents Behind Bars: What Happens to Their Children?" *Child Trends,* 2015, https://www.childtrends.org/publications/parents-behind-bars-what-happens-to-their-children.

112. A. Geller, C. E. Cooper, I. Garfinkel, O. Schwartz-Soicher, and R. B. Mincy, "Beyond Absenteeism: Father Incarceration and Child Development," *Demography* 49, no. 1 (2012): 49–76.

113. N. Freudenberg, "Jails, Prisons, and the Health of Urban Populations: A Review of the Impact of the Correctional System on Community Health," *Journal of Urban Health* 78, no. 2 (2001): 214–235, https://doi.org/10.1093/jurban/78.2.214.

5. History of Contemporary Pandemics and Public Health Emergencies of International Concern

1. Michael B. Prentice and Lila Rahalison, "Plague," *Lancet* 369, no. 9568 (2007): 1196, https://doi.org/10.1016/s0140-6736(07)60566-2.

2. G. L. Campbell and J. M. Hughes, "Plague in India: A New Warning from an Old Nemesis," *Annals of Internal Medicine* 122, no. 2 (1995): 151, https://doi.org/10.7326/0003-4819-122-2-199501150-00014.

3. Michael B. Prentice and Lila Rahalison, "Plague," *Lancet* 369, no. 9568 (2007): 1196, https://doi.org/10.1016/s0140-6736(07)60566-2.

4. Centers for Disease Control and Prevention, "Human Plague—U.S., 1993–1994," *Morbidity and Mortality Weekly Report* 8, no. 43 (1994): 242.

5. L. D. Crook and B. Tempest, "Plague: A Clinical Review of 27 Cases," *Archives of Internal Medicine* 152, no. 6 (1992): 1253, https://doi.org/10.1001/archinte.152.6.1253.

6. B. G. Weniger, "Human Bubonic Plague Transmitted by a Domestic Cat Scratch," *JAMA* 17, no. 251 (1984): 927, https://doi.org/10.1001/jama.1984.03340310041017.

7. Centers for Disease Control and Prevention, "Fatal Laboratory-Acquired Infection with an Attenuated Yersinia Pestis Strain—Chicago, Illinois, 2009," *Morbidity and Mortality Weekly Report* 60, no. 7 (2011): 201, https://www.cdc.gov/mmwr/preview/mmwrhtml/mm6007a1.htm.

8. Niels Høiby, "Pandemics: Past, Present, Future," *APMIS* 129, no. 7 (2021), https://doi.org/10.1111%2Fapm.13098.

9. M. A. Spyrou, L. Musralina, G. A. Gnecchi Ruscone, et al., "The Source of the Black Death in Fourteenth-Century Central Eurasia," *Nature* 606 (2022): 718–724, https://doi.org/10.1038/s41586-022-04800-3.

10. C. Benedict, *Bubonic Plague in Nineteenth-Century China* (Stanford University Press, 1996).

11. Barbara Bramanti et al., "The Third Plague Pandemic in Europe," *Proceedings of the Royal Society B: Biological Sciences* 286, no. 1901 (2019): 20182429, https://doi.org/10.1098%2Frspb.2018.2429.

12. Srilata Chatterjee, "Plague and Politics in Bengal, 1896 to 1898," *Proceedings of the Indian History Congress* 66 (2005): 1194–1201, https://www.jstor.org/stable/44145931.

13. Maynard W. Swanson, "The Sanitation Syndrome: Bubonic Plague and Urban Native Policy in the Cape Colony, 1900–1909," *Journal of African History* 18, no. 3 (1977): 387–410, https://doi.org/10.1017/S0021853700027328.

14. M. Lee, "When Chinese Americans Were Scapegoated for Bubonic Plague," History, October 11, 2022, https://www.history.com/news/bubonic-plague-honolulu-fire-san-francisco.

15. Sheldon Watts, *Epidemics and History—Disease, Power and Imperialism* (Yale University Press, 1997), https://www.scribd.com/document/609486002/Dr-Sheldon-Watts-Epidemics-and-History-Disease-Power-and-Imperialism-1997-Yale-University-Press-Libgen-li.

16. Ana A. Weil et al., "Clinical Outcomes in Household Contacts of Patients with Cholera in Bangladesh," *Clinical Infectious Diseases* 49, no. 10 (2009): 1473–1479, https://doi.org/10.1086/644779.

17. Jason B. Harris et al., "Cholera," *Lancet* 379, no. 9835 (2012): 2466, https://doi.org/10.1016/S0140-6736(12)60436-X.

18. N. Hirschhorn et al., "Decrease in Net Stool Output in Cholera During Intestinal Perfusion with Glucose-Containing Solutions," *New England Journal of Medicine* 279, no. 4 (1968): 176, https://doi.org/10.1056/nejm196807252790402.

19. R. A. Cash et al., "Response of Man to Infection with *Vibrio cholerae*. I. Clinical, Serologic, and Bacteriologic Responses to a Known Inoculum," *Journal of Infectious Diseases* 129, no. 1 (1974): 45, https://doi.org/10.1093/infdis/129.1.45.

20. R. B. Hornick et al., "The Broad Street Pump Revisited: Response of Volunteers to Ingested Cholera Vibrios," *Bulletin of the New York Academy of Medicine* 47, no. 10 (1971): 1181.

21. R. Oseasohn et al., "Clinical and Bacteriological Findings Among Families of Cholera Patients," *Lancet* 1, no. 7433 (1966): 340, https://doi.org/10.1016/s0140-6736(66)91322-5.

22. Centers for Disease Control and Prevention, "Update: Outbreak of Cholera—Haiti, 2010," *Morbidity and Mortality Weekly Report* 59, no. 48 (2010): 1586, https://www.cdc.gov/mmwr/preview/mmwrhtml/mm5948a4.htm.

23. Jason B. Harris et al., "Cholera," *Lancet* 379, no. 9835 (2012): 2466–2476, https://doi.org/10.1016/S0140-6736(12)60436-X.

24. D. Scott Merrell et al., "Host-Induced Epidemic Spread of the Cholera Bacterium," *Nature* 417, no. 6889 (2002): 642, https://doi.org/10.1038/nature00778.

25. David M. Hartley, J. Glenn Morris Jr., and David L. Smith, "Hyperinfectivity: A Critical Element in the Ability of *V. Cholerae* to Cause Epidemics?," *PLoS Med* 3, no. 1 (2006): e7, https://doi.org/10.1371/journal.pmed.0030007.

26. Katia Koelle et al., "Refractory Periods and Climate Forcing in Cholera Dynamics," *Nature* 436, no. 7051 (2005): 696–700, https://doi.org/10.1038/nature03820.

27. J. L. Deen, L. von Seidlein, D. Sur, M. Agtini, M. E. S. Lucas, et al., "The High Burden of Cholera in Children: Comparison of Incidence from Endemic Areas in Asia and Africa," *PLOS Neglected Tropical Diseases* 2, no. 2 (2008): e173, https://doi.org/10.1371/journal.pntd.0000173.

28. A. Richterman et al., "Individual and Household Risk Factors for Symptomatic Cholera Infection: A Systematic Review and Meta-Analysis," *Journal of Infectious Diseases* 218, suppl 3 (2018): S154.

29. Amir M. Mohareb and Louise C. Ivers, "Disease and Famine as Weapons of War in Yemen," *New England Journal of Medicine* 380, no. 2 (2019): 109, https://doi.org/10.1056/nejmp1813831.

30. A. K. Siddique et al., "Why Treatment Centres Failed to Prevent Cholera Deaths Among Rwandan Refugees in Goma, Zaire," *Lancet* 345, no. 8946 (1995): 359, https://doi.org/10.1016/s0140-6736(95)90344-5.

31. J. Lindenbaum, W. B. Greenough, and M. R. Islam, "Antibiotic Therapy of Cholera," *Bulletin of the World Health Organization* 36, no. 6 (1967): 871, http://www.ncbi.nlm.nih.gov/pmc/articles/pmc2476357/.

32. John D Clemens et al., " Cholera," https://pubmed.ncbi.nlm.nih.gov/28302312/.

33. W. H. Mosley, A. S. Benenson, and R. Barui, "A Serological Survey for Cholera Antibodies in Rural East Pakistan," *Bulletin of the World Health Organization* 38, no. 3 (1968): 327, https://pubmed.ncbi.nlm.nih.gov/5302327.

34. N. Hirschhorn, A. K Chowdhury, and J. Lindenbaum, "Cholera in Pregnant Women," *Lancet* 1, no. 7608 (1969): 1230, https://doi.org/10.1016/s0140-6736(69)92115-1.

35. "Cholera," World Health Organization, December 11, 2023, https://www.who.int/news-room/fact-sheets/detail/cholera.

36. M. H. Azizi and F. Azizi, "History of Cholera Outbreaks in Iran During the 19th and 20th Centuries," *Middle East Journal of Digestive Diseases* 2, no. 1 (2010): 51–55.

37. R. Pollitzer, "Cholera Studies," *Bulletin of the World Health Organization*, 1954, 452, https://www.ncbi.nlm.nih.gov/pmc/articles/PMC2542143/pdf/bullwho00557-0108.pdf.

38. "Cholera," World Health Organization, December 11, 2023, https://www.who.int/news-room/fact-sheets/detail/cholera.

39. Archived April 20, 2005, at the Wayback Machine," Society of Philippines Health History "Health in the 1900s: The Epidemic Years History," accessed August 18, 2022, https://web.archive.org/web/20050420083132/http://www.doh.gov.ph/sphh/1900.htm.

40. James Pettifer and Tom Buchanan, *War in the Balkans* (I. B. Tauris & Co, 2016), https://unipub.uni-graz.at/obvugroa/content/titleinfo/4363082/full.pdf.

41. Franklin MacVeagh, "The Cholera Situation," *Public Health Reports* 26, no. 29 (1911), https://doi.org/10.2307/4566506.

42. M. Phelps, M. L. Perner, V. E. Pitzer, V. Andreasen, P. K. M. Jensen, and L. Simonsen, "Cholera Epidemics of the Past Offer New Insights into an Old Enemy," *Journal of Infectious Diseases* 217, no. 4 (2018): 641–649, https://doi.org/10.1093/infdis/jix602.

43. Jacqueline Deen, Martin A. Mengel, and John D. Clemens, "Epidemiology of Cholera," suppl., *Science Direct* 38, no. S1 (2020): A36, https://doi.org/10.1016/j.vaccine.2019.07.078.

44. D. V. Colombara, K. D. Cowgill, and A. S. G. Faruque, "Risk Factors for Severe Cholera Among Children Under Five in Rural and Urban Bangladesh, 2000–2008: Hospital-Based Surveillance Study," *PLOS One* 8, no. 1 (2013): e54395, https://doi.org/10.1371/journal.pone.0054395.

45. "Copepod," ScienceDirect, accessed September 14, 2023, https://www.sciencedirect.com/topics/immunology-and-microbiology/copepod.

46. M. A. Mengel, I. Delrieu, L. Heyerdahl, and B. D. Gessner, "Cholera Outbreaks in Africa," *Current Topics in Microbiology and Immunology* 379 (2014): 117–144, https://doi.org/10.1007/82_2014_369.

47. "Pulse Survey on Continuity of Essential Health Services During the COVID-19 Pandemic," World Health Organization, August 27, 2020, https://iris.who

.int/bitstream/handle/10665/334048/WHO-2019-nCoV-EHS_continuity-survey
-2020.1-eng.pdf.

48. Timothy M. Uyeki and Malik Peiris, "Novel Avian Influenza A Virus Infections of Humans," *Infectious Disease Clinics of North America* 33, no. 4 (2019): 907, https://doi.org/10.1016/j.idc.2019.07.003.

49. Kumnuan Ungchusak et al., "Probable Person-to-Person Transmission of Avian Influenza A (H5N1)," *New England Journal of Medicine* 352, no. 4 (2005): 333, https://doi.org/10.1056/nejmoa044021.

50. Hua Wang et al., "Probable Limited Person-to-Person Transmission of Highly Pathogenic Avian Influenza A (H5N1) Virus in China," *Lancet* 371, no. 9622 (2008): 1427, https://doi.org/10.1016/s0140-6736(08)60493-6.

51. Max Roser, "The Spanish Flu: The Global Impact of the Largest Influenza Pandemic in History," Our World in Data, March 4, 2020, https://ourworldindata.org/spanish-flu-largest-influenza-pandemic-in-history.

52. Jeffery K. Taubenberger and David M. Morens, "1918 Influenza: The Mother of All Pandemics," *Emerging Infectious Diseases* 12, no. 1 (2006): 15, https://doi.org/10.3201/eid1201.050979.

53. Max Roser, "The Spanish Flu: The Global Impact of the Largest Influenza Pandemic in History," Our World in Data, March 4, 2020, https://ourworldindata.org/spanish-flu-largest-influenza-pandemic-in-history.

54. J. R. McLane, "Paradise Locked: The 1918 Influenza Pandemic in American Samoa," *Sites: A Journal of Social Anthropology and Cultural Studies*, December 20, 2013, https://doi.org/10.11157/sites-vol10iss2id215.

55. "How Flu Viruses Can Change: 'Drift' and 'Shift,'" Centers for Disease Control and Prevention, December 12, 2020, https://www.cdc.gov/flu/about/viruses/change.htm.

56. Eugene L. Opie et al., "Pneumonia," *JAMA*, 1919, https://jamanetwork.com/journals/jama/article-abstract/220026.

57. Margaret Humphreys, "The Influenza of 1918," *Evolution, Medicine, and Public Health* 2018, no. 1 (2018): 219–221, https://doi.org/10.1093/emph/eoy024.

58. Angela D'Adamo et al., "Health Disparities in Past Influenza Pandemics: A Scoping Review of the Literature," *SSM—Population Health* 21 (2023), https://doi.org/10.1016/j.ssmph.2022.101314.

59. K. H. Grantz, M. S. Rane, H. Salje, G. E. Glass, S. E. Schachterle, and D. A. Cummings, "Disparities in Influenza Mortality and Transmission Related to Sociodemographic Factors Within Chicago in the Pandemic of 1918," *Proceedings of the National Academy of Sciences* 113, no. 48 (2016): 13839–13844, https://doi.org/10.1073/pnas.1612838113.

60. A. D'Adamo, A. Schnake-Mahl, P. H. Mullachery, M. Lazo, A. V. Diez Roux, and U. Bilal, "Health Disparities in Past Influenza Pandemics: A Scoping Review of the Literature," *SSM—Population Health* 21 (2023): 101314, https://doi.org/10.1016/j.ssmph.2022.101314.

61. H. Okland and S. E. Mamelund, "Race and 1918 Influenza Pandemic in the United States: A Review of the Literature," *International Journal of Environmental Research and Public Health* 16, no. 14 (July 2019): 2487, https://pmc.ncbi.nlm.nih.gov/articles/PMC6678782/.

62. Sriram Tiruvadi-Krishnan et al., "Coupling Between DNA Replication, Segregation, and the Onset of Constriction in Escherichia Coli," *Cell Report* 38 (2022), https://doi.org/10.1016/j.celrep.2022.110539.

63. M. Eiermann, E. Wrigley-Field, J. J. Feigenbaum, J. Helgertz, E. Hernandez, and C. E. Boen, "Racial Disparities in Mortality During the 1918 Influenza Pandemic in United States Cities," *Demography* 59, no. 5 (2022): 1953–1979, https://doi.org/10.1215/00703370-10235825.

64. Timothy M. Uyeki and Malik Peiris, "Novel Avian Influenza A Virus Infections of Humans," *Infectious Disease Clinics of North America* 33, no. 4 (2019): 907, https://doi.org/10.1016/j.idc.2019.07.003.

65. "1957–1958 Pandemic (H2N2 virus)," Centers for Disease Control and Prevention, accessed September 12, 2023, https://www.cdc.gov/flu/pandemic-resources/1957-1958-pandemic.html.

66. Edwin D. Kilbourne, "Influenza Pandemics of the 20th Century," *Emerging Infectious Diseases* 12, no. 1 (2006): 9–14, https://doi.org/10.3201%2Feid1201.051254.

67. Edwin D. Kilbourne, "Influenza Pandemics of the 20th Century," *Emerging Infectious Diseases* 12, no. 1 (2006): 9–14, https://doi.org/10.3201%2Feid1201.051254.

68. Edwin D. Kilbourne, "Influenza Pandemics of the 20th Century," *Emerging Infectious Diseases* 12, no. 1 (2006): 9–14, https://doi.org/10.3201%2Feid1201.051254.

69. William R. Clark, *Bracing for Armageddon? The Science and Politics of Bioterrorism in America* (Oxford University Press, 2008), 72.

70. "About WHO in China," World Health Organization, accessed August 25, 2023, https://www.who.int/china/about-us.

71. Ying Qing et al., "History of Influenza Pandemics in China During the Past Century," *Chinese Journal of Epidemiology* [in Chinese] 39, no. 8 (2018), https://doi.org/10.3760/cma.j.issn.0254-6450.2018.08.003.

72. "Weekly Epidemiological Record," *Weekly Epidemiological Record* 32, no. 19 (1957): 231–244.

73. "Symposium on the Asian Influenza Epidemic, 1957," *Proceedings of the Royal Society of Medicine* 51, no. 12 (1958): 1009–1018, https://doi.org/10.1177/003591575805101205.

74. Mark Honigsbaum, "Revisiting the 1957 and 1968 Influenza Pandemics," *Lancet* 395, no. 10240 (2020): 1824–1826, https://doi.org/10.1016/S0140-6736(20)31201-0.

75. I. G. Menon, "The 1957 Pandemic of Influenza in India," *Bulletin of the World Health Organization* 20, no. 2–3 (1959): 199–224.

76. Claire Jackson, "History Lessons: The Asian Flu Pandemic," *British Journal of General Practice* 59, no. 565 (2009): 622–623, https://doi.org/10.3399/bjgp09X453882.

77. Herschel E. Griffin, "Influenza Control in the Armed Forces," *Public Health Reports* 73, no. 2 (1958): 145–148, https://doi.org/10.2307/4590064.

78. Fred M. Davenport, "Role of the Commission on Influenza: Studies of Epidemiology and Prevention," *Public Health Reports* 73, no. 2 (1958): 133–139, https://doi.org/10.2307/4590062.

79. Herschel E. Griffin, "Influenza Control in the Armed Forces," *Public Health Reports* 73, no. 2 (1958): 145–148, https://doi.org/10.2307/4590064.

80. Stephen B. Thacker, Andrew L. Dannenberg, and Douglas H. Hamilton, "Epidemic Intelligence Service of the Centers for Disease Control and Prevention: 50 Years of Training and Service in Applied Epidemiology," *American Journal of Epidemiology* 154, no. 11 (2001): 985–992, https://doi.org/10.1093/aje/154.11.985.

81. N. Nathanson, W. J. Hall, L. D. Thrupp, and H. Forester, "Surveillance of Poliomyelitis in the U.S. in 1956," *Public Health Reports*, May 1957, https://pubmed.ncbi.nlm.nih.gov/13432107.

82. W. H. Lawrence, "Mrs. Hobby Quits as Welfare Head; Folsom Is Named," *New York Times*, July 26, 1955, https://www.nytimes.com/1955/07/14/archives/mrs-hobby-quits-as-welfare-head-folsom-is-named-she-cites-husbands.html.

83. "Hong Kong Battling Influenza Epidemic," *New York Times*, April 17, 1957, https://www.nytimes.com/1957/04/17/archives/hong-kong-battling-influenza-epidemic.html.

84. "1957 Asian Flu Pandemic," The History of Vaccines, accessed October 01, 2023, https://historyofvaccines.org/.

85. Justin M. Andrews, "Research Programs on Asian Influenza," *Public Health Reports* 73, no. 2 (1958): 159–164, https://doi.org/10.2307/4590070.

86. "Asian Strain of Influenza A," *Public Health Reports* 72, no. 9 (1957): 768–770, https://pubmed.ncbi.nlm.nih.gov/13465935.

87. M. Honigsbaum, "Revisiting the 1957 and 1968 Influenza Pandemics," *Lancet* 395, no. 10240 (2020): 1824–1826, https://doi.org/10.1016/S0140-6736(20)31201-0.

88. C. Jackson, "History Lessons: The Asian Flu Pandemic," *British Journal of General Practice* 59, no. 565 (2009): 622–623, https://doi.org/10.3399/bjgp09X453882.

89. Edwin D. Kilbourne, "Influenza Pandemics of the 20th Century," *Emerging Infectious Diseases* 12, no. 1 (2006): 9–14, https://doi.org/10.3201%2Feid1201.051254.

90. *Global Influenza Programme*, World Health Organization, n.d., https://www.who.int/teams/global-influenza-programme.

91. D. A. Henderson, B. Courtney, T. V. Inglesby, E. Toner, and J. B. Nuzzo, "Public Health and Medical Responses to the 1957–58 Influenza Pandemic," *Biosecurity and Bioterrorism: Biodefense Strategy, Practice, and Science* 7, no. 3 (2009): 265–273, https://doi.org/10.1089/bsp.2009.0729.

92. J. Pinkowski, *The History of the Forgotten Pandemic*, Yale Insights, January 7, 2021, https://insights.som.yale.edu/insights/the-history-of-the-forgotten-pandemic.

93. C. Viboud, L. Simonsen, R. Fuentes, J. Flores, M. A. Miller, and G. Chowell, "Global Mortality Impact of the 1957–1959 Influenza Pandemic," *Journal of Infectious Diseases* 213, no. 5 (2016): 738–745, https://doi.org/10.1093/infdis/jiv534.

94. C. Viboud, R. F. Grais, B. A. Lafont, M. A. Miller, L. Simonsen, and Multinational Influenza Seasonal Mortality Study Group, "Multinational Impact of the 1968 Hong Kong Influenza Pandemic: Evidence for a Smoldering Pandemic," *Journal of Infectious Diseases* 192, no. 2 (2005): 233–248, https://doi.org/10.1086/431150.

95. R. B. Belshe, "The Origins of Pandemic Influenza—Lessons from the 1918 Virus," *New England Journal of Medicine* 353, no. 21 (2005): 2209–2211, https://doi.org/10.1056/NEJMp058281.

96. Barbara J. Jester, Timothy M. Uyeki, and Daniel B. Jernigan, "Fifty Years of Influenza A(H3N2) Following the Pandemic of 1968," *American Journal of Public Health* 110, no. 5 (2020): 669–676, https://doi.org/10.2105%2FAJPH.2019.305557.

97. "1968 Pandemic (H3N2 virus)," Centers for Disease Control and Prevention, accessed February 7, 2022, https://www.cdc.gov/flu/pandemic-resources/1968 -pandemic.html.

98. Edwin D. Kilbourne, "Influenza Pandemics of the 20th Century," *Emerging Infectious Diseases* 12, no. 1 (2006): 9–14, https://doi.org/10.3201%2Feid1201.051254.

99. W. C. Cockburn, P. J. Delon, and W. Ferreira. "Origin and Progress of the 1968–69 Hong Kong Influenza Epidemic," *Bulletin of the World Health Organization* 41, no. 3 (1969): 345–348.

100. W. K. Chang, "National Influenza Experience in Hong Kong, 1968," *Bulletin of the World Health Organization*, 1969.

101. W. K. Chang, "National Influenza Experience in Hong Kong, 1968," *Bulletin of the World Health Organization*, 1969.

102. Ying Qing et al., "History of Influenza Pandemics in China During the Past Century," *Chinese Journal of Epidemiology* (in Chinese) 39, no. 8 (2018), https://doi .org/10.3760/cma.j.issn.0254-6450.2018.08.003.

103. Mark Honigsbaum, "Revisiting the 1957 and 1968 Influenza Pandemics," *Lancet* 395, no. 10240 (2020): 1824–1826, https://doi.org/10.1016/S0140-6736(20) 31201-0.

104. "The 'Hong Kong Flu' Began in Red China," *New York Times*, December 15, 1968, https://www.nytimes.com/1968/12/15/archives/the-hong-kong-flu-began-in -red-china.html.

105. W. C. Cockburn, P. J. Delon, and W. Ferreira, "Origin and Progress of the 1968–69 Hong Kong Influenza Epidemic," *Bulletin of the World Health Organization* 41, no. 3 (1969): 345–348.

106. Barbara J. Jester et al., "Fifty Years of Influenza A(H3N2) Following the Pandemic of 1968," *American Journal of Public Health* 110, no. 5 (2020), https://doi.org /10.2105%2FAJPH.2019.305557.

107. Vernon J. Lee et al., "Influenza Pandemics in Singapore, a Tropical, Globally Connected City," *Emerging Infectious Diseases* 13, no. 7 (2007), https://doi.org /10.3201%2Feid1307.061313.

108. R. F. Grais, J. H. Ellis, and G. E. Glass, "Assessing the Impact of Airline Travel on the Geographic Spread of Pandemic Influenza," *European Journal of Epidemiology* 18, no. 11 (2003): 1065–1072, https://doi.org/10.1023/a:1026140019146.

109. B. H. Kean, "Turista in Teheran: Travellers' Diarrhoea at the Eighth International Congresses of Tropical Medicine and Malaria," *Lancet*, September 13, 1969, https://pubmed.ncbi.nlm.nih.gov/4185545/.

110. W. O. Williams, "H.K. Influenza 1969–70: A Practice Study," *Journal of the Royal College of General Practitioners* 21, no. 107 (1971): 325–335.

111. F. Avery Jones, "Winter Epidemics," *British Medical Journal* 68, no. 4 (1968): 327, https://doi.org/10.1136/bmj.4.5626.327-c.

112. Bojan Pancevski, "Forgotten Pandemic Offers Contrast to Today's Coronavirus Lockdowns," *Wall Street Journal*, April 24, 2020.

113. R. G. Sharrar, "National Influenza Experience in the USA, 1968–69," *Bulletin of the World Health Organization* 41, no. 3 (1969): 361–366.

114. R. G. Sharrar, "National Influenza Experience in the USA, 1968–69," *Bulletin of the World Health Organization* 41, no. 3 (1969): 361–366.

115. A. Noymer and A. M. Nguyen, "Influenza as a Proportion of Pneumonia Mortality: United States, 1959–2009," *Biodemography and Social Biology* 59, no. 2 (2013): 178–190, https://doi.org/10.1080/19485565.2013.833816.

116. "Immunization Against Infectious Disease 1968," Stephen B. Thacker CDC Library Collection, Centers for Disease Control and Prevention, 168, accessed August 25, 2023, https://stacks.cdc.gov/view/cdc/60811.

117. "Influenza Vaccine," *New York Times*, July 7, 1957, accessed February 3, 2022.

118. Roderick Murray, "Production and Testing in the USA of Influenza Virus Vaccine Made from the Hong Kong Variant in 1968–69," *Bulletin of the World Health Organization* 41 (1969): 493–496.

119. Mark Honigsbaum, "Revisiting the 1957 and 1968 Influenza Pandemics," *Lancet* 395, no. 10240 (2020): 1824–1826, https://doi.org/10.1016/S0140-6736(20)31201-0.

120. Patrick R. Saunders-Hastings and Daniel Krewski, "Reviewing the History of Pandemic Influenza: Understanding Patterns of Emergence and Transmission," *Pathogens* 5, no. 4 (2016): 66, https://doi.org/10.3390/pathogens5040066.

121. Patrick R. Saunders-Hastings and Daniel Krewski, "Reviewing the History of Pandemic Influenza: Understanding Patterns of Emergence and Transmission," *Pathogens* 5, no. 4 (2016): 66, https://doi.org/10.3390/pathogens5040066.

122. Sami Al Hajjara and Kenneth McIntosh, "The First Influenza Pandemic of the 21st Century," *Annals of Saudi Medicine* 30, no. 1 (2010): 1–10, https://doi.org/10.4103%2F0256-4947.59365.

123. "2009 H1N1 Pandemic (H1N1pdm09 Virus)," Centers for Disease Control and Prevention, accessed February 7, 2022, https://www.cdc.gov/flu/pandemic-resources/2009-h1n1-pandemic.html.

124. "Updated Interim Recommendations for the Use of Antiviral Medications in the Treatment and Prevention of Influenza for the 2009–2010 Season," Centers for

Disease Control and Prevention, last modified December 7, 2009, https://www.cdc
.gov/h1n1flu/recommendations.htm.

125. Sami Al Hajjara and Kenneth McIntosh, "The First Influenza Pandemic of the
21st Century," *Annals of Saudi Medicine* 30, no. 1 (2010): 1–10, https://doi.org
/10.4103%2F0256-4947.59365.

126. Michael A. Jhung, David Swerdlow, Sonja J. Olsen, Daniel Jernigan, Matthew
Biggerstaff, Laurie Kamimoto, Krista Kniss, Carrie Reed, Alicia Fry, Lynnette
Brammer, et al., "Epidemiology of 2009 Pandemic Influenza A (H1N1) in the United
States," suppl., *Clinical Infectious Diseases* 52, no. S1 (2011): S13–S26, https://doi.org
/10.1093/cid/ciq008.

127. Fatimah S. Dawood et al., "Estimated Global Mortality Associated with the
First 12 Months of 2009 Pandemic Influenza A H1N1 Virus Circulation: A Modelling
Study," *Lancet Infections Diseases* 12, no. 9 (2012): 687–95, https://doi.org/10.1016
/s1473-3099(12)70121-4.

128. I. Batta, T. Kaur, and D. K. Agrawal, "Distinguishing Swine Flu (H1N1) from
COVID-19: Clinical, Virological, and Immunological Perspectives," *Archives of
Microbiology & Immunology* 7, no. 4 (2023): 271–280, https://doi.org/10.26502
/ami.936500125.

129. S. S. Shrestha, D. L. Swerdlow, R. H. Borse, V. S. Prabhu, L. Finelli,
C. Y. Atkins, K. Owusu-Edusei, B. Bell, P. S. Mead, M. Biggerstaff, et al., "Estimating the Burden of 2009 Pandemic Influenza A (H1N1) in the United States
(April 2009–April 2010)," suppl., *Clinical Infectious Diseases* 52, no. S1 (2011): S75–S82,
https://doi.org/10.1093/cid/ciq012.

130. "Swine Influenza A (H1N1) Infection in Two Children—Southern California,
March—April 2009," Centers for Disease Control and Prevention, April 24, 2009,
https://www.cdc.gov/mmwr/preview/mmwrhtml/mm5815a5.htm.

131. P. R. Saunders-Hastings and D. Krewski, "Reviewing the History of Pandemic
Influenza: Understanding Patterns of Emergence and Transmission," *Pathogens* 5,
no. 4 (2016): 66, https://doi.org/10.3390/pathogens5040066.

132. Rebekah H. Borse et al., "Effects of Vaccine Program Against Pandemic
Influenza A(H1N1) Virus, U.S., 2009–2010," *Emerging Infectious Diseases* 19, no. 3
(2013): 439–448, https://doi.org/10.3201%2Feid1903.120394.

133. S. Balter, L. S. Gupta, S. Lim, J. Fu, S. E. Perlman, and New York City 2009
H1N1 Flu Investigation Team, "Pandemic (H1N1) 2009 Surveillance for Severe Illness
and Response, New York, New York, USA, April–July 2009," *Emerging Infectious
Diseases* 16, no. 8 (2010): 1259–1264, https://doi.org/10.3201/eid1608.091847.

134. R. Ridzon et al., "Simultaneous Transmission of Human Immunodeficiency
Virus and Hepatitis C Virus from a Needle-Stick Injury," *New England Journal of
Medicine* 336, no. 13 (1997): 919–922, https://doi.org/10.1056/nejm199703273361304.

135. P. Sax, "Acute and Early HIV Infection: Clinical Manifestations and Diagnosis," Up to Date, May 24, 2024, https://www.uptodate.com/contents/acute-and-early
-hiv-infection-clinical-manifestations-and-diagnosis/print.

136. Merlin L. Robb et al., "Prospective Study of Acute HIV-1 Infection in Adults in East Africa and Thailand," *New England Journal of Medicine* 374, no. 22 (2016): 2120–2130, https://doi.org/10.1056/nejmoa1508952.

137. Hassen Kared et al., "HIV-Specific Regulatory T Cells Are Associated with Higher CD4 Cell Counts in Primary Infection," *AIDS* 22, no. 18 (2008): 2451–2460, https://doi.org/10.1097/qad.0b013e328319edc0.

138. M. T. Niu, D. S. Stein, and S. M. Schnittman, "Primary Human Immunodeficiency Virus Type 1 Infection: Review of Pathogenesis and Early Treatment Intervention in Humans and Animal Retrovirus Infections," *Journal of Infectious Diseases* 16, no. 6 (1993): 1490–1501, https://doi.org/10.1093/infdis/168.6.1490.

139. E. S. Daar et al., "Diagnosis of Primary HIV-1 Infection: Los Angeles County Primary HIV Infection Recruitment Network," *Annals of Internal Medicine* 134, no. 1 (2001): 25–29, https://doi.org/10.7326/0003-4819-134-1-200101020-00010.

140. Dominique L. Braun et al., "Frequency and Spectrum of Unexpected Clinical Manifestations of Primary HIV-1 Infection," *Clinical Infectious Diseases* 61, no. 6 (2015): 1013–1021, https://doi.org/10.1093/cid/civ398.

141. Trevor A. Crowell et al., "Acute Retroviral Syndrome Is Associated with High Viral Burden, CD4 Depletion, and Immune Activation in Systemic and Tissue Compartments," *Clinical Infectious Diseases* 66, no. 10 (2018): 1540–1549, https://doi.org/10.1093/cid/cix1063.

142. G. P. Rizzardi, G. Tambussi, and A. Lazzarin, "Acute Pancreatitis During Primary HIV-1 Infection," *New England Journal of Medicine* 336, no. 25 (1997): 1836–1837, https://doi.org/10.1056/nejm199706193362516.

143. J. M. Molina et al., "Hepatitis Associated with Primary HIV Infection," *Gastroenterology* 102, no. 2 (1992): 739, https://doi.org/10.1016/0016-5085(92)90138-0.

144. P. D. Rutter, O. T. Mytton, M. Mak, and L. J. Donaldson, "Socio-Economic Disparities in Mortality Due to Pandemic Influenza in England," *International Journal of Public Health* 57, no. 4 (2012): 745–750, https://doi.org/10.1007/s00038-012-0337-1.

145. R. Yarchoan et al., "CD4 Count and the Risk for Death in Patients Infected with HIV Receiving Antiretroviral Therapy," *Annals of Internal Medicine* 115, no. 3 (1991): 184–189, https://doi.org/10.7326/0003-4819-115-3-184.

146. A. N. Phillips et al., "Immunodeficiency and the Risk of Death in HIV Infection," *JAMA* 268, no. 19 (2018): 2662–2666.

147. "Global AIDS Update 2022—in Danger," UNAIDS, accessed September 9, 2022, https://www.unaids.org/sites/default/files/media_asset/2022-global-aids-update_en.pdf.

148. "Global HIV & AIDS Statistics—Fact Sheet—2022," UNAIDS, accessed September 9, 2022, https://www.unaids.org/en/resources/fact-sheet.

149. A. B. Kharsany and Q. A. Karim, "HIV Infection and AIDS in Sub-Saharan Africa: Current Status, Challenges and Opportunities," *Open AIDS Journal* 10 (2016): 34–48, https://doi.org/10.2174/1874613601610010034.

150. "HIV Prevention 2025 Road Map—Getting on Track to End AIDS as a Public Health Threat by 2030," UNAIDS, accessed September 9, 2022, https://www.unaids .org/sites/default/files/media_asset/prevention-2025-roadmap_en.pdf.

151. GBD 2017 HIV Collaborators, "Global, Regional, and National Incidence, Prevalence, and Mortality of HIV, 1980–2017, and Forecasts to 2030, for 195 Countries and Territories: A Systematic Analysis for the Global Burden of Diseases, Injuries, and Risk Factors Study 2017," *Lancet HIV* 6, no. 12 (2019): e831–e859, https://doi.org/10.1016/s2352-3018(19)30196-1.

152. "World AIDS Day—December 1, 2019," *Morbidity and Mortality Weekly Report* 68, no. 47 (2019): 1089, https://doi.org/10.15585%2Fmmwr.mm6847a1.

153. "HIV/AIDS Surveillance in Europe, 2019," European Centre for Disease Prevention and Control and the World Health Organization, accessed April 29, 2021, https://www.ecdc.europa.eu/sites/default/files/documents/hiv-surveillance-report -2019.pdf.

154. Myron S. Cohen, Olivia D. Council, and Jane S. Chen, "Sexually Transmitted Infections and HIV in the Era of Antiretroviral Treatment and Prevention: The Biologic Basis for Epidemiologic Synergy," suppl., *Journal of the International AIDS Society* 22, no. S6 (2019): e25355, https://doi.org/10.1002/jia2.25355.

155. "Gini Coefficient by Country 2023," World Population Review, accessed September 10, 2023, https://worldpopulationreview.com/country-rankings/gini -coefficient-by-country.

156. "Women and Girls and HIV," UNAIDS, accessed April 3, 2018, http://www .unaids.org/sites/default/files/media_asset/women_girls_hiv_en.pdf.

157. Chris Beyrer, "HIV Epidemiology Update and Transmission Factors: Risks and Risk Contexts—16th International AIDS Conference Epidemiology Plenary," *Clinical Infectious Diseases* 1, no. 44 (2007): 981–987, https://doi.org/10.1086/512371.

158. "Global AIDS Update 2019—Communities at the Centre," UNAIDS, accessed April 30, 2021, https://www.unaids.org/sites/default/files/media_asset/2019-global -AIDS-update_en.pdf.

159. C. Zhong, M. Sun, and W. Yao, "A Hybrid Model for HIV Transmission Among Men Who Have Sex with Men," *Infectious Disease Modelling* 5 (2020): 814–826, https://doi.org/10.1016/j.idm.2020.08.015

160. Kamyar Arasteh and Don C. Des Jarlais, "Injecting Drug Use, HIV, and What to Do About It," *Lancet* 372, no. 9651 (2008): 1709–1710, https://doi.org/10.1016 /s0140-6736(08)61312-4.

161. Michael Worobey et al., "Direct Evidence of Extensive Diversity of HIV-1 in Kinshasa by 1960," *Nature* 455, no. 7213 (2008): 661, https://doi.org/10.1038 /nature07390.

162. Nuno R. Faria et al., "HIV Epidemiology: The Early Spread and Epidemic Ignition of HIV-1 in Human Populations," *Science* 346, no. 6205 (2014): 56–61, https://doi.org/10.1126/science.1256739.

163. Jonathan L. Heeney, Angus G. Dalgleish, and Robin A. Weiss, "Origins of HIV and the Evolution of Resistance to AIDS," *Science* 313, no. 5786 (2006): 462, https://doi.org/10.1126/science.1123016.

164. Michael Worobey et al., "Island Biogeography Reveals the Deep History of SIV," *Science* 329, no. 5998 (2010): 1487, https://doi.org/10.1126/science.1193550.

165. Gillette Conner et al., "Aids Knowledge and Homophobia Among French and American University Students," *Sage Journals* 67, no. 3 (1990), https://doi.org/10.2466/pro.1990.67.3f.1147.

166. Tony Barnett and Alan Whiteside, *AIDS in the Twenty-First Century: Disease and Globalization* (Palgrave Macmillan, 2002), https://link.springer.com/book/10.1057/9780230599208.

167. Laurie Garrett, *The Coming Plague: Newly Emerging Diseases in a World Out of Balance* (Farrar, Straus and Giroux, 1994), https://www.lauriegarrett.com/the-coming-plague.

168. C. Rosenberg, "What Is an Epidemic? AIDS in Historical Perspective," *Daedalus: Living with AIDS* 118, no. 2 (1989): 1–17 https://edisciplinas.usp.br/pluginfile.php/3785122/mod_resource/content/1/Rosenberg_What%20is%20an%20epidemic.pdf.

169. Adrian D. Smith et al., "Men Who Have Sex with Men and HIV/AIDS in Sub-Saharan Africa," *Lancet* 374, no. 9687 (2009): 416, https://doi.org/10.1016/s0140-6736(09)61118-1.

170. *Gender-Based Violence—AIDS 2020*, UNAIDS, n.d., https://aids2020.unaids.org/chapter/chapter-4-securing-rights/gender-based-violence/.

171. F. Lloyd-Davies, "Why Eastern DR Congo Is 'Rape Capital of the World,'" November 25, 2011, https://www.cnn.com/2011/11/24/world/africa/democratic-congo-rape/index.html.

172. Robert Steinbrook, "HIV in India—a Complex Epidemic," *New England Journal of Medicine* 356, no. 11 (2007): 1089, https://doi.org/10.1056/nejmp078009.

173. Tie-Jian Feng et al., "Prevalence of Syphilis and Human Immunodeficiency Virus Infections Among Men Who Have Sex with Men in Shenzhen, China: 2005 to 2007," *Sex Transmissible Diseases* 35, no. 12 (2008): 1022, https://doi.org/10.1097/olq.0b013e3181860of4.

174. A. E. Siddiqi, X. Hu, H. I. Hall, and Centers for Disease Control and Prevention, "Mortality Among Blacks or African Americans with HIV Infection—United States, 2008–2012," *Morbidity and Mortality Weekly Report* 64, no. 4 (2015): 81–86.

175. Centers for Disease Control and Prevention, *HIV Surveillance Report, 2018*, vol. 31, May 2020, http://www.cdc.gov/hiv/library/reports/hiv-surveillance.html.

176. "History," Republic of South Africa Official Information and Services, 2024, https://www.gov.za/about-sa/history.

177. Mamphela Ramphele, *A Bed Called Home: Life in the Migrant Labour Hostels of Cape Town* (Ohio University Press, 1993), https://books.google.com/books?hl=en&lr

=&id=I4_kNb9CWtIC&oi=fnd&pg=PA4&dq=Ramphele,+1993&ots=foixnfmbMJ&sig
=rsF1vzXJb12Vawje5datt6-ss5U#v=onepage&q=Ramphele%2C%201993&f=false.

178. Mark Hunter, "Beyond the Male-Migrant: South Africa's Long History of Health Geography and the Contemporary AIDS Pandemic," *Health & Place* 16 (2009): 25–33, https://doi.org/10.1016/j.healthplace.2009.08.003.

179. Ndangwa Noyoo, "Social Policy and Welfare Regimes Typologies: Any Relevance to South Africa?," *Sozialpolitik.ch.* 2 (2017), https://doi.org/10.18753/2297-8224-91.

180. Greg Behrman, *The Invisible People* (Simon and Schuster, 2004), https://www.simonandschuster.com/books/The-Invisible-People/Greg-Behrman/9781439157350.

181. John S. Schieffelin et al., "Clinical Illness and Outcomes in Patients with Ebola in Sierra Leone," *New England Journal of Medicine* 371, no. 22 (2014): 2092, https://doi.org/10.1056/nejmoa1411680.

182. Daniel S. Chertow et al., "Ebola Virus Disease in West Africa—Clinical Manifestations and Management," *New England Journal of Medicine* 371, no. 22 (2014): 2054, https://doi.org/10.1056/nejmp1413084.

183. Elhadj Ibrahima Bah et al., "Clinical Presentation of Patients with Ebola Virus Disease in Conakry, Guinea," 372, no. 1 (2015): 40, https://doi.org/10.1056/nejmoa1411249.

184. John S. Schieffelin et al., "Clinical Illness and Outcomes in Patients with Ebola in Sierra Leone," *New England Journal of Medicine* 371, no. 22 (2014): 2092, https://doi.org/10.1056/nejmoa1411680.

185. Daniel S. Chertow et al., "Ebola Virus Disease in West Africa—Clinical Manifestations and Management," *New England Journal of Medicine* 371, no. 22 (2014): 2054, https://doi.org/10.1056/nejmp1413084.

186. Elhadj Ibrahima Bah et al., "Clinical Presentation of Patients with Ebola Virus Disease in Conakry, Guinea," 372, no. 1 (2015): 40, https://doi.org/10.1056/nejmoa1411249.

187. Rashid Ansumana et al., "Ebola in Freetown Area, Sierra Leone—a Case Study of 581 Patients," *New England Journal of Medicine* 372, no. 6 (2015): 587, https://doi.org/10.1056/nejmc1413685.

188. M. Bray and D. Chertow, "Filoviruses," in *Clinical Virology*, 4th ed. (American Society of Microbiology, 2016).

189. Nicholas Di Paola et al., "Viral Genomics in Ebola Virus Research," *Nature Reviews Microbiology* 18, no. 7 (2018): 365, https://doi.org/10.1038/s41579-020-0354-7.

190. Heinz Feldmann, Armand Sprecher, and Thomas W Geisbert, "Ebola," *New England Journal of Medicine* 382, no. 19 (2020): 1832, https://doi.org/10.1056/nejmra1901594.

191. Tracey Goldstein et al., "The Discovery of Bombali Virus Adds Further Support for Bats as Hosts of Ebolaviruses," *Nature Microbiology* 3, no. 10 (2018): 1084, https://doi.org/10.1038/s41564-018-0227-2.

192. Report of an International Commission, "Ebola Haemorrhagic Fever in Zaire, 1976," *Bulletin of the World Health Organization* 56, no. 2 (1978): 271.

193. Cordelia E. M. Coltart, "The Ebola Outbreak, 2013–2016: Old Lessons for New Epidemics," *Philosophical Transactions of the Royal Society B: Biological Sciences* 26, no. 372 (2017): 20160297, https://doi.org/10.1098/rstb.2016.0297.

194. Aaron Aruna et al., "Ebola Virus Disease Outbreak—Democratic Republic of the Congo, August 2018–November 2019," *Morbidity and Mortality Weekly Report* 68, no. 50 (2019): 1162, https://doi.org/10.15585/mmwr.mm6850a3.

195. Julie Erb-Alvarez, Aaron M. Wendelboe, and Daniel S. Chertow, "Ebola Virus in the Democratic Republic of the Congo: Advances and Remaining Obstacles in Epidemic Control, Clinical Care, and Biomedical Research," *Chest* 157, no. 1 (2020): 42, https://doi.org/10.1016/j.chest.2019.08.2183.

196. Boyo C. Pare et al., "Ebola Outbreak in Guinea, 2021: Clinical Care of Patients with Ebola Virus Disease," *South African Journal of Infectious Diseases* 38, no. 1 (2023): 454, https://doi.org/10.4102/sajid.v38i1.454.

197. Alpha Kabinet Keita et al., "Resurgence of Ebola Virus in 2021 in Guinea Suggests a New Paradigm for Outbreaks," *Nature* 597, no. 7877 (2017): 539, https://doi.org/10.1038/s41586-021-03901-9.

198. World Health Organization/International Study Team, "Ebola Haemorrhagic Fever in Sudan, 1976. Report of a WHO/International Study Team," *Bulletin of the World Health Organization* 56, no. 2 (1978): 247.

199. Jonathan S. Towner et al., "Newly Discovered Ebola Virus Associated with Hemorrhagic Fever Outbreak in Uganda," *PLoS Pathogens* 4, no. 11 (2008): e1000212, https://doi.org/10.1371/journal.ppat.1000212.

200. P. Formenty et al., "Ebola Virus Outbreak Among Wild Chimpanzees Living in a Rain Forest of Côte d'Ivoire," suppl., *Journal of Infectious Diseases* 179, no. S1 (1999): S120, https://doi.org/10.1086/514296.

201. M. Bray and D. Chertow, "Filoviruses," in *Clinical Virology*, 4th ed. (American Society of Microbiology, 2016).

202. Heinz Feldmann, Armand Sprecher, and Thomas W Geisbert, "Ebola," *New England Journal of Medicine* 382, no. 19 (2020): 1832, https://doi.org/10.1056/nejmra1901594.

203. Alpha Kabinet Keita et al., "Resurgence of Ebola Virus in 2021 in Guinea Suggests a New Paradigm for Outbreaks," *Nature* 597, no. 7877 (2017): 539, https://doi.org/10.1038/s41586-021-03901-9.

204. Placide Mbala-Kingebeni et al., "Ebola Virus Transmission Initiated by Relapse of Systemic Ebola Virus Disease," *New England Journal of Medicine* 384, no. 13 (2021): 1240, https://doi.org/10.1056/nejmoa2024670.

205. Boubacar Diallo et al., "Resurgence of Ebola Virus Disease in Guinea Linked to a Survivor with Virus Persistence in Seminal Fluid for More Than 500 Days," *Clinical Infectious Diseases* 63, no. 10 (2016): 1353, https://doi.org/10.1093/cid/ciw601.

206. Emily Kainne Dokubo et al., "Persistence of Ebola Virus After the End of Widespread Transmission in Liberia: An Outbreak Report," *Lancet Infectious Diseases* 18, no. 9 (2018): 1015, https://doi.org/10.1016/s1473-3099(18)30417-1.

207. S. F. Dowell et al., "Transmission of Ebola Hemorrhagic Fever: A Study of Risk Factors in Family Members, Kikwit, Democratic Republic of the Congo, 1995. Commission de Lutte contre les Epidémies à Kikwit," suppl., *Journal of Infectious Diseases* 179, no. S1 (1999): S87, https://doi.org/10.1086/514284.

208. Mary R. Reichler et al., "Household Transmission of Ebola Virus: Risks and Preventive Factors, Freetown, Sierra Leone, 2015," *Journal of Infectious Diseases* 218, no. 5 (2018): 757, https://doi.org/10.1093/infdis/jiy204.

209. Benno Kreuels et al., "A Case of Severe Ebola Virus Infection Complicated by Gram-Negative Septicemia," *New England Journal of Medicine* 371, no 251 (2014): 2394, https://doi.org/10.1056/nejmoa1411677.

210. A. K. Rowe et al., "Clinical, Virologic, and Immunologic Follow-Up of Convalescent Ebola Hemorrhagic Fever Patients and Their Household Contacts, Kikwit, Democratic Republic of the Congo. Commission de Lutte Contre les Epidémies à Kikwit," suppl., *Journal of Infectious Diseases* 179, no. S1 (1999): S28, https://doi.org/10.1086/514318.

211. Daniel G. Bausch et al., "Assessment of the Risk of Ebola Virus Transmission from Bodily Fluids and Fomites," suppl., *Journal of Infectious Diseases* 196, no. S2 (2007): S142–S147, https://doi.org/10.1086/520545.

212. Jay B. Varkey, "Persistence of Ebola Virus in Ocular Fluid During Convalescence," *New England Journal of Medicine* 372, no. 25 (2015): 2423, https://doi.org/10.1056/nejmoa1500306.

213. Helena Nordenstedt et al., "Ebola Virus in Breast Milk in an Ebola Virus-Positive Mother with Twin Babies, Guinea, 2015," *Emerging Infectious Diseases* 22, no. 4 (2016): 759–760, https://doi.org/10.3201/eid2204.151880.

214. Report of an International Commission, "Ebola Haemorrhagic Fever in Zaire, 1976," *Bulletin of the World Health Organization* 56, no. 2 (1978): 271.

215. World Health Organization/International Study Team, "Ebola Haemorrhagic Fever in Sudan, 1976. Report of a WHO/International Study Team," *Bulletin of the World Health Organization* 56, no. 2 (1978): 247.

216. A. S. Khan et al., "The Reemergence of Ebola Hemorrhagic Fever, Democratic Republic of the Congo, 1995. Commission de Lutte contre les Epidémies à Kikwit," suppl., *Journal of Infectious Diseases* 179, no. S1 (1999): S76, https://doi.org/10.1086/514306.

217. Placide Mbala-Kingebeni et al., "2018 Ebola Virus Disease Outbreak in Équateur Province, Democratic Republic of the Congo: A Retrospective Genomic Characterisation," *Lancet Infectious Diseases* 19, no. 6 (2019): 641, https://doi.org/10.1016/s1473-3099(19)30124-0.

218. Aaron Aruna et al., "Ebola Virus Disease Outbreak—Democratic Republic of the Congo, August 2018–November 2019," *Morbidity and Mortality Weekly Report* 68, no. 50 (2019): 1162, https://doi.org/10.15585/mmwr.mm6850a3.

219. Oly Ilunga Kalenga et al., "The Ongoing Ebola Epidemic in the Democratic Republic of Congo, 2018–2019," *New England Journal of Medicine* 381, no. 4 (2019): 373, https://doi.org/10.1056/nejmsr1904253.

220. Kai Kupferschmidt et al., "Ebola Virus May Lurk in Survivors for Many Years," *Science* 371, no. 6535 (2021): 1188, https://doi.org/10.1126/science.371 .6535.1188.

221. "Ebola Virus Disease—Democratic Republic of the Congo," World Health Organization, accessed October 10, 2021, https://www.who.int/emergencies/disease -outbreak-news/item/ebola-virus-disease-democratic-republic-of-the-congo_1.

222. Centers for Disease Control and Prevention, "Outbreak of Ebola Hemor-rhagic Fever Uganda, August 2000–January 2001," *Morbidity and Mortality Weekly Report* 50, no. 5 (2001): 73, https://pubmed.ncbi.nlm.nih.gov/?term =Centers+for+Disease+Control+and+Prevention+%28CDC%29%5BCorporate+ Author%5D.

223. Anthony Sanchez et al., "Analysis of Human Peripheral Blood Samples from Fatal and Nonfatal Cases of Ebola (Sudan) Hemorrhagic Fever: Cellular Responses, Virus Load, and Nitric Oxide Levels," *Journal of Virology* 78, no. 19 (2004): 10370, https://doi.org/10.1128/jvi.78.19.10370-10377.2004.

224. "Ebola Disease Caused by Sudan Virus—Uganda," World Health Organization, accessed September 28, 2022, https://www.who.int/emergencies /disease-outbreak-news/item/2022-DON410.

225. Sylvain Baize et al., "Emergence of Zaire Ebola Virus Disease in Guinea," *New England Journal of Medicine* 371, no. 15 (2014): 1418, https://doi.org/10.1056 /nejmoa1404505.

226. Miles W. Carroll et al., "Temporal and Spatial Analysis of the 2014–2015 Ebola Virus Outbreak in West Africa," *Nature* 524, no. 7563 (2015): 97, https://doi.org /10.1038/nature14594.

227. Edward C. Holmes et al., "The Evolution of Ebola Virus: Insights from the 2013–2016 Epidemic," *Nature* 538, no. 7624 (2016): 193, https://doi.org/10.1038 /nature19790.

228. David J. Blackley et al., "Reduced Evolutionary Rate in Reemerged Ebola Virus Transmission Chains," *Science Advances* 2, no. 4 (2016): e1600378, https://doi .org/10.1126/sciadv.1600378.

229. Benno Kreuels et al., "A Case of Severe Ebola Virus Infection Complicated by Gram-Negative Septicemia," *New England Journal of Medicine* 371, no 251 (2014): 2394, https://doi.org/10.1056/nejmoa1411677.

230. G. Marshall Lyon et al., "Clinical Care of Two Patients with Ebola Virus Disease in the U.S.," *New England Journal of Medicine* 371, no. 25 (2014): 2402, https://doi.org/10.1056/nejmoa1409838.

231. Timothy M. Uyeki et al., "Clinical Management of Ebola Virus Disease in the U.S. and Europe," *New England Journal of Medicine* 374, no. 7 (2016): 636, https://doi .org/10.1056/nejmoa1504874.

232. Robert Roos, "1982 Study Suggested Ebola Was in Liberia Then," April 7, 2015, https://www.cidrap.umn.edu/ebola/1982-study-suggested-ebola-was-liberia-then.

233. "Ebola Situation Report," World Health Organization, accessed May 31, 2015, http://apps.who.int/ebola/en/current-situation/ebola-situation-report-27 -may-2015.

234. "At a Glance: Sierra Leone," UNICEF, accessed June 1, 2015, http://www .unicef.org/infobycountry/sierraleone_statistics.html (link no longer active as of this writing).

235. "Missing Dimensions Projects," Oxford Poverty and Human Development Initiative, accessed September 14, 2023, https://ophi.org.uk/research/missing -dimensions/projects/.

236. L. Gberie, *A Dirty War in West Africa: The RUF and the Destruction of Sierra Leone* (Indiana University Press, 2005).

237. "Tiffany & Co Enters into a $50 Million Term Loan Facility Agreement with Koidu Holdings S.A.," *Fasken Martineau*, May 25, 2015, http://www.fasken.com/en /tiffany-co-enters-into-a-us50-million-term-loan-facility-agreement-with-koidu -holdings-sa/.

238. "Hezbollah Profiting from American Diamonds," *Washington Post*, June 29, 2004, http://www.washingtonpost.com/wp-dyn/articles/A15153-2004Jun29_2.html.

239. Miners, personal interview with author.

240. "Ebola Crisis: Sierra Leone Bodies Found Piled Up in Kono," BBC News, December 11, 2014, http://www.bbc.com/news/world-africa-30429360.

241. Qun Li et al., "Early Transmission Dynamics in Wuhan, China, of Novel Coronavirus-Infected Pneumonia," *New England Journal of Medicine* 382, no. 13 (2020): 1199, https://doi.org/10.1056/nejmoa2001316.

242. Wei-Jie Guan et al., "Clinical Characteristics of Coronavirus Disease 2019 in China," *New England Journal of Medicine* 382, no. 18 (2020): 1708, https://doi.org /10.1056/nejmoa2002032.

243. Yu Wu et al., "Incubation Period of COVID-19 Caused by Unique SARS-CoV-2 Strains: A Systematic Review and Meta-analysis," *JAMA Network Open* 5, no. 8 (2022): e2228008, https://doi.org/10.1001/jamanetworkopen.2022.28008.

244. Souheil Zayet et al., "Clinical Features of COVID-19 and Influenza: A Comparative Study on Nord Franche-Comte Cluster," *Microbes and Infection* 22, no. 9 (2020): 481, https://doi.org/10.1016/j.micinf.2020.05.016.

245. Thomas Struyf et al., "Signs and Symptoms to Determine If a Patient Presenting in Primary Care or Hospital Outpatient Settings Has COVID-19 Disease," *Cochrane Database of Systemic Reviews* 7, no. 7 (2020): CD013665, https://doi.org /10.1002/14651858.cd013665.

246. Chen Chen et al., "Global Prevalence of Post-Coronavirus Disease 2019 (COVID-19) Condition or Long COVID: A Meta-Analysis and Systematic Review," *Journal of Infectious Diseases* 226, no. 9 (2022): 1593, https://doi.org/10.1093/infdis/jiac136.

247. Yiying Huang et al., "Impact of Coronavirus Disease 2019 on Pulmonary Function in Early Convalescence Phase," *Respiratory Research* 21, no. 29 (2020): 163, https://doi.org/10.1186/s12931-020-01429-6.

248. Jingjing You et al., "Abnormal Pulmonary Function and Residual CT Abnormalities in Rehabilitating COVID-19 Patients After Discharge," *Journal of Infectious Diseases* 81, no. 2 (2020): e150, https://doi.org/10.1016/j.jinf.2020 .06.003.

249. Xiaoneng Mo et al., "Abnormal Pulmonary Function in COVID-19 Patients at Time of Hospital Discharge," *European Respiratory Journal* 55, no. 6 (2020): 2001217, https://doi.org/10.1183/13993003.01217-2020.

250. Bram van den Borst et al., "Comprehensive Health Assessment 3 Months After Recovery from Acute Coronavirus Disease 2019 (COVID-19)," *Clinical Infectious Diseases* 73, no. 5 (2021): e1089, https://doi.org/10.1093/cid/ciaa1750.

251. Bram van den Borst et al., "Comprehensive Health Assessment 3 Months After Recovery from Acute Coronavirus Disease 2019 (COVID-19)," *Clinical Infectious Diseases* 73, no. 5 (2021): e1089, https://doi.org/10.1093/cid/ciaa1750.

252. Saurabh Rajpal et al., "Cardiovascular Magnetic Resonance Findings in Competitive Athletes Recovering from COVID-19 Infection," *JAMA* 6, no. 1 (2021): 116, https://doi.org/10.1001/jamacardio.2020.4916.

253. Coronaviridae Study Group of the International Committee on Taxonomy of Viruses, "The Species Severe Acute Respiratory Syndrome-Related Coronavirus: Classifying 2019-nCoV and Naming It SARS-CoV-2," *Nature Microbiology* 5, no. 4 (2020): 536, https://doi.org/10.1038/s41564-020-0695-z.

254. Na Zhu et al., "A Novel Coronavirus from Patients with Pneumonia in China, 2019," *New England Journal of Medicine* 382, no. 8 (2020): 727, https://doi.org /10.1056/nejmoa2001017.

255. Roujian Lu et al., "Genomic Characterisation and Epidemiology of 2019 Novel Coronavirus: Implications for Virus Origins and Receptor Binding," *Lancet* 395, no. 10224 (2020): 565, https://doi.org/10.1016/s0140-6736(20)30251-8.

256. "WHO-Convened Global Study of Origins of SARS-CoV-2: China Part," World Health Organization, March 30, 2021, https://www.who.int/publications/i/item/who -convened-global-study-of-origins-of-sars-cov-2-china-part.

257. Jonathan Pekar, "The Molecular Epidemiology of Multiple Zoonotic Origins of SARS-CoV-2," *Science* 377, no. 6609 (2022): 960–966, https://doi.org/10.1126 /science.abp8337.

258. "Climate Change May Have Driven the Emergence of SARS-CoV-2," University of Cambridge, February 5, 2021, https://www.cam.ac.uk/research/news/climate -change-may-have-driven-the-emergence-of-sars-cov-2.

259. Julian E. Barnes, "Lab Leak Most Likely Caused Pandemic, Energy Dept. Says," *New York Times*, February 26, 2023, https://www.nytimes.com/2023/02/26/us /politics/china-lab-leak-coronavirus-pandemic.html.

260. Paul LeBlanc, "New Assessment on the Origins of Covid-19 Adds to the Confusion," CNN Politics, February 27, 2023, https://www.cnn.com/2023/02/27/politics/covid-origins-doe-assessment-what-matters/index.html.

261. Z. B. Wolf, "Analysis: Why Scientists Are Suddenly More Interested in the Lab-Leak Theory of Covid's Origin," CNN, May 25, 2021, https://www.cnn.com/2021/05/25/politics/wuhan-lab-covid-origin-theory/index.html.

262. E. C. Holmes et al., "The Origins of SARS-CoV-2: A Critical Review," *Cell (Review)* 184, no. 19 (2021): 4848–4856, https://doi.org/10.1016/j.cell.2021.08.017.

263. Yang Cao, "COVID-19 Case-Fatality Rate and Demographic and Socioeconomic Influencers: Worldwide Spatial Regression Analysis Based on Country-Level Data," *BMJ Open* 10, no. 11, https://bmjopen.bmj.com/content/10/11/e043560.abstract.

264. Kangqi Ng et al., "COVID-19 and the Risk to Healthcare Workers: A Case Report," *Annals of Internal Medicine* 172, no. 11 (2020): 766, https://doi.org/10.7326/l20-0175.

265. S. C. Y. Wong et al., "Risk of Nosocomial Transmission of Coronavirus Disease 2019: An Experience in a General Ward Setting in Hong Kong," *Journal of Hospital Infection* 105, no. 2 (2020): 119, https://doi.org/10.1016/j.jhin.2020.03.036.

266. Weilie Chen et al., "Detectable 2019-nCoV Viral RNA in Blood Is a Strong Indicator for the Further Clinical Severity," *Emerging Microbes & Infections* 9, no. 1 (2020): 469, https://doi.org/10.1080/22221751.2020.1732837.

267. Wenling Wang et al., "Detection of SARS-CoV-2 in Different Types of Clinical Specimens," *JAMA* 323, no. 18 (2020): 1843, https://doi.org/10.1001/jama.2020.3786.

268. Ka Shing Cheung et al., "Gastrointestinal Manifestations of SARS-CoV-2 Infection and Virus Load in Fecal Samples from a Hong Kong Cohort: Systematic Review and Meta-analysis," *Gastroenterology* 159, no. 1 (2020): 81, https://doi.org/10.1053/j.gastro.2020.03.065.

269. Shufa Zheng et al., "Viral Load Dynamics and Disease Severity in Patients Infected with SARS-CoV-2 in Zhejiang Province, China, January–March 2020: Retrospective Cohort Study," *BMJ* 369 (2020): m1443, https://doi.org/10.1136/bmj.m1443.

270. Diangeng Li et al., "Clinical Characteristics and Results of Semen Tests Among Men with Coronavirus Disease 2019," *JAMA Network Open* 3, no. 5 (2020): e208292, https://doi.org/10.1001/jamanetworkopen.2020.8292.

271. Kangqi Ng et al., "COVID-19 and the Risk to Healthcare Workers: A Case Report," *Annals of Internal Medicine* 172, no. 11 (2020): 766, https://doi.org/10.7326/l20-0175.

272. S. C. Y. Wong et al., "Risk of Nosocomial Transmission of Coronavirus Disease 2019: An Experience in a General Ward Setting in Hong Kong," *Journal of Hospital Infection* 105, no. 2 (2020): 119, https://doi.org/10.1016/j.jhin.2020.03.036.

273. Francesca Colavita et al., "SARS-CoV-2 Isolation from Ocular Secretions of a Patient with COVID-19 in Italy with Prolonged Viral RNA Detection," *Annals of Internal Medicine* 173, no. 3 (2020): 242, https://doi.org/10.7326/m20-1176.

274. Jun Yuan et al., "Sewage as a Possible Transmission Vehicle During a Coronavirus Disease 2019 Outbreak in a Densely Populated Community: Guangzhou, China, April 2020," *Clinical Infectious Diseases* 73, no. 7 (2021): e1487, https://doi.org/10.1093/cid/ciaa1494.

275. "Report of the WHO-China Joint Mission on Coronavirus Disease 2019 (COVID-2019)," World Health Organization, accessed March 4, 2020, http://www.who.int/docs/default-source/coronaviruse/who-china-joint-mission-on-covid-19-final-report.pdf.

276. I. J. Onakpoya, C. J. Heneghan, E. A. Spencer, J. Brassey, A. Plüddemann, D. H. Evans, J. M. Conly, and T. Jefferson, "SARS-CoV-2 and the Role of Close Contact in Transmission: A Systematic Review," *F1000Research* 10, no. 280 (2021), https://doi.org/10.12688/f1000research.52439.3.

277. G. Viceconte and N. Petrosillo, "COVID-19 R0: Magic Number or Conundrum?," *Infectious Disease Reports* 12, no. 1 (2020): 8516, https://doi.org/10.4081/idr.2020.8516.

278. S. Sanche, Y. Lin, C. Xu, E. Romero-Severson, N. Hengartner, and R. Ke, "High Contagiousness and Rapid Spread of Severe Acute Respiratory Syndrome Coronavirus 2," *Emerging Infectious Diseases* 26, no. 7 (2020): 1470–1477, https://doi.org/10.3201/eid2607.200282.

279. Daphne Duval et al., "Long Distance Airborne Transmission of SARS-CoV-2: Rapid Systematic Review," *BMJ* 377 (2022): e068743, https://doi.org/10.1136/bmj-2021-068743.

280. Jonathan Steinberg et al., "COVID-19 Outbreak Among Employees at a Meat Processing Facility—South Dakota, March–April 2020," *Morbidity and Mortality Weekly Report* 69, no. 31 (2020): 1015, https://doi.org/10.15585/mmwr.mm6931a2.

281. Jonathan W. Dyal et al., "COVID-19 Among Workers in Meat and Poultry Processing Facilities—19 States, April 2020," *Morbidity and Mortality Weekly Report* 69, no. 18 (2020), https://doi.org/10.15585/mmwr.mm6918e3.

282. Isaac Ghinai et al., "Community Transmission of SARS-CoV-2 at Two Family Gatherings—Chicago, Illinois, February–March 2020," *Morbidity and Mortality Weekly Report* 69, no. 15 (2020): 446, https://doi.org/10.15585/mmwr.mm6915e1.

283. Hassan Tarhini et al., "Long-Term Severe Acute Respiratory Syndrome Coronavirus 2 (SARS-CoV-2) Infectiousness Among Three Immunocompromised Patients: From Prolonged Viral Shedding to SARS-CoV-2 Superinfection," *Journal of Infectious Diseases* 223, no. 9 (2021): 1552, https://doi.org/10.1093/infdis/jiab075.

284. Ji Hoon Baang et al., "Prolonged Severe Acute Respiratory Syndrome Coronavirus 2 Replication in an Immunocompromised Patient," *Journal of Infectious Diseases* 223, no. 1 (2021): 23, https://doi.org/10.1093/infdis/jiaa666.

285. Kiva A. Fisher et al., "Community and Close Contact Exposures Associated with COVID-19 Among Symptomatic Adults ≥ 18 Years in 11 Outpatient Healthcare Facilities—U.S., July 2020," *Morbidity and Mortality Weekly Report* 69, no. 36 (2020): 1258, https://doi.org/10.15585/mmwr.mm6936a5.

286. Maogui Hu et al., "Risk of Coronavirus Disease 2019 Transmission in Train Passengers: An Epidemiological and Modeling Study," *Clinical Infectious Diseases* 72, no. 4 (2021): 604, https://doi.org/10.1093/cid/ciaa1057.

287. J. Bryner, "1st Known Case of Coronavirus Traced Back to November in China," Livescience.com, March 14, 2020, https://www.livescience.com/first-case -coronavirus-found.html.

288. "Tracing the New Coronavirus Gene Sequencing: When Did the Alarm Sound," *Caixin* (in Chinese), April 26, 2020, https://web.archive.org/web/202002270 94018/https://china.caixin.com/2020-02-26/101520972.html.

289. Lu Zikang, "How Did She, the First Person to Report the Epidemic, Discover This Different Kind of Pneumonia," *China News*, accessed September 15, 2023, https://web.archive.org/web/20200302165302.

290. Tanu Singhal, "A Review of Coronavirus Disease-2019 (COVID-19)," *Indian Journal of Pediatrics* 87, no. 4 (2020), https://doi.org/10.1007%2Fs12098-020-03263-6.

291. Hannah Ritchie, "Coronavirus Pandemic (COVID-19)," Our World in Data, 2020–2022, https://ourworldindata.org/coronavirus.

292. "China Delayed Releasing Coronavirus Info, Frustrating WHO," Associated Press, June 2 2020, https://apnews.com/article/united-nations-health-ap-top-news -virus-outbreak-public-health-3c061794970661042b18d5aeaaed9fae.

293. "Coronavirus: Primi due casi in Italia" (Coronavirus: First two cases in Italy), *Corriere della sera* (in Italian), January 31, 2020, https://www.corriere.it/cronache/20 _gennaio_30/coronavirus-italia-corona-9d6dc436-4343-11ea-bdc8-faf1f56f19b7.shtml.

294. "Coronavirus: Number of COVID-19 Deaths in Italy Surpasses China as Total Reaches 3,405," *Sky News*, accessed October 1, 2023, https://news.sky.com/story /coronavirus-number-of-covid-19-deaths-in-italy-surpasses-china-as-total-reaches-3 -405-11960412.

295. D. G. McNeil Jr., "The U.S. Now Leads the World in Confirmed Coronavirus Cases," *New York Times*, March 26, 2020, https://www.nytimes.com/2020/03/26 /health/usa-coronavirus-cases.html.

296. "Studies Show N.Y. Outbreak Originated in Europe," *New York Times*, April 8, 2020, https://www.nytimes.com/2020/03/26/health/usa-coronavirus-cases.html.

297. "The Pandemic's True Death Toll," *Economist*, August 28, 2023, https://www .economist.com/graphic-detail/coronavirus-excess-deaths-estimates.

298. M. Stobbe, "US Deaths in 2020 Top 3 Million, by Far Most Ever Counted," Associated Press, December 21, 2020, https://apnews.com/article/us-coronavirus -deaths-top-3-million-e2bc856b6ec45563b84ee2e87ae8d5e7.

299. M. Nedelman, "South Carolina Detects First US Cases of Coronavirus Strain First Seen in South Africa," CNN, January 28, 2021, https://www.cnn.com/2021/01 /28/health/south-carolina-variant-south-africa/index.html.

300. "Countries Evaluate Evacuation of Citizens Amid Wuhan Coronavirus Panic," Associated Press, 2020, https://thediplomat.com/2020/01/countries-evaluate -evacuation-of-citizens-amid-wuhan-coronavirus-panic/.

301. Haiqian Chen et al., "Response to the COVID-19 Pandemic: Comparison of Strategies in Six Countries," *Front Public Health* 9 (2021), https://doi.org/10.3389%2Ffpubh.2021.708496.

302. Andrew Taylor, "Trump Signs $8.3B Bill to Combat Coronavirus Outbreak in US," Associated Press, March 5, 2020, https://apnews.com/article/donald-trump-ap-top-news-virus-outbreak-politics-public-health-3ofcoaf2ffb9320e1d8fa6bb6d8b23a1.

303. "COVID-19 Cases Are Skyrocketing, but Deaths Are Flat—So Far. These 5 Charts Explain Why," *Time* magazine, accessed October 1, 2023, https://time.com/5903590/coronavirus-covid-19-third-wave/.

304. "Proclamation on Declaring a National Emergency Concerning the Novel Coronavirus Disease (COVID-19) Outbreak," Trump White House Archives, March 13, 2020, https://trumpwhitehouse.archives.gov/presidential-actions/proclamation-declaring-national-emergency-concerning-novel-coronavirus-disease-covid-19-outbreak/.

305. L. Robertson, "Trump's Snowballing China Travel Claim," FactCheck.org, April 15, 2020, https://www.factcheck.org/2020/04/trumps-snowballing-china-travel-claim.

306. S. Moon, "A Seemingly Healthy Woman's Sudden Death Is Now the First Known US Coronavirus-Related Fatality," CNN, April 24, 2020, https://www.cnn.com/2020/04/23/us/california-woman-first-coronavirus-death/index.html.

307. D. Debolt, "29 People Had Flu-Like Symptoms When They Died in Santa Clara County: Nine Tested Positive for Coronavirus," *Mercury News*, April 25, 2020, https://www.mercurynews.com/2020/04/25/9-santa-clara-deaths-reclassified-as-covid-19-related.

308. M. Taylor, "Exclusive: U.S. Axed CDC Expert Job in China Months Before Virus Outbreak," Reuters, March 22, 2020, https://www.reuters.com/article/us-health-coronavirus-china-cdc-exclusiv/exclusive-u-s-axed-cdc-expert-job-in-china-months-before-virus-outbreak-idUSKBN21910S.

309. "Lawrence Garbuz, NY's First Known COVID-19 Case, Reveals What He Learned About Attorney Well-Being from the Virus," New York State Bar Association, accessed October 1, 2023, https://nysba.org/lawrence-garbuz-new-yorks-first-known-covid-19-case-reveals-what-he-learned-about-attorney-well-being-from-the-virus/.

310. G. Hauck, "More Contagious COVID-19 Strain Identified in 3 States and 33 Countries: What to Know," *USA Today*, January 15, 2021, https://www.usatoday.com/story/news/health/2021/01/02/new-covid-strain-b-117-explained/4112125001/.

311. Nate Rattner, "U.S. Sets Fresh Records for COVID Hospitalizations and Cases with 1.5 Million New Infections," CNBC, January 11, 2022, https://www.cnbc.com/2022/01/11/omicron-variant-us-sets-fresh-records-for-covid-hospitalizations-and-cases-with-1point5-million-new-infections.html.

312. Marita Vlachou, "CDC Estimates How Many Americans Hadn't Had COVID by End of 2022," *HuffPost*, July 4, 2023, https://www.huffpost.com/entry/covid-americans-study-seroprevalence_n_64a3f2bfe4b030efa12297ca.

313. "The 4 Key Reasons the U.S. Is So Behind on Coronavirus Testing," *Atlantic*, accessed October 1, 2023, https://www.theatlantic.com/health/archive/2020/03/why-coronavirus-testing-us-so-delayed/607954/.

314. Aja Seldon, "Passengers from Cruise Ship with Coronavirus-Like Symptoms Relocating to San Carlos Hotel," *Fox KTVU*, March 11, 2020, https://www.ktvu.com/news/passengers-from-cruise-ship-with-coronavirus-like-symptoms-relocating-to-san-carlos-hotel.

315. "Can You Be Forced to Quarantine or Stay Home? Your Questions, Answers," *New York Times*, accessed September 11, 2023, https://www.nytimes.com/article/coronavirus-quarantine-questions.html.

316. C. Norwood, "Most States Have Issued Stay-at-Home Orders, but Enforcement Varies Widely," PBS, April 3, 2020, https://www.pbs.org/newshour/politics/most-states-have-issued-stay-at-home-orders-but-enforcement-varies-widely.

317. "U.S. Coronavirus Deaths Top 20,000, Highest in World Exceeding Italy: Reuters Tally," Reuters, April 11, 2020, https://www.reuters.com/article/us-health-coronavirus-usa-casualties-idUSKCN21T0NA.

318. Steve Almasy, Christina Maxouris, and Nicole Chavez, "Us Coronavirus Cases Surpass 1 Million and the Death Toll Is Greater than US Losses in Vietnam War," CNN, accessed October 1, 2023, https://www.cnn.com/2020/04/28/health/us-coronavirus-tuesday/index.html.

319. M. Fisher, "U.S. Coronavirus Death Toll Surpasses 100,000, Exposing Nation's Vulnerabilities," *Washington Post*, May 27, 2020, https://www.washingtonpost.com/graphics/2020/national/100000-deaths-american-coronavirus/.

320. A. F. Noori et al., "U.S. Surpasses 2 Million Coronavirus Cases," *Washington Post*, June 11, 2020, https://www.washingtonpost.com/nation/2020/06/11/coronavirus-update-us/.

321. A. Joseph, "Actual COVID-19 Case Count Could Be 6 to 24 Times Higher Than Official Estimates, CDC Study Shows," *Statnews*, July 21, 2020, https://www.washingtonpost.com/nation/2020/06/11/coronavirus-update-us/.

322. "Briefing on the U.S. Government's Next Steps with Regard to Withdrawal from the World Health Organization," US Department of State, September 2, 2020, https://www.state.gov/briefing-with-nerissa-cook-deputy-assistant-secretary-of-state-bureau-of-international-organization-affairs-garrett-grigsby-director-of-the-office-of-global-affairs-department-of-health-and-human/.

323. *COVID-19 Pandemic Planning Scenarios*, Centers for Disease Control and Prevention, July 10, 2020, https://www.cdc.gov/coronavirus/2019-ncov/hcp/planning-scenarios-archive/planning-scenarios-2020-09-10.pdf.

324. B. Chappel, "'Enormous and Tragic': U.S. Has Lost More Than 200,000 People to COVID-19," NPR, September 22, 2020, https://www.npr.org/sections/coronavirus-live-updates/2020/09/22/911934489/enormous-and-tragic-u-s-has-lost-more-than-200-000-people-to-covid-19.

325. M. Haberman, "Trump Says He'll Begin 'Quarantine Process' After Hope Hicks Tests Positive for Coronavirus," *New York Times*, October 1, 2020.

326. J. Dawsey and C. Itkowitz, "Trump Says He and the First Lady Have Tested Positive for Coronavirus," *Washington Post*, accessed October 1, 2023, ISSN 0190–8286.

327. K. Liptak, "Trump Taken to Walter Reed Medical Center and Will Be Hospitalized 'for the Next Few Days," CNN, October 3, 2020, https://www.cnn.com /2020/10/02/politics/president-donald-trump-walter-reed-coronavirus/index.html.

328. A. E. Cha and A. Goldstein, "Prospect of Trump's Early Hospital Discharge Mystifies Doctors," *Washington Post*, October 4, 2020, https://www.washingtonpost .com/health/2020/10/04/trump-covid-19-discharge/.

329. S. H. Shahcheraghi, J. Ayatollahi, A. A. Aljabali, M. D. Shastri, S. D. Shukla, D. K. Chellappan, N. K. Jha, K. Anand, N. K. Katari, M. Mehta, et al., "An Overview of Vaccine Development for COVID-19," *Therapeutic Delivery* 12, no. 3 (2021): 235–244, https://doi.org/10.4155/tde-2020-0129.

330. S. Gottlieb, "America Needs to Win the Coronavirus Vaccine Race," U.S. Senate Committee on Small Business and Entrepreneurship, accessed October 1, 2023, https://www.wsj.com/articles/america-needs-to-win-the-coronavirus-vaccine -race-11587924258.

331. Michael Erman, "U.S. to Pay $1 Billion for 100 Million Doses of Johnson & Johnson's COVID-19 Vaccine Candidate," Reuters, August 5, 2020, https://www .reuters.com/article/us-health-coronavirus-usa-johnsonandjohn/u-s-to-pay-1 -billion-for-100-million-doses-of-johnson-johnsons-covid-19-vaccine-candidate -idUSKCN2511VH.

332. J. Corum, S. L. Wee, and C. Zimmer, "Coronavirus Vaccine Tracker," *New York Times*, October 2020.

333. Office of the Commissioner, "Coronavirus (COVID-19) Update: FDA Authorizes Pfizer-BioNTech COVID-19 Vaccine for Emergency Use in Adolescents in Another Important Action in Fight Against Pandemic," US Food and Drug Administration, May 13, 2021.

334. "Vaccines and Related Biological Products Advisory Committee December 10, 2020 Meeting Announcement," US Food and Drug Administration, accessed November 30, 2020.

335. "Coronavirus (COVID-19) Update: FDA Announces Advisory Committee Meeting to Discuss COVID-19 Vaccine Candidate," US Food and Drug Administration, press release, November 20, 2020.

336. B. Bryant and S. Gimont, "Biden-Harris Transition Team Announces COVID-19 Advisory Board," *National Association of Counties* (blog), November 18, 2020, https://www.naco.org/blog/biden-harris-transition-team-announces-covid-19 -advisory-board.

337. "10 Million People Have Tested Positive for Coronavirus in the United States," *Time* magazine, November 9, 2020.

338. R. Alonso-Zalidivar, "Feds Announce COVID-19 Vaccine Agreement with Drug Stores," Associated Press, November 12, 2020.

339. S. E. Oliver, J. W. Gargano, M. Marin, M. Wallace, K. G. Curran, M. Chamberland, et al., "The Advisory Committee on Immunization Practices' Interim Recommendation for Use of Moderna COVID-19 Vaccine—United States, December 2020," *Morbidity and Mortality Weekly Report* 69, no. 5152 (2021): 1653–1656, https://doi.org/10.15585/mmwr.mm695152e1.

340. K. Thomas, S. LaFraniere, N. Weiland, A. Goodnough, and M. Haberman, "F.D.A. Clears Pfizer Vaccine, and Millions of Doses Will Be Shipped Right Away," *New York Times*, December 12, 2020.

341. I. Stanley-Becker, Y. Abutaleb, L. H. Sun, and J. Dawsey, "States Report Confusion as Government Reduces Vaccine Shipments, While Pfizer Says It Has 'Millions' of Unclaimed Doses," *Washington Post*, December 17, 2020.

342. S. E. Oliver, J. W. Gargano, M. Marin, M. Wallace, K. G. Curran, M. Chamberland, et al., "The Advisory Committee on Immunization Practices' Interim Recommendation for Use of Moderna COVID-19 Vaccine—United States, December 2020," *Morbidity and Mortality Weekly Report* 69, no. 5152 (2021): 1653–1656, https://doi.org/10.15585/mmwr.mm695152e1.

343. "Moderna Applies for Emergency F.D.A. Approval for Its Coronavirus Vaccine," *New York Times*, November 30, 2020.

344. B. Lovelace Jr, "FDA Approves Second COVID Vaccine for Emergency Use as It Clears Moderna's for U.S. Distribution," CNBC, accessed December 19, 2020.

345. E. Dubé et al., "Vaccine Hesitancy: An Overview," *Human Vaccines & Immunotherapeutics* 9, no. 8 (2013): 1763–1773, https://doi.org/10.4161/hv.24657.

346. M. O'Brien, "Many Americans Flying for Thanksgiving Despite CDC Pleas," *Republican*, November 23, 2020, https://www.masslive.com/coronavirus/2020/11/thanksgiving-travel-many-americans-flying-for-holiday-despite-cdcs-pleas-not-to-due-to-covid-19-transmission-risk.html.

347. J. Bacon, E. Aspegren, and G. Hauck, "Coronavirus Updates: Joe Biden Pledges to Deliver 100M Doses in 100 Days; US Reaches 15M Infections; Ohio-State Michigan Football Game Off," *USA Today*, December 8, 2020, https://www.usatoday.com/story/news/health/2020/12/08/covid-news-britain-vaccine-wyoming-california-donald-trump/6481339002/.

348. H. Yan, "COVID-19 Now Kills More Than 1 American Every Minute and the Rate Keeps Accelerating as the Death Toll Tops 300,000," CNN, December 14, 2020, https://www.cnn.com/2020/12/14/health/us-covid-deaths-300k/index.html.

349. S. Tavernise and R. A. Oppel Jr., "Spit On, Yelled At, Attacked: Chinese-Americans Fear for Their Safety," *New York Times*, March 23, 2020, https://www.nytimes.com/2020/03/23/us/chinese-coronavirus-racist-attacks.html.

350. "How George Floyd Died, and What Happened Next," *New York Times*, July 29, 2022, https://www.nytimes.com/article/george-floyd.html

351. Paul Farmer, *Infectious and Inequalities* (University of California Press, 2001), https://www.ucpress.edu/book/9780520229136/infections-and-inequalities/.

352. Paul Farmer, *Pathologies of Power* (University of California Press, 2004), https://www.ucpress.edu/book/9780520243262/pathologies-of-power.

353. Clyde W. Yancy, "COVID-19 and African Americans," *JAMA* 323, no. 19 (2020), https://doi.org/10.1001/jama.2020.6548.

354. Manny Fernandez and Audra D. S. Burch, "George Floyd from 'I Want to Touch the World' to 'I Can't Breathe,'" *New York Times*, April 20, 2021, https://www.nytimes.com/article/george-floyd-who-is.html.

355. Elizabeth Arias, Betzaida Tejada-Vera, and Farida Ahmad, "Provisional Life Expectancy Estimates for 2020," Vital Statistics Rapid Release, July 2021, https://www.cdc.gov/nchs/data/vsrr/vsrr015-508.pdf.

356. "The Color of Coronavirus: COVID-19 Deaths by Race and Ethnicity in the U.S.," *APM Research Lab: American Public Media*, June 27, 2023, https://www.apmresearchlab.org/covid/deaths-by-race.

357. J. Bosman, S. Kasakove, and D. Victor, "U.S. Life Expectancy Plunged in 2020, Especially for Black and Hispanic Americans," *New York Times*, July 21, 2021, https://www.nytimes.com/2021/07/21/us/american-life-expectancy-report.html.

358. Clyde W. Yancy, "COVID-19 and African Americans," *JAMA* 323, no. 19 (2020): 1891–1892, https://doi.org/10.1001/jama.2020.6548.

359. Reis Thebault, Andrew Ba Tran, and Vanessa Williams, "The Coronavirus Is Infecting and Killing Black Americans at an Alarmingly High Rate," *Washington Post*, April 7, 2020.

360. Roni Caryn Rabin, "U.S. Life Expectancy Falls Again in 'Historic' Setback," *New York Times*, August 31, 2022, https://web.archive.org/web/20220831133930/https://www.nytimes.com/2022/08/31/health/life-expectancy-covid-pandemic.html.

361. Marco Morabito et al., "Heat Warning and Public and Workers' Health at the Time of COVID-19 Pandemic," *ScienceDirect* 738, no. 10 (2020), https://doi.org/10.1016/j.scitotenv.2020.140347.

362. Sweta Haldar, "Latest Data on COVID-19 Vaccinations by Race/Ethnicity," KFF, July 14, 2022, https://www.kff.org/coronavirus-covid-19/issue-brief/latest-data-on-covid-19-vaccinations-by-race-ethnicity/.

363. Jasmine Soriano, Haylea Hannah, and Karina Arambula, "COVID-19 Vaccine Perceptions Survey for Real-Time Vaccine Outreach in Marin County, California," *Cureus*, March 23, 2023, https://doi.org/10.7759/cureus.36583.

364. "The US Public Health Service Syphilis Study at Tuskegee," Centers for Disease Control and Prevention, modified December 5, 2022, https://www.cdc.gov/tuskegee/timeline.htm.

365. Zselykw Csaky and Nate Schenkkan, "Confronting Illiberalism," Freedom House, 2018, https://freedomhouse.org/report/nations-transit/2018/confronting-illiberalism.

366. Lola Butcher, "Pandemic Puts All Eyes on Public Health," *Knowable Magazine*, November 17, 2020, https://doi.org/10.1146/knowable-111720-1.

367. "Pulse Survey on Continuity of Essential Health Services During the COVID-19 Pandemic," World Health Organization, August 27, 2020, https://iris.who .int/bitstream/handle/10665/334048/WHO-2019-nCoV-EHS_continuity-survey -2020.1-eng.pdf.

368. Syed A. K. Shifat Ahmed, "Impact of the Societal Response to COVID-19 on Access to Healthcare for Non-COVID-19 Health Issues in Slum Communities of Bangladesh, Kenya, Nigeria and Pakistan: Results of Pre-COVID and COVID-19 Lockdown Stakeholder Engagements," *BMJ GLobal Health* 5, no. 8, http://dx.doi.org /10.1136/bmjgh-2020-003042.

369. Robin Williams et al., "Diagnosis of Physical and Mental Health Conditions in Primary Care During the COVID-19 Pandemic: A Retrospective Cohort Study," *Lancet Public Health* 5, no. 10 (2020), https://doi.org/10.1016/S2468-2667(20)30201-2.

370. "With Almost Half of World's Population Still Offline, Digital Divide Risks Becoming 'New Face of Inequality,' Deputy Secretary-General Warns General Assembly," United Nations, April 2021, https://press.un.org/en/2021/dsgsm1579.doc .htm.

371. "COVID-19 and the Social Determinants of Health and Health Equity," World Health Organization, October 2021, https://iris.who.int/bitstream/handle/10665 /348333/9789240038387-eng.pdf.

372. "With Almost Half of World's Population Still Offline, Digital Divide Risks Becoming 'New Face of Inequality,' Deputy Secretary-General Warns General Assembly," United Nations, April 2021, https://press.un.org/en/2021/dsgsm1579.doc .htm.

373. Juan C. Palomino, Juan G. Rodríguez, and Raquel Sebastian, "Wage Inequality and Poverty Effects of Lockdown and Social Distancing in Europe," *Elsevier* 129 (2020), https://doi.org/10.1016/j.euroecorev.2020.103564.

374. Julia Raifman, Jacob Bor, and Atheendar Venkataramani, "Association Between Receipt of Unemployment Insurance and Food Insecurity Among People Who Lost Employment During the COVID-19 Pandemic in the U.S.," *JAMA Network Open* 4, no. 1 (2021): e2035884, https://doi.org/10.1001/jamanetworkopen .2020.35884.

375. Min Zhou and Wei Guo, "Social Factors and Worry Associated with COVID-19: Evidence from a Large Survey in China," *Elsevier* 277 (2021), https://doi .org/10.1016/j.socscimed.2021.113934.

376. "COVID-19 and the Social Determinants of Health and Health Equity," World Health Organization, October 2021, https://iris.who.int/bitstream/handle/10665 /348333/9789240038387-eng.pdf.

377. "Health Workforce," World Health Organization, accessed July 25, 2022, https://www.who.int/health-topics/health-workforce.

6. The Most Prevalent Infectious Disease Killers Today

1. "The Top 10 Causes of Death," World Health Organization, December 9, 2020, https://www.who.int/news-room/fact-sheets/detail/the-top-10-causes-of-death.

2. A. H. Baykan, H. S. Sayiner, E. Aydin, M. Koc, I. Inan, and S. M. Erturk, "Extrapulmonary Tuberculosis: An Old but Resurgent Problem," *Insights into Imaging* 13, no. 1 (2022): 39, https://doi.org/10.1186/s13244-022-01172-0.

3. *Global Tuberculosis Report 2020*, World Health Organization, October 15, 2020, https://www.who.int/publications/i/item/9789240013131.

4. "Tuberculosis," World Health Organization, 2021, https://www.who.int/health-topics/tuberculosis#tab=tab_1.

5. R. M. Houben and P. J. Dodd, "The Global Burden of Latent Tuberculosis Infection: A Re-Estimation Using Mathematical Modelling," *PLOS Medicine* 13, no. 10 (2016): e1002152, https://doi.org/10.1371/journal.pmed.1002152.

6. *Global Tuberculosis Report 2020*, World Health Organization, 2020, https://www.who.int/publications/i/item/9789240013131.

7. E. L. Corbett et al., "Tuberculosis in Sub-Saharan Africa: Opportunities, Challenges, and Change in the Era of Antiretroviral Treatment," *Lancet* 367, no. 9514 (2006): 926–937, https://doi.org/10.1016/S0140-6736(06)68383-9.

8. A. Wright et al., "Global Project on Anti-Tuberculosis Drug Resistance Surveillance. Epidemiology of Antituberculosis Drug Resistance, 2002–07: An Updated Analysis of the Global Project on Anti-Tuberculosis Drug Resistance Surveillance," *Lancet* 373, no. 9678 (2009): 1861–1873, https://doi.org/10.1016/S0140-6736(09)60331-7.

9. C. Dye et al., "Trends in Tuberculosis Incidence and Their Determinants in 134 Countries," *Bulletin of the World Health Organization* 87, no. 9 (2009): 683–691, https://doi.org/10.2471/blt.08.058453.

10. J. R. Hargreaves, D. Boccia, C. A. Evans, M. Adato, M. Petticrew, and J. D. Porter, "The Social Determinants of Tuberculosis: From Evidence to Action," *American Journal of Public Health* 101, no. 4 (2011): 654–662, https://doi.org/10.2105/AJPH.2010.199505.

11. D. Pedrazzoli et al., "Modelling the Social and Structural Determinants of Tuberculosis: Opportunities and Challenges," *International Journal of Tuberculosis and Lung Disease* 21, no. 9 (2017): 957–964, https://doi.org/10.5588/ijtld.16.0906.

12. P. C. Hill et al., "Risk Factors for Pulmonary Tuberculosis: A Clinic-Based Case Control Study in The Gambia," *BMC Public Health* 6, no. 156 (2006), https://doi.org/10.1186/1471-2458-6-156.

13. D. P. Boccia et al., "Tuberculosis Infection in Zambia: The Association with Relative Wealth," *American Journal of Tropical Medicine and Hygiene* 80, no. 6 (2009): 1004–1011.

14. M. Baker et al., "Tuberculosis Associated with Household Crowding in a Developed Country," *Journal of Epidemiology and Community Health* 62, no. 8 (2008): 715–721.

15. M. Van Lettow et al., "Malnutrition and the Severity of Lung Disease in Adults with Pulmonary Tuberculosis in Malawi," *International Journal of Tuberculosis and Lung Disease* 8, no. 2 (2004): 211–217.

16. N. Kanara et al., "Association Between Distance to HIV Testing Site and Uptake of HIV Testing for Tuberculosis Patients in Cambodia," *International Journal of Tuberculosis and Lung Disease* 13, no. 2 (2009): 226–231.

17. D. Somma et al., "Gender and Socio-Cultural Determinants of TB-Related Stigma in Bangladesh, India, Malawi and Colombia," *International Journal of Tuberculosis and Lung Disease* 12, no. 7 (2008): 856–866.

18. L. Gilbert and L. Walker, "Treading the Path of Least Resistance: HIV/AIDS and Social Inequalities a South African Case Study," *Social Science & Medicine* 54, no. 7 (2002): 1093–1110.

19. J. E. Svenson et al., "Imported Malaria: Clinical Presentation and Examination of Symptomatic Travelers," *Archives of Internal Medicine* 155, no. 8 (1995): 861–868, https://doi.org/10.1001/archinte.155.8.861.

20. E. A. Ashley and N. J. White, "Harrison's Principles of Internal Medicine," ed. I. L. Jameson, A. S. Fauci, and D. L. Kasper, 20th ed. (McGraw Hill, 2018).

21. *WHO Guidelines for Malaria 2022*, World Health Organization, accessed April 1, 2022, https://www.who.int/publications/i/item/guidelines-for-malaria.

22. *World Malaria Report 2021*, World Health Organization, accessed February 7, 2022, https://www.who.int/teams/global-malaria-programme/reports/world-malaria-report-2021.

23. *World Malaria Report 2021*, World Health Organization, accessed February 7, 2022, https://www.who.int/teams/global-malaria-programme/reports/world-malaria-report-2021.

24. A. K. Owusu-Ofori et al., "Transfusion-Transmitted Malaria in Ghana," *Clinical Infectious Diseases* 56, no. 12 (2013): 1735–1741, https://doi.org/10.1093/cid/cit130.

25. H. Gruell et al., "On Taking a Different Route: An Unlikely Case of Malaria by Nosocomial Transmission," *Clinical Infectious Diseases* 65, no. 8 (2017): 1404–1406, https://doi.org/10.1093/cid/cix520.

26. K. E. Mace et al., "Malaria Surveillance—U.S., 2017," *MMWR Surveillance Summaries* 70, no. 2 (2021): 1–35, https://doi.org/10.15585/mmwr.ss7002a1.

27. *World Malaria Report 2021*, World Health Organization, 2021, https://www.who.int/teams/global-malaria-programme/reports/world-malaria-report-2021.

28. W. Haileselassie, D. M. Parker, B. Taye, et al. "Burden of Malaria, Impact of Interventions and Climate Variability in Western Ethiopia: An Area with Large Irrigation Based Farming," *BMC Public Health* 22, no. 196 (2022), https://doi.org/10.1186/s12889-022-12571-9.

29. Christopher J. L. Murray et al., "Global Malaria Mortality Between 1980 and 2010: A Systematic Analysis," accessed August 11, 2011, https://pubmed.ncbi.nlm.nih.gov/22305225.

30. *World Malaria Report 2018*, World Health Organization, 2018, accessed August 11, 2021, https://apps.who.int/iris/handle/10665/275867.

31. D. Gwatkin and M. Guillot, *The Burden of Disease Among the Global Poor: Current Situations, Future Trends, and Implications for Strategy* (World Bank, 2000).

32. A. Degarege, K. Fennie, D. Degarege, S. Chennupati, and P. Madhivanan, "Improving Socioeconomic Status May Reduce the Burden of Malaria in Sub-Saharan Africa: A Systematic Review and Meta-Analysis," *PloS One* 14, no. 1 (2019): e0211205, https://doi.org/10.1371/journal.pone.0211205.

33. F. M. Mburu, H. C. Spencer, and D. C. O. Kaseje, "Changes in Sources of Treatment Occurring After Inception of a Community-Based Malaria Control Programme in Saradidi, Kenya," suppl., *Annals of Tropical Medicine & Parasitology* 81, no. S1 (1987): 105–110, https://doi.org/10.1080/00034983.1987.11812195.

34. Elizabeth H. Shayo, Susan F. Rumisha, Malongo R. S. Mlozi, Veneranda M. Bwana, Benjamin K. Mayala, Robert C. Malima, Tabitha Mlacha, Leonard E. G. Mboera, "Social Determinants of Malaria and Health Care Seeking Patterns Among Rice Farming and Pastoral Communities in Kilosa District in Central Tanzania," *Acta Tropica* 144 (2015): 41–49, https://doi.org/10.1016/j.actatropica.2015.01.003.

35. S. K. Dhiman, "Malaria Control: Behavioural and Social Aspects," *Defense Science Special*, March 2009, 183–186.

36. J. L. Gallup and J. D. Sachs, "The Economic Burden of Malaria," *American Journal of Tropical Medicine and Hygiene* 64, no. 1/2 (2001): 85–96.

37. A. Enayati and J. Hemingway, "Malaria Management: Past, Present and Future," *Annual Review of Entomology* 55 (2010): 569–591.

38. R. G. Feachem, A. A. Phillips, J. Hwang, C. Cotter, B. Wielgosz, B. M. Greenwood, O. Sabot, M. H. Rodriguez, R. R. Abeyasinghe, T. A. Ghebreyesus, and R. W. Snow, "Shrinking the Malaria Map: Progress and Prospects," *Lancet (London)* 376, no. 9752 (2010): 1566–1578, https://doi.org/10.1016/S0140-6736(10)61270-6.

39. R. G. Feachem, A. A. Phillips, J. Hwang, C. Cotter, B. Wielgosz, B. M. Greenwood, O. Sabot, M. H. Rodriguez, R. R. Abeyasinghe, T. A. Ghebreyesus, and R. W. Snow, "Shrinking the Malaria Map: Progress and Prospects," *Lancet (London)* 376, no. 9752 (2010): 1566–1578, https://doi.org/10.1016/S0140-6736(10)61270-6.

40. "Malaria: Control vs Elimination vs Eradication," *Lancet*, September 24, 2011, https://www.thelancet.com/journals/lancet/article/PIIS0140-6736(11)61489-X/fulltext.

41. H. Erdem et al., "Central Nervous System Infections in the Absence of Cerebrospinal Fluid Pleocytosis," *International Journal of Infectious Diseases* 65 (2017): 107–109, https://doi.org/10.1016/j.ijid.2017.10.011.

42. M. W. Bijlsma et al., "Community-Acquired Bacterial Meningitis in Adults in the Netherlands, 2006–14: A Prospective Cohort Study," *Lancet Infectious Diseases* 16, no. 3 (2016): 339–347, https://doi.org/10.1016/S1473-3099(15)00430-2.

43. M. L. Durand et al., "Acute Bacterial Meningitis in Adults. A Review of 493 Episodes," *New England Journal of Medicine* 328, no. 1 (1993): 21–28, https://doi.org/10.1056/NEJM199301073280104.

44. H. Erdem et al., "Central Nervous System Infections in the Absence of Cerebrospinal Fluid Pleocytosis," *International Journal of Infectious Diseases* 65 (2017): 107–109, https://doi.org/10.1016/j.ijid.2017.10.011.

45. M. N. Swartz, "Bacterial Meningitis—a View of the Past 90 Years," *New England Journal of Medicine* 351, no. 18 (2004): 1826–1828, https://doi.org/10.1056/NEJMp048246.

46. M. C. Thigpen et al., "Bacterial Meningitis in the U.S., 1998–2007," *New England Journal of Medicine* 364, no. 21 (2011): 2016–2025, https://doi.org/10.1056/NEJMoa1005384.

47. C. J. T Sai et al., "Changing Epidemiology of Pneumococcal Meningitis After the Introduction of Pneumococcal Conjugate Vaccine in the U.S.," *Clinical Infectious Diseases* 46, no. 11 (2008): 1664–1672, https://doi.org/10.1086/587897.

48. A. M. Oordt-Speets et al., "Global Etiology of Bacterial Meningitis: A Systematic Review and Meta-Analysis," *PLoS One* 13, no. 6 (2018): e0198772, https://doi.org/10.1371/journal.pone.0198772.

49. C. L. Trotter et al., "Impact of MenAfriVac in Nine Countries of the African Meningitis Belt, 2010–15: An Analysis of Surveillance Data," *Lancet Infectious Diseases* 17 (2017): 867–872, https://doi.org/10.1016/S1473-3099(17)30301-8.

50. R. Verma and P. Khanna, "Meningococcal Vaccine," *Human Vaccines and Immunotherapeutics* 8 (2012): 1904–1906, https://doi.org/10.4161/hv.21666.

51. "Managing Epidemics," World Health Organization, accessed May 9, 2019, http://www.who.int/emergencies/diseases/managing-epidemics/en.

52. H. Broutin et al., "Comparative Study of Meningitis Dynamics Across Nine African Countries: A Global Perspective," *International Journal of Health Geographics* 6 (2007): 29, https://doi.org/10.1186/1476-072X-6-29.

53. C. L. Trotter et al., "Impact of MenAfriVac in Nine Countries of the African Meningitis Belt, 2010–15: An Analysis of Surveillance Data," *Lancet Infectious Diseases* 17 (2017): 867–872, https://doi.org/10.1016/S1473-3099(17)30301-8.

54. F. Sidikou et al., "Emergence of Epidemic *Neisseria meningitidis* Serogroup C in Niger, 2015: An Analysis of National Surveillance Data," *Lancet Infectious Diseases* 16 (2016): 1288–1294, https://doi.org/10.1016/S1473-3099(16)30253-5.

55. B. A. Kwambana-Adams et al., "Meningococcus Serogroup C Clonal Complex ST-10217 Outbreak in Zamfara State, Northern Nigeria," *Scientific Reports*, 2018, https://doi.org/10.1038/s41598-018-32475-2.

56. N. Luo et al., "Spread of *Neisseria meningitidis* Group A Clone III–I Meningitis Epidemic into Zambia," *Journal of Infection*, 1998, https://www.journalofinfection.com/article/S0163-4453(98)80002-9/pdf.

57. M. Ceyhan et al., "Meningococcal Disease in the Middle East and North Africa: An Important Public Health Consideration That Requires Further Attention," *International Journal of Infectious Diseases* 16 (2012): e574–e582, https://doi.org/10.1016/j.ijid.2012.03.011.

58. "Meningococcal Disease," World Health Organization, accessed September 5, 2019, http://www.who.int/csr/don/archive/disease/meningococcal_disease/en/.

59. C. L. Trotter et al., "Impact of MenAfriVac in Nine Countries of the African Meningitis Belt, 2010–15: An Analysis of Surveillance Data," *Lancet Infectious Diseases* 17 (2017): 867–872, https://doi.org/10.1016/S1473-3099(17)30301-8.

60. J. de Gans and D. van de Beek, "European Dexamethasone in Adulthood Bacterial Meningitis Study Investigators. Dexamethasone in Adults with Bacterial Meningitis," *New England Journal of Medicine* 347, no. 20 (2002): 1549–1556, https://doi.org/10.1056/NEJMoa021334.

61. M. K. Taha, F. Martinon-Torres, R. Köllges, P. Bonanni, M. A. P. Safadi, R. Booy, and V. Abitbol, "Equity in Vaccination Policies to Overcome Social Deprivation as a Risk Factor for Invasive Meningococcal Disease," *Expert Review of Vaccines* 21, no. 5 (2022): 659–674, https://doi.org/10.1080/14760584.2022.2052048.

62. M. M. Mustapha and L. H. Harrison, "Vaccine Prevention of Meningococcal Disease in Africa: Major Advances, Remaining Challenges," *Human Vaccines & Immunotherapeutics* 14, no. 5 (2018): 1107–1115, https://doi.org/10.1080/21645515.2017.1412020.

63. H. Broutin et al., "Comparative Study of Meningitis Dynamics Across Nine African Countries: A Global Perspective," *International Journal of Health Geographics* 6 (2007): 29, https://doi.org/10.1186/1476-072X-6-29.

64. "For Healthcare Providers," Centers for Disease Control and Prevention, accessed on December 17, 2021, https://www.cdc.gov/measles/hcp/index.html.

65. M. Richardson et al., "Evidence Base of Incubation Periods, Periods of Infectiousness and Exclusion Policies for the Control of Communicable Diseases in Schools and Preschools," *Pediatric Infectious Disease Journal* 20, no. 4 (2001): 380–391, https://doi.org/10.1097/00006454-200104000-00004.

66. *Guide for Clinical Case Management and Infection Prevention and Control During a Measles Outbreak*, World Health Organization, accessed February 16, 2022, https://apps.who.int/iris/handle/10665/331599.

67. J. M. Hübschen et al., "Measles," *Lancet* 399, no. 10325 (2022): 678–690, https://doi.org/10.1016/S0140-6736(21)02004-3.

68. C. E. Stein et al., "The Global Burden of Measles in the Year 2000: A Model That Uses Country-Specific Indicators," suppl., *Journal of Infectious Diseases* 187, no. S1 (2003): S8–S14, https://doi.org/10.1086/368114.

69. Centers for Disease Control and Prevention. "Global Measles Mortality, 2000–2008," *Morbidity and Mortality Weekly Report* 58, no. 47 (2009): 1321–1326.

70. "Measles," Pan American Health Organization. accessed on February 21, 2019, https://www.paho.org/hq/index.php?option=com_topics&view=article&id=255&Itemid=40899&lang=en.

71. A. Dabbagh et al., "Progress Toward Regional Measles Elimination—Worldwide, 2000–2017," *Morbidity and Mortality Weekly Report* 67, no. 47 (2018): 1323–1329, https://doi.org/10.15585/mmwr.mm6747a6.

72. R. E. Simpson, "Infectiousness of Communicable Diseases in the Household (Measles, Chickenpox, and Mumps)," *Lancet* 2, no. 6734 (1952): 549–554, https://doi.org/10.1016/s0140-6736(52)91357-3.

73. Centers for Disease Control and Prevention, *Epidemiology and Prevention of Vaccine-Preventable Diseases*, ed. W. Atkinson, C. Wolfe, and J. Hamborsky, 12th ed. (Public Health Foundation, 2012).

74. A. B. Bloch et al., "Measles Outbreak in a Pediatric Practice: Airborne Transmission in an Office Setting," *Pediatrics* 75, no. 4 (1985): 676–683.

75. Centers for Disease Control and Prevention, "Notes from the Field: Multiple Cases of Measles After Exposure During Air Travel—Australia and New Zealand, January 2011," *Morbidity and Mortality Weekly Report* 60, no. 25 (2011): 851.

76. J. C. Bester, "Measles and Measles Vaccination: A Review," *JAMA Pediatrics* 170, no. 12, (2016): 1209–1215, https://doi.org/10.1001/jamapediatrics.2016.1787.

77. E. Banerjee et al., "Notes from the Field: Measles Transmission in an International Airport at a Domestic Terminal Gate—April–May 2014," *Morbidity and Mortality Weekly Report* 64, no. 24 (2015): 679.

78. GBD 2019 Diseases and Injuries Collaborators, "Global Burden of 369 Diseases and Injuries in 204 Countries and Territories, 1990–2019: A Systematic Analysis for the Global Burden of Disease Study 2019," *Lancet Global Health Metrics* 396, no. 10258 (2020): 1204–1222, https://doi.org/10.1016/S0140-6736(20)30925-9.

79. Global Vaccine Action Plan, "Decade of Vaccine Collaboration," suppl., *Vaccine* 31, no. S2 (2013): B5–B31, https://doi.org/10.1016/j.vaccine.2013.02.015.

80. GBD 2019 Diseases and Injuries Collaborators, "Global Burden of 369 Diseases and Injuries in 204 Countries and Territories, 1990–2019: A Systematic Analysis for the Global Burden of Disease Study 2019," *Lancet Global Health Metrics* 396, no. 10258 (2020): 1204–1222, https://doi.org/10.1016/S0140-6736(20)30925-9.

81. P. J. Hotez et al., "Combating Vaccine Hesitancy and Other 21st Century Social Determinants in the Global Fight Against Measles," *Current Opinion in Virology* 41 (2020): 1–7, https://doi.org/10.1016/j.coviro.2020.01.001.

82. M. K. Patel et al., "Progress Toward Regional Measles Elimination—Worldwide, 2000–2019," *Morbidity and Mortality Weekly Report* 69, no. 45 (2020): 1700–1705, https://doi.org/10.15585/mmwr.mm6945a6.

83. P. J. Hotez et al., "Combating Vaccine Hesitancy and Other 21st Century Social Determinants in the Global Fight Against Measles," *Current Opinion in Virology* 41 (2020): 1–7, https://doi.org/10.1016/j.coviro.2020.01.001.

84. M. K. Patel et al., "Progress Toward Regional Measles Elimination—Worldwide, 2000–2019," *Morbidity and Mortality Weekly Report* 69, no. 45 (2020): 1700–1705. https://doi.org/10.15585/mmwr.mm6945a6.

85. P. J. Hotez et al., "Combating Vaccine Hesitancy and Other 21st Century Social Determinants in the Global Fight Against Measles," *Current Opinion in Virology* 41 (2020): 1–7, https://doi.org/10.1016/j.coviro.2020.01.001.

86. A. E. Paniz-Mondolfi, A. Tami, M. E. Grillet, M. Márquez, J. Hernández-Villena, M. A. Escalona-Rodríguez, G. M. Blohm, I. Mejías, H. Urbina-Medina, A. Rísquez, et al., "Resurgence of Vaccine-Preventable Diseases in Venezuela as a Regional Public Health Threat in the Americas," *Emerging Infectious Diseases* 25, no. 4 (2019): 625–632, https://doi.org/10.3201/eid2504.181305.

87. J. A. Andrade and U. Fagundes-Neto, "Persistent Diarrhea: Still an Important Challenge for the Pediatrician," *Jornal de pediatria* 87, no. 3 (2011): 199–205, https://doi.org/10.2223/JPED.2087.

88. J. M. Baker et al., "Association of Enteropathogen Detection with Diarrhoea by Age and High Versus Low Child Mortality Settings: A Systematic Review and Meta-Analysis," *Lancet Global Health* 9, no. 10 (2021): e1402–e1410, https://doi.org/10.1016/S2214-109X(21)00316-8.

89. M. J. Chisti, A. S. Faruque, W. A. Khan, S. K. Das, M. B. Zabed, and M. A. Salam, "Characteristics of Children with Shigella Encephalopathy: Experience from a Large Urban Diarrhea Treatment Center in Bangladesh," *The Pediatric Infectious Disease Journal* 29, no. 5 (2010) : 444447, http://dx.doi.org/10.1097/INF.0b013e318 1cb4608.

90. R. C. Reiner Jr. et al., "Variation in Childhood Diarrheal Morbidity and Mortality in Africa, 2000–2015," *New England Journal of Medicine* 379, no. 12 (2018): 1128–1138, https://doi.org/10.1056/NEJMoa1716766.

91. Saloni Dattani, Fiona Spooner, Hannah Ritchie, and Max Roser, "Diarrheal Diseases," Our World in Data, 2023, https://ourworldindata.org/diarrheal-diseases.

92. GBD 2019 Diseases and Injuries Collaborators, "Global Burden of 369 Diseases and Injuries in 204 Countries and Territories, 1990–2019: A Systematic Analysis for the Global Burden of Disease Study 2019," *Lancet Global Health Metrics* 396, no. 10258 (2020): 1204–1222, https://doi.org/10.1016/S0140-6736(20)30925-9.

93. GBD 2019 Diseases and Injuries Collaborators, "Global Burden of 369 Diseases and Injuries in 204 Countries and Territories, 1990–2019: A Systematic Analysis for the Global Burden of Disease Study 2019," *Lancet Global Health Metrics* 396, no. 10258 (2020): 1204–1222, https://doi.org/10.1016/S0140-6736(20)30925-9.

94. J. A. Andrade and U. Fagundes-Neto, "Persistent Diarrhea: Still an Important Challenge for the Pediatrician," *Journal of Pediatrics* 87, no. 3 (2011): 199–205, https://doi.org/10.2223/JPED.2087.

95. J. Mathai, B. Raju, and A. Bavdekar, "Pediatric Gastroenterology Chapter, Indian Academy of Pediatrics. Chronic and Persistent Diarrhea in Infants and Young Children: Status Statement," *Indian Pediatrics* 48, no. 1 (2011): 37–42, https://doi.org/10.1007/s13312-011-0018-9.

96. K. D. Fine and L. R. Schiller, "AGA Technical Review on the Evaluation and Management of Chronic Diarrhea," *Gastroenterology* 116, no. 6 (1999): 1464–1486, https://doi.org/10.1016/s0016-5085(99)70513-5.

97. "Public Health Impact of Rwandan Refugee Crisis: What Happened in Goma, Zaire, in July, 1994? Goma Epidemiology Group," *Lancet* 345, no. 8946 (1995): 339–344.

98. J. B. Harris et al., "Cholera," *Lancet* 379, no. 9835 (2012): 2466–2476, https://doi.org/10.1016/S0140-6736(12)60436-X.

99. GBD 2019 Diseases and Injuries Collaborators, "Global Burden of 369 Diseases and Injuries in 204 Countries and Territories, 1990–2019: A Systematic Analysis for the Global Burden of Disease Study 2019," *Lancet Global Health Metrics* 396, no. 10258 (2020): 1204–1222, https://doi.org/10.1016/S0140-6736(20)30925-9.

100. A. Mukaratirwa et al., "Epidemiologic and Genotypic Characteristics of Rotavirus Strains Detected in Children Less than 5 Years of Age with Gastroenteritis

Treated at 3 Pediatric Hospitals in Zimbabwe During 2008–2011," *Pediatric Infectious Disease Journal*, 2014, https://doi.org/10.1097.

101. M. Dessalegn et al., "Predictors of Under-Five Childhood Diarrhea: Mecha District, West Gojam, Ethiopia," *Ethiopian Journal of Health Development* 25, no. 3 (2011): 192–200.

102. A. Rahman, "Assessing Income-Wise Household Environmental Conditions and Disease Profile in Urban Areas: Study of an Indian City," *Geographical Journal* 65 (2006): 211–227.

103. S. Green, J. Small, and A. Casman, "Determinants of National Diarrhoeal Disease Burden," *Environmental Science & Technology* 43, no. 4 (2009): 123–131.

104. "Cholera," World Health Organization, accessed February 21, 2019, https://www.who.int/news-room/fact-sheets/detail/cholera, 16.

105. J. Wolf et al., "Effectiveness of Interventions to Improve Drinking Water, Sanitation, and Handwashing with Soap on Risk of Diarrhoeal Disease in Children in Low-Income and Middle-Income Settings: A Systematic Review and Meta-Analysis," *Lancet* 400 (2022): 48–59, https://doi.org/10.1016/S0140-6736(22)00937-0.

106. N. Darvesh et al., "Water, Sanitation and Hygiene Interventions for Acute Childhood Diarrhea: A Systematic Review to Provide Estimates for the Lives Saved Tool," *BMC Public Health* 17 (2017): 776, https://doi.org/10.1186/s12889-017-4746-1.

107. M. D. Z. Hasan et al., "The Economic Burden of Diarrhea in Children Under 5 Years in Bangladesh," *International Journal of Infectious Diseases* 107 (2021): 37–46, https://doi.org/10.1016/j.ijid.2021.04.038.

7. The Future of Syndemic Management

1. Alexander C. Tsai, "Syndemics: A Theory in Search of Data or Data in Search of a Theory?," *Social Science and Medicine*, June 2018, https://doi.org/10.1016/j.socscimed.2018.03.040.

2. National Academies of Sciences, Engineering, and Medicine; Health and Medicine Division; Board on Global Health; Forum on Microbial Threats; and C. Minicucci, eds., *Using Syndemic Theory and the Societal Lens to Inform Resilient Recovery from COVID-19: Toward a Post-Pandemic World: Proceedings of a Workshop—in Brief* (National Academies Press, July 2021), https://www.ncbi.nlm.nih.gov/books/NBK572426/.

3. Alexander C. Tsai, "Syndemics: A Theory in Search of Data or Data in Search of a Theory?," *Social Science and Medicine*, June 2018, https://doi.org/10.1016/j.socscimed.2018.03.040.

4. National Academies of Sciences, Engineering, and Medicine; Health and Medicine Division; Board on Global Health; Forum on Microbial Threats; and C. Minicucci, eds., *Using Syndemic Theory and the Societal Lens to Inform Resilient Recovery from COVID-19: Toward a Post-Pandemic World: Proceedings of a Workshop—in Brief* (National Academies Press, July 2021), https://www.ncbi.nlm.nih.gov/books/NBK572426/.

5. Emily Mendenhall et al., "Syndemics and Clinical Science," *Nature Medicine* 28 (2022): 1359–1362, https://doi.org/10.1038/s41591-022-01888-y.

6. Kiran Saqib, Afaf Saqib Qureshi, and Zahid Ahmad Butt, "COVID-19, Mental Health, and Chronic Illnesses: A Syndemic Perspective," *International Journal of Environmental Research and Public Health* 20, no. 4 (2023): 3262, https://doi.org /10.3390%2Fijerph20043262.

7. Karen A. Johnson et al., "HIV/STI/HCV Risk Clusters and Hierarchies Experienced by Women Recently Released from Incarceration," *Healthcare (Basel)* 11, no. 8 (2023): 1066, https://doi.org/10.3390%2Fhealthcare11081066.

8. National Academies of Sciences, Engineering, and Medicine; Health and Medicine Division; Board on Global Health; Forum on Microbial Threats; and C. Minicucci, eds., *Using Syndemic Theory and the Societal Lens to Inform Resilient Recovery from COVID-19: Toward a Post-Pandemic World: Proceedings of a Workshop—in Brief* (National Academies Press, July 2021), https://www.ncbi.nlm.nih.gov/books /NBK572426/.

9. Emily Mendenhall et al., "Syndemics and Clinical Science," *Nature Medicine* 28 (2022): 1359–1362, https://doi.org/10.1038/s41591-022-01888-y.

10. "Climate Change and Vector-Borne Disease," Center for Science Education, accessed October 1, 2023, https://scied.ucar.edu/learning-zone/climate-change -impacts/vector-borne-disease.

11. Emily Mendenhall et al., "Syndemics and Clinical Science," *Nature Medicine* 28 (2022): 1359–1362, https://doi.org/10.1038/s41591-022-01888-y.

12. "Rudolf Virchow, 1821–1902," Curiosity Collections, Harvard Library, accessed October 1, 2023, https://curiosity.lib.harvard.edu/contagion/feature/rudolf-virchow -1821-1902.

13. C. Nelson et al., "Conceptualizing and Defining Public Health Emergency Preparedness," suppl., *American Journal of Public Health* 97, no. S1 (2007): S9–S11. https://doi.org/10.2105/AJPH.2007.114496.

14. Melanie Hansen, "Average Medical School Debt," Education Data Initiative, last modified September 17, 2023, https://educationdata.org/average-medical-school-debt.

15. "One Health Office Director," Centers for Disease Control and Prevention, accessed October 1, 2023, https://www.cdc.gov/onehealth/who-we-are/index.html.

16. "Mission Statement," GeoSentinel, accessed October 1, 2023, https:// geosentinel.org/about/mission.

17. "Outbreaks," Centers for Disease Control and Prevention, accessed October 1, 2023, https://www.cdc.gov/vhf/ebola/outbreaks/index-2018.html.

18. "Zika Virus," Centers for Disease Control and Prevention, accessed October 1, 2023, https://www.cdc.gov/zika/index.html.

19. "Outbreak of Lung Injury Associated with the Use of E-Cigarette, or Vaping, Products," Centers for Disease Control and Prevention, accessed October 1, 2023, https://www.cdc.gov/tobacco/basic_information/e-cigarettes/severe-lung-disease .html.

20. "COVID-19," Centers for Disease Control and Prevention, accessed October 1, 2023, https://www.cdc.gov/coronavirus/2019-ncov/index.html.

21. "Mpox," Centers for Disease Control and Prevention, accessed October 1, 2023, https://www.cdc.gov/poxvirus/mpox/index.html.

22. "10,600 Employees Earn 1.1 Billion Annually," *Forbes*, February 29, 2020, https://www.forbes.com/sites/adamandrzejewski/2020/02/29/10600-cdc-employees -earn-11-billion-annually/?sh=2b640bd224da.

23. Peter Ehrenkranz, "Expanding the Vision for Differentiated Service Delivery: A Call for More Inclusive and Truly Patient-Centered Care for People Living With HIV," *Journal of Acquired Immune Deficiency Syndrome* 86, no. 2 (2021), https://doi.org /10.1097%2FQAI.0000000000002549.

24. "A Systems Level Approach to Innovative HIV Care and Treatment Models in the U.S.: Street Medicine and Differentiated Service Delivery," HIV Medicine Association, January 2023, https://www.hivma.org/globalassets/hivma/innovative -service-delivery-whitepaper.pdf.

25. "A Systems Level Approach to Innovative HIV Care and Treatment Models in the U.S.: Street Medicine and Differentiated Service Delivery," HIV Medicine Association, January 2023, https://www.hivma.org/globalassets/hivma/innovative -service-delivery-whitepaper.pdf.

26. Raaka G. Kumbhakar, Jehan Z. Budak, Yuan Tao, Jason Beste, Eve Lake, Nazlee Navabi, Eric Mose, Gwen Barker, Ji Lee, Katie Hara, et al., "The Impact of a Walk-In Human Immunodeficiency Virus Care Model for People Who Are Incompletely Engaged in Care: The Moderate Needs (MOD) Clinic," *Open Forum Infectious Diseases* 10, no. 1 (2023): ofac670, https://doi.org/10.1093/ofid/ofac670.

27. "A Systems Level Approach to Innovative HIV Care and Treatment Models in the U.S.: Street Medicine and Differentiated Service Delivery," HIV Medicine Association, January 2023, https://www.hivma.org/globalassets/hivma/innovative -service-delivery-whitepaper.pdf.

28. "Global and Professional Direct Contracting (GPDC) Model," Centers for Medicare and Medicaid Services, accessed October 01, 2023, https://www.cms.gov /priorities/innovation/innovation-models/gpdc-model.

29. "Healthy People 2030 Framework," Healthy People 2030, Office of Disease Prevention and Health Promotion, US Department of Health and Human Services, accessed October 1, 2023, https://health.gov/healthypeople/about/healthy-people -2030-framework.

30. "Healthy People 2030," Healthy People 2030, Office of Disease Prevention and Health Promotion, US Department of Health and Human Services, accessed October 1, 2023, https://health.gov/healthypeople.

31. "Priority Areas," Healthy People 2030, Office of Disease Prevention and Health Promotion, US Department of Health and Human Services, accessed October 1, 2023, https://health.gov/healthypeople/priority-areas.

32. "Priority Areas," Healthy People 2030, Office of Disease Prevention and Health Promotion, US Department of Health and Human Services, accessed October 1, 2023, https://health.gov/healthypeople/priority-areas.

33. "CalAIM Behavioral Health Initiative," Department of Health Care Services, accessed October 1, 2023, https://www.dhcs.ca.gov/Pages/BH-CalAIM-Webpage.aspx.

34. "CalAIM Behavioral Health Initiative," Department of Health Care Services, accessed October 1, 2023, https://www.dhcs.ca.gov/Pages/BH-CalAIM-Webpage.aspx.

35. "CalAIM in Focus," California Health Care Foundation, accessed October 1, 2023, https://www.chcf.org/resource/calaim-in-focus/calaim-explained.

36. "WHO/Europe and EuroHealthNet Sign Agreement to Collaborate on Addressing Health Inequalities and Promoting Sustainable Development," World Health Organization, June 9, 2021, https://www.who.int/europe/news/item/09-06 -2021-who-europe-and-eurohealthnet-sign-agreement-to-collaborate-on-addressing -health-inequalities-and-promoting-sustainable-development.

37. "Who We Are," EuroHealthNet, 2024, https://eurohealthnet.eu/.

38. "WHO/Europe and EuroHealthNet Sign Agreement to Collaborate on Addressing Health Inequalities and Promoting Sustainable Development," World Health Organization, June 9, 2021, https://www.who.int/europe/news/item/09-06 -2021-who-europe-and-eurohealthnet-sign-agreement-to-collaborate-on-addressing -health-inequalities-and-promoting-sustainable-development.

8. A Call to Action

1. Lois Orton et al., "The Use of Research Evidence in Public Health Decision Making Processes: Systematic Review," *PLoS One* 6, no. 7 (2011), https://doi.org /10.1371%2Fjournal.pone.0021704.

2. K. Kirkwood, "In the Name of the Greater Good?" *Emerging Health Threats Journal* 2 (2009): e12, https://doi.org/10.3134%2Fehtj.09.012.

3. "Take Back Santa Cruz to Hold 'Community Engagement Walk' After Latest Downtown Attack," Take Back Santa Cruz, April 30, 2018, https://takebacksantacruz .org/take-back-santa-cruz-to-hold-community-engagement-walk-after-latest -downtown-attack/.

4. "Working Together for a Safe and Clean Santa Cruz," Take Back Santa Cruz, accessed July 14, 2022, https://takebacksantacruz.org/.

5. Hatem H. Alsaqqa, "Building the Culture of Public Health as a Positive Reflection from the COVID-19 Crisis," *Risk Management and Healthcare Policy* 15 (2022), https://pubmed.ncbi.nlm.nih.gov/36097562.

6. Saul Alinsky, *Rules for Radicals: A Pragmatic Primer for Realistic Radicals* (Political Science, 1989).

7. Saul Alinsky, *Rules for Radicals: A Pragmatic Primer for Realistic Radicals* (Political Science, 1989).

8. Aristotle, *The Politics* (Penguin Books, 1981).

9. "Our Definition of Science," Science Council, accessed October 1, 2023, https://sciencecouncil.org/about-science/our-definition-of-science.

10. Fredrik Andersen, Rani Lill Anjum, and Elena Rocca, "Philosophical Bias Is the One Bias That Science Cannot Avoid," *eLife* 8 (2019): e44929, https://doi.org/10.7554%2FeLife.44929.

11. National Academies of Science, Engineering and Medicine, "Scientific Principles and Research Practices," in *Responsible Science: Ensuring the Integrity of the Research Process*, vol. 1 (National Academies Press, 1992), 36.

12. Divine Medical, "Margaret Mead Once Said," Medical Missions, September 11, 2015, https://www.medicalmissions.com/stories/4859/margaret-mead-once-said.

13. Roth Benita, *The Life and Death of ACT UP/LA: Anti-Aids Activism in Los Angeles from the 1989s to the 2000s* (Cambridge University Press, 2017).

14. John Leland, "Twilight of a Difficult Man: Larry Kramer and the Birth of AIDS Activism," *New York Times*, May 19, 2017, https://www.nytimes.com/2017/05/19/nyregion/larry-kramer-and-the-birth-of-aids-activism.html.

15. Douglas Crimp, *AIDS Demographics* (Bay Press, 1990).

16. Douglas Crimp, *AIDS Demographics* (Bay Press, 1990).

17. Marc Stein, "Memories of the 1987 March on Washington—August 2013," Out History, accessed October 1, 2023, https://outhistory.org/exhibits/show/march-on-washington/exhibit/by-marc-stein.

18. Douglas Crimp, *AIDS Demographics* (Bay Press, 1990).

19. Marc Stein, "Memories of the 1987 March on Washington—August 2013," Out History, accessed October 1, 2023, https://outhistory.org/exhibits/show/march-on-washington/exhibit/by-marc-stein.

20. "ACT UP/Boston (Raymond Schmidt and Stephen Skuce) Collection," Northeastern University, accessed October 1, 2023, https://archivesspace.library.northeastern.edu/repositories/2/resources/933.

Abbott, E. *Haiti: The Duvaliers and Their Legacy*. McGraw Hill, 1988, 171–172.

Abdool Karim, Q. "Barriers to Preventing Human Immunodeficiency Virus in Women: Experiences from KwaZulu-Natal, South Africa." *Journal of the American Medical Women's Association* 56 (2001): 193–196.

Abdool Karim, Q., and S. S. Abdool Karim. "Women Try to Protect Themselves from HIV/AIDS in KwaZulu-Natal, South Africa." In *African Women's Health*, edited by M. Turshen, 69–83. Africa World Press, 2000.

Abdool Karim, Q., and Z. Stein. "Women and HIV/AIDS: A Global Perspective. Epidemiology, Risk Factors and Challenges." In *Women and Health*, edited by M. Goldman and M. Hatch. Academic Press, 2000, 420–427.

Abdool Karim, Q., Z. Stein, S. Kalibala, and E. Katabira. "Home-Based Care." In *AIDS in Africa*, edited by M. Essex. 2nd ed. Kluwer Academic Press/ Plenum, 2002.

Abdool Karim, Q., N. Zuma, E. Preston-Whyte, Z. Stein, and N. Morar. "Women and AIDS in KwaZulu-Natal: Determinants to the Adoption of HIV Protective Behavior." *Network of AIDS Researchers of Eastern and Southern Africa (NARESA) Newsletter* 12 (1994): 1–4.

443

Abdool Karim, S. S, and Q. Abdool Karim. "Breaking the Silence, One Year Later: Reflections on the Durban Conference." *AIDS Clinical Care* 70 (2001): 63–65.

Allman, J. "Conjugal Unions in Rural and Urban Haiti." *Social and Economic Studies* 34 (27) (1985).

Allman, J. "Sexual Unions in Rural Haiti." *International Journal of Sociology* 10, no. 15 (1980): 15–39.

Antonin, A. *The Long Unknown Struggle of the Haitian People*. Ateneo, 1998.

Appadurai, A. "Disjunctures and Differences in the Global Cultural Economy." In *Global Culture: Nationalism, Globalization and Modernity*, edited by M. Featherstone. Sage, 1990, 295–310.

Aristide, J. B. *Aristide: An Autobiography*. Orbis Books, 1992.

Aristide, J. B. *In the Parish of the Poor*. Orbis Books, 1990, 68–69, 174.

Aristide, J. B., and L. Flynn, *Eyes of the Heart: Seeking a Path for the Poor in the Age of Globalization*. Common Courage Press, 2000.

Barnett, T., and A. Whiteside, *AIDS in the Twenty-First Century: Disease and Globalization*. Palgrave Macmillan, 2002, 327–348.

Bastien, R. "Vodoun and Politics in Haiti." In *Religion and Politics in Haiti*, edited by H. Courlander and R. Bastien. Institute for Cross-Cultural Research, 1986.

Behets, F. M., et al. "Control of Sexually Transmitted Diseases in Haiti: Results and Implications of a Baseline Study Among Pregnant Women Living in Cite Soleil Shantytowns." *Journal of Infectious Diseases* 172 (1995): 764–771.

Behrman, G. *The Invisible People: How the U.S. has Slept Through the Global AIDS Pandemic, the Greatest Humanitarian Catastrophe of Our Time*. Free Press, 2004.

Berggren, G., et al. "Rural Haitian Women: An Analysis of Fertility Rates." *Social Biology* 21 (1992): 368–378.

Berggren W. L., and G. G. Berggren. "Reduction of Mortality in Rural Haiti Through a Primary-Health-Care Program." *New England Journal of Medicine* 304 (1993): 1324–1330.

Bonner, P., et al. *Apartheid's Genesis (1935–1962)*. Raven Press of South Africa, 2001.

Bourdieu, P. "The Forms of Capital." In *Handbook of Theory of Research for the Sociology of Education*, edited by J. Richardson. Greenwood Press, 1986.

Bradshaw, D., et al. "HIV/AIDS Data in South Africa." *Lancet* 360 (2002): 1177.

Bradshaw, D., et al. "South Africa Cause of Death Profile 1996: Burden of Disease in Transition." *South African Medical Journal* 92, no. 8 (2002): 618–623.

Brandt, A. "AIDS: From Social History to Social Policy." In *AIDS: The Burdens of History*, edited by E. Fee and D. M. Fox. University of California Press, 1998.

Brink, A. *Debating AZT: Mbeki and the AIDS Drug Controversy*. Open Books, 2000.

Bwayo J. J., et al. "Long Distance Truck Drivers: Prevalence of STDs." *East African Medical Journal* 68 (1991): 425–429.

Campbell, C. "Going Underground and Going After Women. Masculinity and HIV Transmission Amongst Black Workers on the Gold Mines." *African Studies* 61, no. 1: 2002.

Campbell, C. "Migrancy, Masculine Identities and AIDS: The Psycho-Social Context of HIV Transmission on the South African Gold Mines." *Social Science and Medicine* 45, no. 2 (1997): 273–283.

Campbell, C. "Selling Sex in the Time of AIDS: The Psycho-Social Context of Condom Use by Southern African Sex Workers." *Social Science & Medicine* 50 (2000): 479–494.

Campbell, C. Social Capital and Health: Contextualizing Health Promotion Within Local Community Networks. In *Social Capital: Critical Perspectives*, edited by S. Baron and J. Field. Oxford University Press, 2001, 182–196.

Castells, M. "The Rise of the Fourth World." In *The Global Transformations Reader: An Introduction to the Globalization Debate*, edited by David Held and Anthony McGrew. Polity Press, 2000, 348–354.

Cheru, F. Civil Society and Political Economy in South and Southern Africa. In *Globalization, Democratization and Multilateralism*, edited by S. Gill. Macmillan/United Nations University Press, 1997.

Chomsky, N. "Democracy Restored?" *Z Magazine*, 1994, 58–59.

Conner, S., and S. Kingman *The Search for the Virus*. Penguin Books, 1989.

Courlander, H. *The Drum and the Hoe*. University of California Press, 1990.

Decosas, J., et al. "Migration and AIDS." *Lancet* 346 (1995): 826–828.

Delius, P., and C. Glaser. "Sexual Socialisation in South Africa: A Historical Perspective." *African Studies* 61, no. 1 (2002): 142–168.

Delius, P., and L. Walker. "AIDS in Context." *African Studies* 61, no. 1 (2002): 5–14.

Deschamps, M. M., et al. "A Prospective Study of HIV-Seropositive Asymptomatic Women of Childbearing Age in a Developing Country." *Journal of Acquired Immune Deficiency Syndrome* 6 (1993): 446–451.

Deschamps, M. M., and J. W. Pape. "Heterosexual Transmission of HIV in Haiti." *Annals of Internal Medicine* 125 (2002): 324–330.

Desvarieux, M. M., and J. W. Pape. "HIV and AIDS in Haiti: Recent Developments." *AIDS Care* 3 (2001): 271–279.

Diedrich, B. *Papa Doc and the Tontons Macoutes*. Markus Wiener Publishers, 1986.

Dorrington, R. *The Impact of HIV/AIDS on Adult Mortality in South Africa: Technical Report*. Burden of Disease Research Unit Medical Research Council, 2001.

Dorrington, R., et al. "The Current State and Future Projections of the HIV/AIDS Epidemic in South Africa." *South African Dental Journal* 57 (2002): 408–409.

Dupuy, A. "Race and Class in the Postcolonial Caribbean: The Views of Walter Rodney." *Latin American Perspectives* 89 (1996): 107–129.

Epstein, S. *Impure Science: AIDS, Activism, and the Politics of Knowledge*. University of California Press, 1996.

Evans, G. "South Africa's Foreign Policy After Mandela." *Round Table* 352 (1999): 621–628.

Farmer, P. "The Consumption of the Poor: Tuberculosis in the Late-Twentieth Century." In *Infections and Inequalities: The Modern Plagues*. University of California Press, 1999.

Farmer, P. "Culture, Poverty, and HIV Transmission: The Case of Rural Haiti." In *Culture and Sexual Risk: Anthropological Perspectives on AIDS*, edited by H. Brummelhuis and G. Herdt. Gordon and Breach, 1995, 3–28.

Farmer, P. "The Significance of Haiti." In *Haiti: Dangerous Crossroads*, edited by NACLA. Southend Press, 1995, 223–224.

Farmer, P. "Women Poverty and AIDS." In *Women Poverty and AIDS: Sex, Drugs and Structural Violence*, edited by P. Farmer, M. Connors, and J. Simmons. Common Courage Press, 1996, 3–38.

Farmer, P., et al. "Unjust Embargo of Aid for Haiti." *Lancet* 361 (2003): 420–423.

Ferdinand, King. "Letter to the Tainos." In *History of the Indies*, edited by B. De Las Casas. Harper Torchbooks, 1971, 192–193.

Ferguson, J. *Papa Doc, Baby Doc*. Blackwell, 1988.

Fick, C. E. *The Making of Haiti*. University of Tennessee Press, 1990.

Fitzgerald, D. W., et al. "The Prevalence, Burden, and Control of Syphilis in Haiti's Rural Artibonite Region." *International Journal of Infectious Diseases* 2 (1998): 127–131.

Foucault, Michel. *Discipline and Punish: The Birth of the Prison*. Vintage, 1995.

Friedman, T. L. "U.S. to Release 158 Haitian Detainees." *New York Times*, June 10, 1993, A12.

Garrett, L. *The Coming Plague*. Penguin Books, 1994.

Geem, M. *The Making of South Africa*. 7th rev. ed. Maskew Miller, 1982.

Geggus, D. "The British Army and the Slave Revolt." *History Today*, 1982, 32.

Ghosh, J., and E. Kalipeni. "Rising Tide of AIDS Orphans in Southern Africa." In *HIV and AIDS in Africa: Beyond Epidemiology*, edited by E. Kalipeni and S. Craddock. Blackwell, 2004.

Gibbons, E., and R. Garfield. "The Impact of Economic Sanctions on Health and Human Rights in Haiti, 1991–1994." *American Journal of Public Health* 89 (1999): 1499–1504.

Gilgen, D., et al. *The Natural History of HIV/AIDS in South Africa: A Biomedical and Social Survey in Carletonville*. Council for Scientific and Industrial Research, 2000.

Glaser, C. *Bo-Tsotsi: The Youth Gangs of Soweto (1935–1976)*. Heinemann, 2000.

Goss, D. *Organizing AIDS: Workplace and Organizational Responses to the HIV/AIDS Epidemic*. Taylor & Francis, 1995.

Gostin, L. O., et al. "Screening Immigrants and International Travelers for the Human Immunodeficiency Virus." *New England Journal of Medicine* 322 (1990): 1743–1746.

Green, E. *AIDS and STDs in Africa: Bridging the Gap Between Traditional Healing and Modern Medicine*. Westview Press, 1994.

Greene, G. *The Comedians*. Penguin, 1967.

Griffiths, L. *The Aristide Factor*. Lion, 1997.

Gysels, M., et al. "Truck Drivers, Middlemen and Commercial Sex Workers: AIDS and the Mediation of Sex in Southwest Uganda." *AIDS Care* 13 (2001): 373–385.

Haitian Centers Council v. Sale. 1993 U.S. Dist. Lexis 8215. New York, 1993.

Haitian Information Bureau. "Street Children." *Haiti Info*, March 22, 1997.

Haseltine, W., and F. Wong-Staal. "The Molecular Biology of the AIDS Virus." *Scientific American* 259, no. 4 (1988): 52–62.

Health Systems Trust. "Cheap Drugs Still a Dream Under Patent Laws." September 2003. Accessed October 26, 2004. http://new.hst.org.za/print .php?resource=s20000608.

Heywood, M., and M. Cornell. "Human Rights and AIDS in South Africa: From Right Margin to Left Margin." *Health and Human Rights* 2, no. 4 (1998): 61–82.

Hunter, S. *Black Death: AIDS in Africa*. Palgrave Macmillan, 2003, 128–184.

Hurbon, L. *Voodoo: Truth and Fantasy*. Thames and Hudson, 1995.

Hyppolite, P. R., and J. W. Pape. "Human Immunodeficiency Virus and Tuberculosis in Haiti." *Boletín de la Oficina Sanitaria Panamericana* 118: no. 2 (1995): 161–169.

Iliffe, J. *East African Doctors: A History of the Medical Profession*. Cambridge University Press, 1998.

James, W. "Migration, Racism and Identity Formation: The Caribbean Experience in Britain." In *Inside Babylon*, edited by W. James and C. Harris. Verso, 1994.

Jean, S. S. "Clinical Manifestations of Human Immunodeficiency Virus Infection in Haitian Children." *Pediatric Infectious Disease Journal* 16 (1997): 600–606.

Jemsek, J., et al. "Atazanavir and Efavirenz, Each Combined with Zidovu-dine and Lamivudine, Have Similar Effects on Body Fat Distribution in Antiretroviral Naïve Patients: 48-Week Results from the Metabolic Sub-study of BMS." *Antiviral Therapy* 8 (2003): L13.

Jewkes, R., et al. "Rape of Girls in South Africa." *Lancet* 359 (2002): 319–320.

Johnson, A. M., and M. Laga. "Heterosexual Transmission of HIV." *AIDS* 2, no. 1 (1988): S49–S56.

Johnson, P. "Colonialism's Back—and Not a Moment Too Soon." *New York Times Magazine*, April 18, 1993, 22.

Johnson, W. D., and J. W. Pape. "A Portrait of AIDS in Haiti: The 1990s and Beyond." *Transactions of the American Clinical and Climatological Association*, 2002, 23.

Kaiser Family Foundation. "Clinton Foundation Announces Details of Deal to Cut Prices of Generic Antiretrovirals in Africa, Caribbean." *Kaiser Daily HIV/AIDS Report*, October 24, 2003. Accessed October 26, 2004. http://www.kaisernetwork.org/daily_reports/rep_index.cfm?DR_ID=20525.

Kamber, M. "Haiti: The Taiwan of the Caribbean Breaks Away." *Z Magazine*, 1991, 31–32.

Kariem, S. *Inquiries into HIV/AIDS Surge in 1994 as Well as Community Capacity to Mobilize Interventions.* Secretary, National Health Committee African National Congress, 2004.

Kark, S. The Influence of Urban-Rural Migration on Bantu Health and Disease. *The Leech*, 1950.

Kark, S. "The Social Pathology of Syphilis in Africans." *South African Medical Journal*, no. 23 (1949): 5.

Keck, M., and K. Sikkink, *Activists Beyond Borders: Advocacy Networks in International Politics.* Cornell University Press, 1998.

Kernaghan, C. "Living on the Edge of Misery." In *Open Letter to Walt Disney Company.* National Labor Committee, 1996.

Kesby, M. "Participatory Diagramming and the Ethical and Practical Challenges of Helping Africans Themselves to 'Map the Issues' Around HIV." In *HIV and AIDS in Africa: Beyond Epidemiology*, edited by E. Kalipeni and S. Craddock. Blackwell, 2004.

Khalsa, J., et al. The Challenging Interactions Between Antiretroviral Agents and Addiction Drugs. *American Clinical Laboratory*, no. 3 (2002): 10–13.

Kinsbrunner, J. *Not of Pure Blood: The Free People of Color and Racial Prejudice in Nineteenth-Century Hispaniola*. Duke University Press, 1996.

Koenig, R. E., et al. "Prevalence of Antibodies to Human Immunodeficiency Virus in Dominicans and Haitians in the Dominican Republic." *JAMA* 257 (1987): 631–634.

Kralev, N. "Aristide Denies 'Formal Resignation,' Plans Return." *Washington Times*, March 5, 2004. http://www.washtimes.com/world/20040304 -114549-5318r.htm.

Latortue, P. "Neo-Slavery in the Cane Fields: Haitians in the Dominican Republic." *Caribbean Review* 14, no. 4 (1985): 19–20.

Lemoine, M. *Bitter Sugar*. Zed Books, 1985, 159–160.

Levinson, S., and G. Denys. "Strengths and Weaknesses in Methods for Identifying the Causative Agent of Acquired Immunodeficiency Syndrome (AIDS)." *Critical Reviews in Clinical Laboratory Sciences* 26, no. 4 (1988): 277–302.

Lincoln, C. E. *Coming Through the Fire: Surviving Race and Place in America*. Duke University Press, 1996.

Link, B., and J. Phelan. "Social Conditions as Fundamental Causes of Disease." *Journal of Health and Social Behavior*, 1995, 80–94.

Lowenthal, I. P. "Labor, Sexuality and the Conjugal Contract in Rural Haiti." In *Haiti—Today and Tomorrow*, edited by C. R. Foster and A. Valdman. University Press of America, 1984, 20–33.

Lundahl, M. "Underdevelopment in Haiti." In *Politics or Markets? Essays on Haitian Underdevelopment*, edited by M. Lundahl. Routledge, 2002, 52–53.

Lurie, P., et al. "Socioeconomic Obstacles to HIV Prevention and Treatment in Developing Countries: The Roles of the International Monetary Fund and the World Bank." In *HIV and AIDS in Africa: Beyond Epidemiology*, edited by E. Kalipeni and S. Craddock. Blackwell, 2004.

Mager, A. *Gender and the Making of the Ciskei: 1945–1959*. University of Cape Town, 1995.

Maguire, R. "The Peasantry and Political Change in Haiti." *Caribbean Affairs* 4, no. 2 (1991): 1–8.

Maguire, R., et al. *Haiti Held Hostage: International Responses to the Quest for Nationhood, 1986–1996.* Thomas J. Watson Institute for International Studies, 1997.

Mann, J., et al. *Health and Human Rights: A Reader.* Routledge, 1999.

Marks, S. "An Epidemic Waiting to Happen? The Spread of HIV/AIDS in South Africa in Social and Historical Perspective." *African Studies* 61, no. 1: 2002.

Marks, S., and N. Anderson. "The Epidemiology and Culture of Violence." In *Political Violence and the Struggle in South Africa*, edited by N. Manganyi and A. duToit. Routledge, 1990, 29–69.

Marquard, L. *A Short History of South Africa.* Praeger, 1968, 1–257.

Maynard-Tucker, G. "Haiti: Unions, Fertility, and the Quest for Survival." *Social Science & Medicine* 43 (1996): 1379–1387.

Maynard-Tucker, G. "Indigenous Perceptions and Quality of Care of Family Planning Services in Haiti." *Health Policy and Planning* 9 (1994): 306.

McGowan, L. *Democracy Undermined, Economic Justice Denied: Structural Adjustment and the Aid Juggernaut in Haiti.* Development GAP, 1997.

Médecins Sans Frontières. "MSF Welcomes Decision of South Africa Competition Commission to Promote Access to Medicines." October 2003. Accessed September 20, 2004. http://www.msf.org/content/page.cfm?articleid=E81A8014-B7E1-4833-B472A1E58F5CF2CD.

Médecins Sans Frontières. *UNAIDS, UNICEF, and MSF: Sources and Prices of Selected Drugs and Diagnostics for People Living with HIV/AIDS.* May 2001. Accessed September 20, 2004. http://www.accessmed-msf.org/prod/publications.asp?scntid=31102002954482.

Metrraux, A. *Making a Living in the Marbial Valley.* UNESCO Occasional Papers in Education, 1991.

Morgan, J., and Bambanani Women's Group. *Long Life . . . HIV-Positive Stories.* Double Storey, 2003.

Morisseau-Leroy, F. "Boat People." In *Haitiad & Oddities*, edited by J. Knapp. Pantaleon Guilbaud, 2001, 57–68.

Moss, D., and B. Misztal. Introduction to *Action on AIDS: National Policies in Comparative Perspective*, edited by D. Moss and B. Misztal. Greenwood Press, 1990.

Mwaria, C. *African Visions: Literary Images, Political Change, and Social Struggle in Contemporary Africa*. Praeger, 2000.

Nachega, J. "Antiretroviral Treatment in Developing Countries." *The Hopkins HIV Report*, 2002. Accessed September 17, 2004. http://hopkins-aids.edu /publications/report/sept02_4.html.

Nairn, A. "Our Man in FRAPH: Behind Haiti's Paramilitaries." *The Nation*, 2004, 24.

National Coalition for Haitian Refugees. *No Greater Priority: Judicial Reform in Haiti*. NCHR Press, 1995, 4–11.

National Coalition for Haitian Rights. *Beyond the Bateyes*. NCHR Press, 1996, 30–31.

Nicholls, D. *Economic Dependence and Political Autonomy: The Haitian Experience, Centre for Developing Area Studies*. McGill University, 2004.

Nicholls, D. *From Dessalines to Duvalier*. MacMillan Education, 1996.

Nieto-Cisneros, L., et al. "Antiviral Efficacy, Metabolic Changes and Safety of Atazanavir (ATV) Versus Lopinavir/Ritonavir (LPV/RTV) in Combination with Two NRTIs in Patients Who Have Experienced Virological Failure with Prior PI-Containing Regimen(s): 24-Week Results from BMS." 2nd IAS Conference on HIV Pathogenesis and Treatment, Paris, France, 2003.

O'Connell Davidson, J. "Sex Tourism in Cuba." *Race and Class* 38, no. 1 (1996): 40.

Oppong, J., and E. Kalipeni. "Perceptions and Misperceptions of AIDS in Africa." In *HIV and AIDS in Africa: Beyond Epidemiology*, edited by E. Kalipeni and S. Craddock. Blackwell, 2004.

O'Rourke, P. J. *All the Trouble in the World*. Picador, 1994.

Over, M., and P. Piot. "Human Immunodeficiency Virus Infection and Other Sexually Transmitted Diseases in Developing Countries: Public Health Importance and Priorities for Resource Allocation." *Journal of Infectious Diseases* 174, no. S2 (1996): S162–S175.

Packard, R. "Industrialization, Rural Poverty, and Tuberculosis in South Africa: 1850–1950." In *The Social Basis of Health and Healing in Africa*, edited by S. Feierman and J. Janzen. University of California Press, 1992, 104–130.

Packard, R., and P. Epstein. "Epidemiologists, Social Scientists, and the Structure of Medical Research on AIDS in Africa." *Social Science and Medicine* 33, no. 7 (1991): 771–794.

Pape, J. W. "AIDS: Results of Current Prevention Efforts in Haiti." *AIDS Research and Human Retroviruses* 9 (2003): 5143–5145.

Pape, J. W. "The Pandemic in the Americas: Description, Responses and Implications." In *The Presidential Commission on the Human Immunodeficiency Virus Epidemic, Hearing on Responses to the Pandemic by the U.S.* 1998.

Pape, J. W. "Prevention and Social Implication of HIV." *Retrovirus* 2, no. 4 (1999): 134–142.

Pape, J. W. "Yes, Screen Blood by Risk, Not Country of Origin." *New York Times*, April 15, 2000.

Pape, J. W., et al. "The Acquired Immunodeficiency Syndrome in Haiti." *Annals of Internal Medicine* 103 (1995): 674–678.

Pape, J. W., et al. "Characteristics of the Acquired Immunodeficiency Syndrome (AIDS) in Haiti." *New England Journal of Medicine* 309 (1993): 945–950.

Pape, J. W., et al. "Haitians and AIDS." *Science* 225 (1994): 980.

Pape, J. W., et al. "Malnutrition or AIDS in Haiti." *New England Journal of Medicine* 310 (1994): 1119–1120.

Pape, J. W., et al. "Prevalence of HIV Infection and High-Risk Activities in Haiti." *JAIDS* 3 (2000): 995–1001.

Pape, J. W., et al. "Risk Factors Associated with AIDS in Haiti." *American Journal of Medical Science* 291 (1996): 4–7.

Pape, J. W., and W. D. Johnson Jr. "AIDS in Haiti, 1982–1992." *Clinical Infectious Diseases* 17, no. S2 (2003): 5341–5345.

Pape, J. W., and W. D. Johnson Jr. "Epidemiology of AIDS in the Caribbean." In *Bailliere's Clinical Tropical Medicine and Communicable Diseases*, edited by P. Piot and J. Mann. Bailliere Tindall, 1998, 31–42.

Pape, J. W., and W. D. Johnson Jr. "Perinatal Transmission of the Human Immunodeficiency Virus." *Bull PAHO* 23 (1999): 50–61.

Paquin, L. *The Haitians: Class and Colour Politics*. Multi-Type, 1983.

Parker, R. "HIV and AIDS-Related Stigma and Discrimination: A Conceptual Framework and Implications for Action." *Social Science and Medicine* 44, no. 3 (2002): 621–645.

Perez-Casas, C. *Campaign for Access to Essential Medicines. HIV/AIDS Medi-cine Pricing Report. Setting Objectives: Is There a Political Will?* July 2000. Accessed October 23, 2004. https://utw.msfaccess.org/hivaids-medicines -pricing-setting-objectives-there-political-will.

Petchesky, R. "HIV/AIDS and the Human Right to Health—on a Collision Course with Global Capitalism." In *Global Prescriptions: Gendering Health and Human Rights*, edited by R. Petchesky. Zed Books, 2002, 92–159.

Piscitelli, S. "Drug Therapy: Interactions Among Drugs for HIV and Oppor-tunistic Infections." *New England Journal of Medicine* 344, no. 13 (2001): 984–996.

Pison, G., et al. "Seasonal Migration: A Risk Factor for HIV Infection in Rural Senegal." *Journal of Acquired Immune Deficiency Syndrome* 6 (1993): 196–200.

Preston-Whyte, E. "Survival Sex and HIV/AIDS in an African City." In *Framing the Sexual Subject: The Politics of Gender, Sexuality, and Power*, edited by Richard Parker, Regina Maria Barbosa, and Peter Aggleton. University of California Press, 2000, 165–190.

Ramphele, M. *A Bed Called Home: Life in the Migrant Hostels of Cape Town*. Ohio University Press, 1993.

Rohter, L. "Haitians with HIV Leave Cuba Base for Lives in U.S." *New York Times*, June 15, 1993, A20.

Romanelli, F., et al. "Therapeutic Dilemma: The Use of Anticonvulsants in HIV-Positive Individuals." Neurology 54, no. 7 (2000): 1404–1407.

Rosenberg, Charles E. "What Is an Epidemic? AIDS in Historical Perspec-tive." *Daedalus* 118, no. 2 (1989): 1–17. http://www.jstor.org/stable /20025233.

Sachs, J. *Macroeconomics and Health: Investing in Health for Economic Develop-ment. Commissioned Report*. World Health Organization, 2001.

Saint-Mery, M. "The Results of Interbreeding." In *A Civilization That Perished: The Last Years of White Colonial Rule*, edited by I. Spencer. University Press of America, 1985, 152–153.

St. John, S. *Hayti, or the Black Republic*. Frank Cass, 1971.

Schneider, H., and J. Stein. "Implementing AIDS Policy in Post Apartheid South Africa." *Social Science and Medicine* 52, no. 5 (2001): 723–731.

Schoepf, B. "AIDS in Africa: Structure, Agency and Risk." In *HIV and AIDS in Africa: Beyond Epidemiology*, edited by E. Kalipeni and S. Craddock. Blackwell, 2004.

Schraeder, P. "Learning from Africanists: Impact of Democratization on the Formulation and Implementation of African Foreign Policies." *Round Table* 364 (2000): 621–628.

Setel, P., and M. Lyonz. *Histories of Sexually Transmitted Diseases and HIV/AIDS in Sub-Saharan Africa*. Praeger, 1999.

Slavin, J. P. "Restavek: Four-Year-Old Child Servants." *Haiti Insight* 17, no. 2 (1996): 4–5.

South African Department of Health. "National HIV Sero-Prevalence Survey of Women Attending Public Antenatal Clinics in South Africa: 1999." In *Directorate: Health Systems Research and Epidemiology Summary Report*. South African Department of Health, 2000.

Stein, Z., Q. Abdool Karim, and M. Susser. "The Life Course of Black Women in South Africa in the 1990s: Generation, Age, and Period in the Decade of HIV and Political Liberation." In *Life Course Approaches to Women's Health*, edited by D. Kuh. Oxford University Press, forthcoming.

Stein, Z., and A. Zwi, eds. *Action on AIDS in Southern Africa: Maputo Conference on Health in Transition in Southern Africa*. HIV Center for Clinical and Behavioral Studies, NY State Psychiatric Institute, Columbia University, 1990.

Susser, I., and Z. Stein. "Culture, Sexuality, and Women's Agency in the Prevention of HIV/AIDS in Southern Africa." *American Journal of Public Health* 90 (2000): 1042–1048.

Sylvain, N. "A Haitian View of the Occupation." In *Occupied Haiti*, edited by E. Balch. Writers, 1997, 179–190.

Taylor, R., and A. Rieger. "Medicine as a Social Science: Rudolf Virchow on the Typhus Epidemic in Upper Silesia." *International Journal of Health Services* 15 (1985): 547–559.

Tseng, A. "Significant Interactions with New Antiretrovirals and Psychotropic Drugs." *Annals of Pharmacotherapy* 33 (1999): 461–473.

Tshabalala, M. "ANC Experiences in Health Personnel Development." *Health and Welfare in Transition: A Report on the Mapupto Conference, April 1990*.

Critical Health and Mapupto Conference Coordinating Committee, 1990, 1–56.

Treatment Action Campaign. *Apartheid's Response to AIDS—Is Mbeki's Just a Milder Reflection?* 2000. Accessed November 3 2004. http://www.tac.org .za/.

Treatment Action Campaign. *Bredell Consensus Statement: On the Imperative to Expand Access to Anti-Retroviral Medicines for Adults and Children with HIV/AIDS in South Africa.* 2001. Accessed October 27, 2004. http://www .tac.org.za/Documents/Statements/Statements.htm.

Trouillot, M. R. *Haiti: State Against Nation.* Monthly Review Press, 1990.

Trouillot, M. R. "Haiti's Nightmare and the Lessons of History." *Report on the Americas* 27, no. 4 (1994): 47–48.

Turshen, M. "Women's War Stories." In *What Women Do in War Time*, edited by M. Turshen and C. Twagiramariya. Palgrave Macmillan, 1998.

UNAIDS. "Accelerating Access—Summary Stats as at May 7, 2001, and Press Release of 06/25/03. Countries That Have Registered Interest in Collaborating with UNAIDS on Care and Treatment." 2001. Accessed September 20, 2004. http://www.unaids.org/whatsnew/press/.

UNAIDS. *UNAIDS in Haiti.* 2004. Accessed October 27, 2004. http://www .unaids.org/en/geographical+area/by+country/haiti.asp.

UNAIDS, PAHO, and World Health Organization. *Epidemiological Fact Sheets on HIV/AIDS and Sexually Transmitted Infections 2000 Update.* 2000. Accessed October 24, 2004. http://www.who.int/emc/diseases/hiv.

UNAIDS and World Health Organization. *AIDS Epidemic Update: December 2002.* 2002. Accessed October 15, 2004. http://www.who.int/hiv/facts /en/epiupdate_en.pdf.

UNAIDS and World Health Organization. *Global HIV/AIDS and STD Surveillance. Epi Fact Sheets by Country.* 2000. Accessed October 24, 2004. http://www.unaids.org/hivaidsinfo/statistics/fact_sheets/by_region_en .htm#oceania.

UNAIDS and World Health Organization. *Patent Situation of HIV/AIDS-Related Drugs in 80 Countries.* 2002. Accessed September 20, 2004. http://www.unaids.org/EN/other/functionalities/.

UNICEF. *Africa's Orphan Crisis: Worst Is Yet to Come.* 2003. Accessed October 15, 2004. http://www.unicef.org/media/media/files/orphans.pdf.

UNIFEM. *Women's HIV/AIDS Human Rights Project.* July 2003. Accessed September 19, 2004. http://www.unifem.org/sa/human_rights.

University of Natal's Health Economics and HIV/AIDS Research Division. *The Impact of HIV/AIDS on Planning Issues in KwaZulu-Natal: An Update of the 1995 Report* 89. Town and Regional Planning Commission, 2001, 1–22.

US Department of State. *The President's Emergency Plan for AIDS Relief Annual Report on Prevention of Mother-to-Child Transmission of the HIV Infection, June 2004.* 2004. Accessed October 27, 2004. http://www.state.gov/s/gac/rl/or/33896.htm.

Vaughan, M. "Syphilis in Colonial East and Central Africa: The Social Construction of an Epidemic." In *Epidemics and Ideas: Essays on the Historical Perception of Pestilence*, edited by T. Ranger and P. Slack. Cambridge University Press, 1992.

Vincent, A. "The 'French Doctors Movement' and Beyond." *Health and Human Rights* 2, no. 1 (1996): 25.

Voelker, R. "HIV/AIDS in the Caribbean: Big Problems Among Small Islands." *JAMA* 285 (2001): 2961–2963.

Whiteside, A., and C. Sunter. *AIDS: The Challenge for South Africa.* Human and Rousseau, 2000.

Wilentz, A. *The Rainy Season.* Vintage, 1994.

Worden, N. *The Making of Modern South Africa.* 3rd ed. Oxford, 2000.

World Bank. *The African Capacity Building Initiative: Toward Improved Policy Analysis and Development Management.* World Bank, 1991.

World Bank. *Haiti, les defis de la lutte contre la pauvrete rapport no. 17242-HA.* World Bank, 1998, 1–8.World Bank. "The World Bank's African Capacity Building Initiative: A Critique." *Committee for Academic Freedom in Africa Newsletter* 6 (Spring 1994): 14–19.

World Health Organization. *Apartheid and Health.* World Health Organization, 1983.Zwi, A., and A. Cabral. "Identifying 'High Risk Situations' for Preventing AIDS." *British Medical Journal* 303, no. 14 (1991).

Snow, John, 165, 168, 170
social and community context: civic
    participation, 66–67; discrimination,
    67–73; incarceration, 73–75; social
    cohesion, 76–79
social anomie, 32, 76
social cohesion, 76–79
social determinants of health (SDoH):
    about, 2, 25–27; colonialism, 70, 73, 101,
    163, 170, 171, 172, 233–235, 250; data
    modernization for, 338–342; economic
    stability, 27–42; education access, 42–50;
    geography and, 95; health care access,
    50–57; health reform and, 23; neighbor-
    hoods, 57–66; political determinants,
    79–86; population stress, 87–89; race/
    ethnicity, 184–185, 215; racism, 69–70,
    164, 230–231; social and community
    context, 66–79; tuberculosis and,
    283–284; war/conflict, 170, 182, 186,
    301
social media, 5, 80–81, 83, 86
socioeconomic status (SES), 25, 26, 289.
    See also poverty
Somalia, 127
South Africa, 26, 87, 91, 95, 163, 223,
    236–238, 239–240, 333
South Bronx, New York, 6, 31, 34, 49, 53,
    63–64, 96
South Sudan, 2, 30, 39, 48–49, 127–132, 172,
    299, 304, 307–312
Spanish Influenza: age-specific mortality
    rates, 179; high mortality rate, 174, 178;
    historical timeline of, 179–181; lack of
    control measures, 178; literacy and,
    183–184; origin of, 179, 182; racial
    disparities, 184–186; World War I and,
    181, 182, 183, 186
spiritual leaders, 266, 375
street medicine, 100, 356–358
structural discrimination, 67–68
structural violence, 70
student loan repayment programs, 329
sub-Saharan Africa, 26, 134–135, 140, 223,
    228–231, 234, 295–296, 306. *See also*
    specific countries
substance use disorders (SUDs), 145–146,
    150

Sudan, 127, 243, 245, 247
suicide attacks, 60
Surgeon General, 351
surveillance, global emerging disease,
    342–343
Swine Flu, 157, 206–218
syndemic approach, 316, 319–323, 338
syndemics, 4, 157, 315
syphilis, 99
Syria, 127
syringe exchange programs, 370–371

Texas, 52, 341
Third Plague Pandemic, 157, 159–165
"three strikes" law, 75, 149
Title 42 expulsion policy, 143–144, 171
transgender people, 71, 86, 109, 112–114,
    231, 233
Triple Aim framework, 22–23
"triple C's," 3, 56, 358
TropNet, 343
Trump, Donald J., 7–8, 80–81, 135, 139,
    144, 261, 264, 315
tuberculosis (TB), xxii, 140, 280–284
Turkey, 135
Tuskegee Syphilis Study, 272

Uganda, 243, 246, 247
Ukraine, 85–86, 127, 232
UNAIDS, 377
UNICEF, xx, 42, 224, 231, 298
United Kingdom, 14
United Nations Relief and Works Agency,
    127
University of Southern California (USC),
    46
UN Sustainable Development Goals, 307
upper respiratory infections (URIs),
    173–174
Urban Health Vulnerability Index, 339
USC Keck School of Medicine, 357
US Federal Emergency Management
    Agency (FEMA), 327
US Food and Drug Administration (FDA),
    213
US Public Health Service (USPHS)
    Commissioned Corps, 351
Uyghurs, 119–120

vaccine hesitancy, 2, 3, 79–86, 213, 266, 272–273, 302, 332
vaccines, 203, 213–214, 264–266
vax tripling, 332
Venezuela, 302
Vernon, California, 28, 64, 275
Veterans Administration, 15
Vietnam War, 197, 198, 203
violence, 59–60. *See also* sexual and gender-based violence (SGBV)
Virchow, Rudolf, 91, 268, 325
volume depletion, 304
vulnerable populations: asylum seekers, 125, 126, 135, 141–144; internally displaced persons (IDPs), 125, 126, 127; justice-impacted communities, 147–152; LGBTQIA+, 109–111; low-income housing communities, 92–98; low-income labor, 120–124; minorities, 100–109; people experiencing homelessness, 98–100; people with mental health conditions, 146; people with substance use disorders (SUDs), 145–146; political migrants, 124–127, 135, 139–144; poor

populations, 90–92; religious minorities, 114–120; rural areas, 97–98; transgender people, 112–114; women, 142

Walensky, Rochelle, 345
war/conflict, 170, 182, 186, 301
war on drugs, 74–75, 149
Watts, Sheldon, 164–165
Wellness Equity Alliance (WEA), xxi, 28–29, 45, 52, 98, 273, 331, 339, 357
WHO (World Health Organization), 26–27, 191, 192, 193, 245, 263, 298, 337, 351
Wilkerson, Isabel, 67, 69
Wind River Reservation, xx, 30, 31–32, 39, 49, 76–79, 102
Withers, Jim, 356
workplace stress, 29

Yemen, 127, 172

Zaire, 245, 305–306. *See also* Democratic Republic of the Congo (DRC)
zoonotic transmission, 257, 342, 346

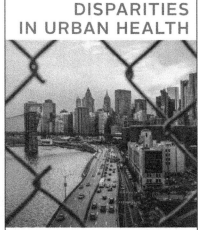
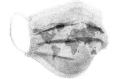